The Psychoanalytic Model
of the Mind

The Psychoanalytic Model of the Mind

By

Elizabeth L. Auchincloss, M.D.

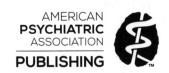

AMERICAN
PSYCHIATRIC
ASSOCIATION
PUBLISHING

Copyright © 2015 American Psychiatric Association
ALL RIGHTS RESERVED

Manufactured in the United States of America on acid-free paper
25   24   23   22   8   7   6   5
First Edition

Typeset in Palatino and Grotesque MT Std.

American Psychiatric Association Publishing
1000 Wilson Boulevard
Arlington, VA 22209-3901
www.appi.org

Library of Congress Cataloging-in-Publication Data
Auchincloss, Elizabeth L., 1951– , author.
  The psychoanalytic model of the mind / by Elizabeth L. Auchincloss.
    p. ; cm.
  Includes bibliographical references and index.
  ISBN 978-1-58562-471-3 (pbk. : alk. paper)
  I. Title.
  [DNLM: 1. Psychoanalytic Theory. WM 460.2]
  RC504
  150.19′5—dc23
                                                              2015002911

British Library Cataloguing in Publication Data
A CIP record is available from the British Library.

For my students

Contents

Part I
Foundations

Part II
The Topographic Model

Part III

The Structural Model

Part IV

Object Relations Theory
and Self Psychology

Part V

Integration and Application

Part VI

Appendixes

About the Author

Elizabeth L. Auchincloss, M.D., is Vice-Chair for Education, Director of the Institute for Psychodynamic Medicine, DeWitt Wallace Senior Scholar, and Professor of Clinical Psychiatry in the Department of Psychiatry at Weill Cornell Medical College in New York City. She is also Senior Associate Director, and Training and Supervising Analyst, at the Columbia University Center for Psychoanalytic Training and Research.

Foreword

Otto F. Kernberg, M.D.

To carry out a clear, comprehensive, in-depth overview of contemporary psychoanalytic theory, including its ramifications into divergent ideological approaches to its major components, and, at the same time, to do justice to psychoanalysis' relationships with its boundary sciences, is a major challenge. Elizabeth Auchincloss has achieved it with the present volume. This book permits psychiatrists, psychologists, and mental health professionals to acquire a sophisticated knowledge of the psychoanalytic model of the mind, and to relate it to corresponding scientific developments in the neurosciences and other fields of psychological investigation. For the trained psychoanalyst, this volume presents an original, erudite organizing frame of reference that clarifies the questions and controversies actually being explored and debated by the psychoanalytic community. It also constitutes a natural companion to the impressive *Psychoanalytic Terms and Concepts* published by Samberg and Auchincloss in 2012, in which the entire body of psychoanalytic concepts and terminology so comprehensively synthesized in Auchincloss' present volume is defined in clear and precise terms. This volume may be considered an updated version of—albeit a more sophisticated and comprehensive overview than—Charles Brenner's *An Elementary Textbook of Psychoanalysis* of many years ago.

The basic frame of psychoanalytic theory proposed in this work includes five dimensions: topography, motivation, structure, development, and psychopathology/treatment. These dimensions follow Freud's fundamental discovery of the dynamic unconscious and his theory of unconscious motivational forces—the dual-drive theory of libido and aggression—and their dynamic expression in terms of their conflicts with the demands of reality, represented by defensive operations directed against them. The vicissitudes of the corresponding conflicts, at various unconscious and conscious levels, are expressed in the topographic model; the organization of defensive operations, in the structural model, and particular characteristics in early and later stages of the life span, in the developmental model. The psychoanalytic exploration of psychopathology reveals pathological consequences of those conflicts: in physical and psychological symptoms, in characterological rigidities, and, particularly, in constellations of self-defeating and potentially dangerous limitations in psychosocial functioning. Psychoanalytic psychotherapies facilitate the development of specific approaches to this pathology.

Auchincloss places contemporary developments in psychodynamic theory and treatments within the broad field of general psychoanalytic theory comprehensively explored along those dimensions, combining a historical approach to the evolving formulations with a specific orientation to four currently competing alternative psychoanalytic schools: the early, classical, "Id"-inspired model reflecting mostly the Topographic dimension; the ego psychological school developed mostly within the Structural Model; the revolutionary contemporary Object Relations approaches that center on the structural vicissitudes of development of self and internalized relations with others: and Self Psychology as a particular approach to the vicissitudes of the self.

Auchincloss comes from the background of American Ego Psychology, the prevalent psychoanalytic approach in this country in the second half of the past century, but she pays careful attention to the newer approaches of alternative models, particularly the contemporary Object Relations model represented by the Kleinian school, the Relational approach, and (to some extent) Self Psychology. She also explores the French psychoanalytic approach, quite prevalent in Latin language countries, that stresses Freud's Topographic Model, strongly emphasizes Freud's dual-drive theory, and highlights the dominance of archaic oedipal conflicts. Less well known in the United States than the Relational and the Kleinian approaches, the French psychoanalytic approach has contributed important analyses of the vicissitudes and pathological consequences of infantile sexuality and its relationship to aggression and perversion. French analysts stress the dynamics of synchronic as well as diachronic aspects of psychic functioning, and, within their structural concerns, have highlighted the functions of language as a specific expression of unconscious dynamics.

Throughout the careful description of the multiple aspects of contemporary psychoanalytic theory, Auchincloss stresses the relationship between scientific developments in fields at the boundaries of psychoanalytic observations, particularly the neurosciences, and the sociocultural influences in the early developmental stages of infantile psychic experience. Neurocognitive findings related to or commensurate with psychoanalytic models, and empirical evidence linking them, illustrate Auchincloss' consistent placement of the psychoanalytic view of the mind within present-day scientific progression in related fields.

In agreement with this approach, I would add, as one more important parallel development, the field of affective neuroscience—the contemporary affect theory that considers affect systems as the basic motivational systems of the mind. Neurobiological research of affect activation, expression, and registration involving limbic and related cortical brain structures has provided evidence that early object relations take place in the context of powerful positive and negative affect activation. In fact, affective neuroscience and psychoanalytic object relations theory may turn out to constitute the most important link between neurobiological and psychodynamic development, reflected in current explorations of the relations between affect and drive theory. Are early internalized dynamic relations between self and others the building blocks of the "tripartite" psychic structure? Or are the affective links between self and others the basic components of the psychic drives?

Here we are entering a central territory of contemporary controversies and concerns of psychoanalytic scholars and researchers. *The Psychoanalytic Model of the Mind* provides the reader with a clearly focused orienting frame showing where psychoanalytic theory stands today that illuminates these issues. At the same time, it is a unique introduction to the general psychoanalytic model that should be helpful to all mental health professionals involved in psychotherapeutic treatments, as well as a must for any therapist carrying out psychodynamic psychotherapy.

Preface
and Introduction

The Psychoanalytic Model of the Mind has been written for everyone who wants or needs a way to think about the mind in depth. The model of the mind presented in this book is based on psychoanalytic thinking over the past 120 years. The goal of this book is to explain how the psychoanalytic model of the mind works and how it contributes to the care of people with mental suffering. The psychoanalytic model of the mind attempts to describe mental experiences such as feelings, thoughts, wishes, fears, memories, attitudes, and values. It attempts to understand how these mental experiences interact with and influence each other, how they arise from earlier experiences, and how they are transformed in the course of development. The psychoanalytic model of the mind looks at mental life along parameters such as levels of self-awareness, motivation, structure, and development. It seeks to understand the contribution made by mental experiences to both normal and pathological behavior.

The psychoanalytic account of how the mind works is the most complex model of mental functioning ever invented for clinical purposes. It looks at the mind along parameters such as topography, motivation, structure, and development. It looks at individual symptoms and character traits as well as at the whole person and his or her life. In addition to providing the theoretical scaffolding for psychodynamic psychotherapy, the psychoanalytic model of the mind forms the basis of almost all psychological treatments, or "talking cures," for emotional suffering. Psychological assessment is an important part of the evaluation and treatment of every patient, not just patients treated in psychotherapy. Even in patients whose mental illness has a predominantly biological basis, psychological factors contribute to onset of the illness, improvements in or worsening of the patient's condition, and expression of the illness. Research shows that treatments that focus on symptoms alone, to the exclusion of emotional and interpersonal patterns, are not effective in sustaining change (Westen et al. 2004). Indeed, the outcome of almost every treatment depends on understanding every patient as a psychological being (Lister et al. 1995). Psychological factors also influence the manner in which every patient engages in treatment. Studies show that quality of the therapeutic alliance is the strongest predictor of outcome for all mental illness in all treatment modalities (Krupnick et al. 1996; Zetzel 1956). A strong treatment alliance depends on precise knowledge of the patient as a human being. It also depends on understanding the transference and countertransference reactions that either disrupt or strengthen the clinician–patient bond.

Despite the widespread influence of psychoanalysis in the field of mental health, there is no single book that explains the psychoanalytic model of the mind to the many students and practitioners who want to understand it. Everyone recognizes the face of Sigmund Freud and the symbol of the couch. However, few know what lies behind these icons in the way of either intellectual substance or useful practice. Every student knows that psychoanalysis is at once adored and reviled, eulogized and lampooned. However, few have any idea what the fuss is all about or why the psychoanalytic model of the mind is important. *The Psychoanalytic Model of the Mind* is committed to demonstrating how this model is useful in treating all patients, all of the time.

Although the field of mental health is officially committed to the biopsychosocial model (Engel 1977), we do not often see this model at work. For too many years, our field has been weakened by a polarization of choices to be made along several familiar axes: mental health practitioners are asked to choose between a mind-based and a brain-based point of view; mental health practitioners are asked to choose between either of these points of view and a culturally informed point of view; mental health practitioners are asked to choose between a humanistic and a scientific point of view; mental health practitioners are asked to choose between clinical evidence and empirical evidence; and mental health practitioners are asked to choose between cognitive and psychoanalytic approaches to the mind.

At the same time, the field of psychoanalysis has been beset with its own problems, which interfere with our students' efforts to understand the contributions of psychoanalysis to the understanding of the patient's suffering. These overlapping problems include the isolation of much psychoanalytic thought from ideas emerging from neighboring disciplines; the use of too many terms that are hard to understand, so that students often feel excluded by private, seemingly impenetrable language; the eschewing by some psychoanalysts of the importance of empirical study; the excessive hero-worship felt by many psychoanalysts about Freud the founder; and controversies among psychoanalysts over which is the best model of the mind among competing models, to mention only a few areas of dissent.

The Psychoanalytic Model of the Mind seeks to transcend these many problems with a new approach. This book will be committed to demonstrating that

- The psychoanalytic model of the mind is consistent with a brain-based approach and should never be used separately from such an approach.
- The psychoanalytic model of the mind is consistent with cultural psychiatry.
- The psychoanalytic model of the mind is consistent with other well-known models of the mind, including the cognitive model.
- The psychoanalytic model of the mind can be presented in a way that allows clinicians to use the best aspects of several competing models.
- The basic tenets of the psychoanalytic model of the mind are supported by empirical evidence.

Every chapter of *The Psychoanalytic Model of the Mind* will address these points, avoiding destructive polarization and embracing complexity. In addition, when we talk about Freud, we do so with respect but not with reverence. In other words, when we write that "Freud said...," we do not envision him speaking *ex cathedra*, but rather as speaking with an inquiring mind that seeks to build the best model of the mind using all the evidence. Finally, every effort has been made to explain complicated ideas and concepts in simple language, avoiding jargon whenever possible. However, important terms will be used so that readers can learn what they mean and thereby gain access to what is, and has been, a language-based enterprise. A Glossary has been provided in Appendix C at the end of the book (see Part VI).

This book is divided into six parts. Part I, "Foundations" includes four chapters. Chapter 1 ("Overview: Modeling the Life of the Mind") explores basic questions such as "What is the mind?" "What is psychoanalysis?" and "What is a model?" It also addresses the question "Why do we need a model of the mind in an era of the brain?" Chapter 2 ("Origins of the Psychoanalytic Model of the Mind") tells the back story of how the first psychoanalytic model of the mind was formulated, beginning with a lightning tour of the history of scientific psychology and moving on to the work of Freud himself. Chapter 3 ("Evolution of the Dynamic Unconscious") explores the concept of the dynamic unconscious, which forms the basis of the psychoanalytic model of the mind.

It reviews the history of the concept of the unconscious in Western philosophy and psychology and contrasts the dynamic unconscious with a related but different concept—the cognitive unconscious, developed in the neighboring field of cognitive neuroscience. Chapter 4 ("Core Dimensions of Psychoanalytic Models of the Mind") defines five core dimensions shared by all psychoanalytic models of the mind: topography, motivation, structure/process, development, and theory of psychopathology/treatment (therapeutic action). Each of these dimensions is discussed in relation to similar concepts from neighboring disciplines. This chapter also includes another lightning tour of four foundational psychoanalytic models of the mind: the Topographic Model, the Structural Model, Object Relations Theory, and Self Psychology. These models are presented in the order in which they were developed historically so that readers can see how the psychoanalytic model evolved in response to improvements in clinical understanding and new evidence from other disciplines. As the reader will also see, each of these four psychoanalytic models of the mind has much to say about the core dimensions of mental functioning and psychopathology/treatment. Throughout the book, these four models will be explained in relation to each other and ultimately will be integrated into a single usable and contemporary model of the mind. Finally, Chapter 4 introduces the reader to a chart that will serve as a unifying template for the book's content. In this chart, the core dimensions of mental functioning and psychopathology/treatment are plotted for each of the four foundational psychoanalytic models of the mind. As readers progress through the book, they will see how each successive model conceptualizes each of these key dimensions of mental life and mental illness/treatment. When they reach Part V and the last chapter, the task of understanding the various models will have become much easier.

Parts II through IV are devoted to exploring the four main psychoanalytic models of the mind in depth. Part II, "The Topographic Model," includes three chapters. Chapter 5 ("The Mind's Topography," begins with an overview of the Topographic Model, which postulated conscious, preconscious, and unconscious domains separated by a barrier of repression. Although this model contained rudimentary ideas about motivation, structure, development, and psychopathology/treatment, its main focus was the mind's topography. This chapter highlights the tremendous explanatory value of Freud's Topographic Model, including the important concept of *neurosis*. Indeed, all psychodynamic psychotherapies include the aim of bringing unconscious wishes, fears, and fantasies into awareness. Chapter 6 ("The World of

Dreams") explains how a contemporary psychoanalytic model of dreams works and how dreams are used in psychotherapy. At the same time, it explores theories and empirical evidence from cognitive neuroscience, integrating these theories and findings with the psychoanalytic approach to dreams. Chapter 7 ("The Oedipus Complex") surveys this first important example of unconscious fantasy, developing in childhood and persisting in adult mental life. Although contemporary psychodynamic clinicians no longer believe that the oedipus complex is the cause of all psychopathology, this chapter explores the ways in which oedipal conflict is still important and why it is considered universal.

Part III, "The Structural Model," includes three chapters. Chapter 8 ("A New Configuration and a New Concept: The Ego") provides an overview of the Structural Model with its well-known components: ego, id, and superego. In examining how Freud revised his own model of the mind, the reader will absorb the empowering message that the psychoanalytic model of the mind is "man made" and open to revision. Chapter 8 also describes the concept of the ego in greater detail, examining ideas such as self-regulation/homeostasis and adaptation. Chapter 9 ("The Id and the Superego") considers the concept of the id, as well as the concepts of drive, libido, psychosexuality, and aggression. (In Part VI of this book, Appendix A, "Libido Theory," illustrates how libidinous drives become transformed through defenses into adult sexual behavior, character traits, and neurosis.) Although everyone knows that Freud said, "Everything we do is because of sex," his actual views are poorly understood. Chapter 9 also considers the concept of the superego, examining the important role this structure plays in the experience of moral imperatives. Chapter 10 ("Conflict and Compromise") explains how ego, id, and superego work together in the formation of compromise, forged from the mediation of conflict among their competing aims. The chapter also explores the concept of defense in greater detail. (In Appendix B, "Defenses," common defense mechanisms are classified according to their costs in terms of ego functioning.) Finally, Chapter 10 updates the psychodynamic approach to psychopathology and treatment.

Part IV, "Object Relations Theory and Self Psychology," includes two chapters. Chapter 11 ("Object Relations Theory") explains what Object Relations Theory is and how it developed. The story of how and why this theory was formulated will again remind students that no theory is set in stone. Readers will also learn how Object Relations Theory expands our understanding of clinical problems, making it possible to better understand problems such as borderline psychopathology and problems with intimacy. Chapter 12 ("Self Psychology") traces how Heinz Kohut developed Self Psychology in his work with patients with narcissistic disturbances. This model is based on the observation that certain individuals experience trauma during childhood in the form of a failure of parental empathy. Chapter 12 also explains how Self Psychology can be integrated with other psychoanalytic models of the mind.

Part V ("Integration and Application") consists of a single chapter (Chapter 13, "Toward an Integrated Psychoanalytic Model of the Mind") that explores how the four foundational psychoanalytic models can be integrated into a single approach, while also being used separately. At this point, readers will be able to see a completed version of the chart that has been steadily growing as each model of the mind is introduced. The chart shows the contribution of each of the four models to the core dimensions of mental functioning and psychopathology/ treatment. This chapter will also explore areas of controversy surrounding attempts at integration. Finally, Chapter 13 will show how the psychoanalytic model of the mind coalesces into a complex psychiatry that integrates mind, brain, and culture.

The Psychoanalytic Model of the Mind has been written for students at every level of training, including psychiatry residents, psychology graduate students, social work students, and medical students. It is designed to serve as a resource for undergraduate and graduate students of philosophy, neuroscience, psychology, literature, and all academic disciplines outside of the mental health professions who may want to learn more about what psychoanalysts have to say about the mind. Readers will come away with an appreciation of how psychoanalytic thinking about the mind is useful in understanding patients. At the same time, readers will come away with a deeper understanding of all minds, not just those of patients, but of everyone, including his or her own. Work with patients should be a deep and rewarding experience that affords opportunities for growth, not only for the patients themselves but also for mental health practitioners. These opportunities for growth are most easily found and used by those equipped with the best model of the mind.

References

Engel GL: The need for a new medical model: a challenge for biomedicine. Science 196:129–136, 1977

Krupnick JL, Sotsky SM, Elkin I, et al: Therapeutic alliance in psychotherapy and pharmacotherapy outcome: findings in the National Institute of Mental Health treatment of depression collaborative research program. J Consult Clin Psychol 64:532–539, 1996

Lister EG, Auchincloss EL, Cooper AM: The psychodynamic formulation, in Psychodynamic Concepts in General Psychiatry. Edited by Schwartz H, Bleiberg E, Weissman SH. Arlington, VA, American Psychiatric Publishing, 1995, pp 13–26

Westen D, Novotny CM, Thompson-Brenner H: The empirical status of empirically supported psychotherapies: assumptions, finding and reporting in controlled clinical trials. Psychol Bull 130:631–663, 2004

Zetzel E: Current concepts of transference. International Journal of Psychoanalysis 37:369–375, 1956

Acknowledgments

The Psychoanalytic Model of the Mind is the result of a course by the same name that I have taught to students in the Department of Psychiatry at Weill Cornell Medical School since 1987. I am very grateful to these students for creating wonderful discussions, through which I have learned much.

At Cornell, I also owe special gratitude to Dr. Jack Barchas, Chair of the Department of Psychiatry, whose vision of a world of mental health that includes many points of view has been an inspiration to me. His support, encouragement, and wisdom have been a source of daily sustenance.

I have also been fortunate throughout my career to have worked with fantastic co-teachers in many settings, including Nathan Kravis, George Makari, Helen Meyers, Robert Michels, and especially Arnold Cooper. I have also been lucky to have worked on other projects with extraordinary people, especially Robert Glick and Eslee Samberg, with whom I spent many hours discussing topics related to psychoanalysis.

I am also grateful to many students, teachers, and colleagues in the psychoanalytic world, especially those at the Columbia University Center for Psychoanalytic Training and Research.

Finally, I am grateful to Richard Weiss, who has been my constant intellectual companion.

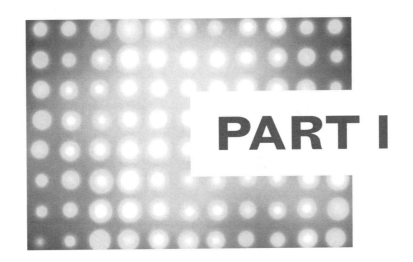

PART I

Foundations

CHAPTER 1

Overview:
Modeling the Life of the Mind

This chapter addresses questions such as the following: "What is the mind?" "What is psychoanalysis?" and "What is a model?" It goes on to explore the question "Why do we need a model of the mind in an era of the brain?" Vocabulary introduced in this chapter includes the following: *computational model of the mind, embodiment, emergent property, mind, mirror neurons, psychoanalysis, psychodynamic,* and *theory of mind.*

This book is based on the premise that each of us behaves and has experiences, makes plans and choices, and lives a life in ways that reflect the operations of something called the *mind*. It begins with the assumption that the experience of having a mind is a special aspect of human existence and that mental events are important determinants of who we are and how we behave in everyday life and in clinical situations. It also begins with the assumption that mental events cannot be reduced to the terms of any other discipline from which psychiatry and psychology draw, but must be described in their own terms.

Merriam-Webster defines the word *mind* as "the complex of elements in an individual that feels, perceives, thinks, wills, and especially reasons." The word includes "the organized conscious and unconscious adaptive mental activity of an organism."[1] The concept of mind can be explored in many different directions. For centuries philosophers of mind such as Plato, Descartes, Leibniz, Kant, Heidegger, Searle, and Dennett, to mention only a few, have debated questions such as "Is there a mind?" "Can mind be reduced to brain?" "What are the properties of mind?" "Do animals or machines have minds?" "Does the mind have causal properties, or is it a mere epiphenomenon of brain processes?" and "What is the relationship between mind and body?" Intellectual historians explore and disagree about how the concept of mind enters discourse about human behavior. Theologians weigh in on the question of the relationship between the mind and God. Of course, psychologists of all stripes offer theories about what kind of mind humans have, and what can be said about this mind.

Mental health professionals may be more or less interested in all of these directions in which the study of mind can lead, most having read enough to know that the philosophy and history of mind is complex (Kendler 2001; Makari 2008). However, we also know that we need a concept of mind to understand our patients. Most clinicians think of mind as an *emergent property* of brain, meaning that it is dependent on the brain but cannot be described in terms or concepts appropriate to the brain (Frith 2007). Indeed, most clinicians function practically as what philosophers call *property dualists,* meaning that even if we understand that mind emerges from brain, we know that we must separate mind and brain for clinical purposes. In other words, we treat the patient's mind and the patient's brain as though they have separate properties, each of which demands a unique kind of thinking and a separate kind of intervention. This way of conceptualizing patients is firmly established in our tradition. It has been written about most clearly in classics such as George Engel's (1977) biopsychosocial model or Paul McHugh and Phillip Slavney's *The Perspectives of Psychiatry* (McHugh and Slavney 1998), both of which assert that mental health professionals need and use several ways of thinking about patients, one of which focuses on psychology, or the study of the mind.

What Is Psychoanalysis?

Psychoanalysis is the branch of psychology that deals most thoroughly and profoundly with understanding human behavior as the result of

---

[1]See http://www.merriam-webster.com/dictionary/mind (accessed April 7, 2013).

the mind. In contrast to neurobiology, which studies behavior and mental experiences from the point of view of brain activity, or to social learning theory and some types of social psychology, which search for the environmental and cultural factors that influence experience and behavior, the psychoanalytic model of the mind attempts to organize our understanding of how mental phenomena such as feelings, thoughts, memories, wishes, and fantasies affect what we experience and do. Traditionally, psychoanalysis has been variously defined as a theory of the mind, as a theory of some aspects of psychopathology, as a treatment, and as a method of investigating the mind (Freud 1923/1962). Throughout this book, the word *psychodynamic,* which literally means "mental forces" (or motivations), will be used interchangeably with *psychoanalytic,* because there are few psychodynamic approaches that are distinct from the psychoanalytic approach.

What Is a Model?

The most common strategy used by psychoanalytic theory makers to organize and explain the mind is the building of what we call *the psychoanalytic model of the mind.* As with all models used in the natural and social sciences, the psychoanalytic model of the mind is an imaginary construction designed to represent a complex system—in this case, the human mind—that cannot be observed directly in its entirety. The purpose of any model is to represent a system in such a way that it is easier to talk about and easier to study. Some scientific models are very abstract, based on the language of mathematics or logical principles. Other models take a more plastic form, constructed by analogy with objects in the physical world that are already well understood. Scientific models are judged by how well they explain the available evidence, predict new findings, and are consistent with other knowledge. Examples of scientific models with which we are all familiar include the Copernican model of the solar system, the Rutherford–Bohr model of the atom, and the "Standard Model" of particle physics (which describes the interactions among the elementary particles that make up all matter). Each of these models attempts to organize available evidence into a representation of some aspect of the natural world.

The psychoanalytic model of the mind attempts to organize the data of the clinical situation—including the patient's life story, the patient's report of his or her inner experience, and the patient's interactions in the treatment setting—into a representation of the human mind as a coherent psychological system. The model describes how psychological phenomena such as feelings, thoughts, wishes, fears, fantasies, memories, attitudes, and values interact in the system and influence each other. It describes the motivations that animate the patient, the structures that organize the patient's mind, and the functions and processes by which the patient's mind works. It also describes how the mind develops. The psychoanalytic model of the mind represents the mind of all human beings in general, as well as the mind of any specific individual, with its unique characteristics. It can be used to describe how mental life is expressed in pathological as well as normal behavior and how treatment is used to influence the mind. The psychoanalytic model is not the first model of the mind. For thousands of years, mankind has been using analogies to represent the mind, drawing upon images such as a theater, an iceberg, a hydraulic system, and (more recently) a computer (McGinn 2013).

The earliest psychoanalytic model of the mind was constructed by Sigmund Freud in his attempt to make sense of his experience with his own patients. In his book *The Interpretation of Dreams* (1900/1962), Freud introduced his first fully developed model of the mind, or what he called the *psychic apparatus*, based on analogies with the science and technology of his day, which included a hodgepodge of neurobiology, reflex arcs, and optical instruments. Freud also borrowed heavily from other fields such as literature and archeology.

Some aspects of Freud's first model, often referred to as the Topographic Model of the mind, survive in the contemporary psychoanalytic model of the mind. Other aspects have been abandoned. Indeed, an important part of Freud's legacy is the reminder that successful model making should always be flexible and open ended. No scientific model is ever complete. For example, we were all taught in childhood that Christopher Columbus' spherical model of the Earth was a brilliant and dramatic improvement over other models popular in his day, which represented the planet as a flat disc, sometimes balanced on the back of a turtle! Columbus' model provided him with the theoretical rationale for his bold plan to sail West in search of "The East." However, Columbus' own failure to properly estimate the size of our planet caused him to be confused about where he was at his journey's end. Later map makers worked with the discoveries of Columbus (and others) to improve on the model of our planet Earth, with its oceans and land masses. Indeed, map makers are still at work charting the unseen depths of the ocean floor. As with our map of the world, the psychoanalytic model of the mind has continued to develop since Freud's first efforts to map the workings of the inner world. Although the contemporary psychoanalytic model of the mind borrows heavily from Freud's first models, it has undergone profound changes in the 100-plus years since the publication of *The Interpretation of Dreams* (Freud 1900/1962), becoming ever more complex in response to new data from clinical exploration and from other sources.

Today, no single psychoanalytic model of the mind is able to account for all data from within and outside of the clinical situation. The contemporary psychoanalytic model of the mind is best described as pluralistic, consisting of not one but several models of the mind, overlapping but distinct, each taking a somewhat different perspective on human mental functioning and each emphasizing a different set of phenomena. Roughly speaking, each contemporary psychoanalytic model of the mind corresponds to a different psychoanalytic "school of thought." Readers have heard of major schools of thought such as Ego Psychology, Object Relations Theory, Attachment Theory, Self Psychology, and Relational Psychoanalysis, to mention a few. These models of the mind (or schools of thought) vary with respect to how they represent the mind, how they understand the patient's suffering, and how they explain the therapeutic action of psychotherapy.

A goal of this book is to combine the major psychoanalytic models of the mind into a single usable contemporary psychoanalytic model of the mind. In the process of integrating these models, we will trace the evolution of efforts to conceptualize the nature of mental life in the work of Freud and of many others. We will describe how the processes of clinical discovery and theoretical formulation interact in the task of model making. We will delineate those elements that are shared by all psychoanalytic models of the mind as well as the important distinctions among competing models. Throughout, we will emphasize the fact that psychoanalytic model making is an ongoing process. Clinicians still face the same questions that challenged Freud: How can we understand patients, and how can we help them change? Our models of the mind are important and useful to the extent that they help us to answer those questions.

Why Do We Need a Model of the Mind?

In the late 1970s, attempts to model the workings of the mind became more interesting with the introduction of a fascinating idea, emerging from cognitive neuroscience, called *theory of mind*. According to this notion, all humans are hardwired with the capacity to develop a theory about how minds work—both our own minds and the minds of other people. If this notion is correct, the question of whether mental health professionals need a model of the mind is moot: As human beings, we already have one, whether we like it or not.

In their groundbreaking paper "Does the chimpanzee have a theory of mind?," cognitive scientists David Premack and Guy Woodruff (1978) used the phrase *theory of mind* for the first time to describe what cognitive psychologists had for a number of years been discussing as a specific capacity possessed by all human beings (and maybe other animals as well). This capacity enables us to 1) understand that others have beliefs, desires, and intentions; 2) realize that others' beliefs, desires, and intentions might be different from our own; and 3) form operational hypotheses, theories, or mental models of what others' beliefs, desires, and intentions might be (Malle 2005). Theory of mind (or ToM, as it is often called) is an innate endowment that equips us to get by in a world where complex interactions with others are part of everyday life. As an evolutionary biologist might put it, ToM is essential to survival in our evolutionary niche. In the psychoanalytic model of the mind, theory of mind is referred to as *mentalization* (see Chapter 12, "Self Psychology," and Appendix C, "Glossary").

Researchers suggest that theory of mind begins as an innate potential in infancy and develops in a facilitating matrix of normal maturation, social interactions, and other experiences. Under normal circumstances, ToM can be shown to be present in children by about the age of 4 years (Bartsch and Wellman 1995; Gopnik and Aslington 1988; Mayes and Cohen 1996). In adults, ToM exists on a continuum ranging from the elaborate, complex, and reasonably accurate to the rudimentary, barely functional, and virtually nonexistent. The ability of each of us to accurately represent what others are feeling or are trying to do predicts how well we perform in a variety of interpersonal tasks. At one end of the spectrum, individuals with autism, who have specific defects in the ToM module, have a very hard time functioning in the social world (Baron-Cohen et al. 1985). At the other end of the spectrum, people with highly developed capacities for ToM can negotiate a range of social and interpersonal transactions, ranging from parenting, friendship, and romantic intimacy to business, teaching, politics, and, of course, working in the field of mental health! Obviously people vary in how well they function in each of these domains.

Cognitive psychologists have developed an array of ingenious experiments to test whether adults, children, or nonhuman primates have a functioning theory of mind. It is very difficult to discern whether preverbal children and animals can imagine the minds of other creatures, and scientists continue to debate this question. The experiments in support of each side of these arguments make for interesting reading (Sperber and Premack 1995). Through use of functional neuroimaging (i.e., functional magnetic resonance imaging [fMRI]) techniques, scientists have been able to illuminate particular brain regions that may play a role in the brain systems responsible for ToM (Frith and Frith 1999). Neuroscientists have demonstrated the existence of *mirror neurons,* widely distributed throughout the primate brain, that fire both when we perform an action and when we see someone else perform the same action (Rizzolatti and Craighero 2004). Scientists believe that these mirror neurons may be a crucial part of the neural substrate for our capacity to envision what others are thinking, feeling, and planning to do. Mirror neurons may allow us to understand the intentions behind others' actions by creating a template for those actions inside our own minds. In fact, some scientists argue that mirror neurons allow us to grasp the minds of other people not through conceptual reasoning at all, but through direct simulation of the other's experience.[2]

The theory of mind hypothesis proposes that most human beings are born with the potential to know and make sense of what goes on in the minds of other people. In other words, our attempts to construct and refine a psychoanalytic model of the mind are not altogether different from mental activities people perform every day. We all use our innate capacity for understanding minds to explain ourselves to ourselves and to understand the behavior of others. In other words, when things go as planned, we are all psychologists.

Modeling the Mind in the Era of the Brain

How does one think about the mind in an era dominated by discoveries about the brain? What role does a model of the mind play in this age of neuroscience? Whereas popular belief often holds that advances in neuroscience and psychopharmacology render thinking about the mind and related "talking cures" obsolete, clinicians know that the opposite is true. Never before has the world of mind science been so lively! As we explore this issue further, recall that Freud's formal education was not in psychology, or even in psychiatry, but almost entirely in the field

---

[2]See also National Institute of Mental Health Research Domain Criteria, domain "Social Processes," construct "Perception and Understanding of Others," subconstruct "understanding mental states" (nimh.nih.gov/research-priorities/rdoc/index.shtml; accessed January 12, 2014).

of neuroscience. Before beginning his work with patients suffering from mental illness, he had a long and successful career as a neuropathologist. Even after Freud became immersed in the study of mental life, his goal was to create a science of the mind that would be based on an understanding of the brain. One of his earliest manuscripts, *The Project for a Scientific Psychology* (Freud 1895/1962), which dates from 1895 (but was not published in his lifetime), records Freud's efforts to create a model for what the brain circuitry of the mind might look like. He abandoned this "Project" only when it became clear to him that the neuroscience of his day was not sophisticated enough to support his plan, so that he found himself engaged in highly speculative "theory making" about neural functioning.

Today, our knowledge of the brain is infinitely more advanced than it was in Freud's time. Although mind science is still far from realizing the dream of a brain-based psychology, we have reached a point where intelligible conversation across the mind–brain barrier is at least possible. In fact, we find ourselves in the early stages of a rapprochement between psychology and neuroscience that sheds new light on the importance of psychology as a basic science and promises a deeper understanding of psychotherapy. Important aspects of our model of the mind that had long been thought to be beyond the scope of systematic inquiry are suddenly of renewed interest. Let me give some examples of what I mean.

The Unconscious

At the turn of the twentieth century, Freud first presented his revolutionary "new psychology" based on the proposition that most of what goes on in the mind occurs outside of awareness (Freud 1896/1962). At the turn of the twenty-first century, it is no longer revolutionary to demand that we take the unconscious into account in our study of psychology. In the exploding world of mind science, nonconscious mental processes are now taken for granted as a basic feature of the mind. The new challenge is to account for consciousness and to explain the purpose it serves (Chalmers 1996; Crick 1994; Damasio 1984, 1999; Dennett 1991; Edelman and Tononi 2000; Gazzaniga et al. 1998; Levine 2001; Thau 2001).

Mind and Body

A second feature of the psychoanalytic model of the mind of new interest to the rest of mind science is its emphasis on *embodiment*. This concept of embodiment includes the idea that the mind is intrinsically shaped by its connection to the body, or that the "hardware" from which the mind emerges—the body—is an essential determinant of the nature of mind. For example, research from the laboratory of University of Southern California neuroscientist Antonio Damasio demonstrates what psychoanalysts have long recognized—that how humans reason cannot be separated from how they feel. In other words, cognition cannot be studied independently from *affects,* the complex emotional/physical states produced by and in the body as part of its system of evaluating the self in relationship to the environment for the purpose of survival (Damasio 1984, 1999). At the same time, from a somewhat different angle, philosophers George Lakoff and Mark Johnson (University of California, Berkeley, and University of Oregon) argue that the whole of the reasoning mind is indelibly shaped by metaphors derived from the experience of the body (Lakoff and Johnson 1980, 1999). As we will see, the psychoanalytic model of the mind has long emphasized the centrality of both affects and bodily determined metaphors as organizers of mental life, introducing ideas about the impact of bodily experience on the organization of mental life very similar to those of Damasio and of Lakoff and Johnson. Concepts of the embodied mind present a major challenge to what has been called the *computational model of the mind,* which asserts that the best model of the mind is offered by the disembodied modern computer. The computational model of the mind has held wide influence in mind science for the past 60 years.

Self and Other

In recent years, cognitive scientists and neuroscientists have demonstrated that mother–baby interactions in earliest infancy help shape the cognitive (and neuronal) structures underlying the infant's capacity to tolerate distress. We are in the early stages of a new biology in which human relationships are recognized as regulating both mind and brain beginning in infancy (Eisenberg 1995; Hofer 1984; Schore 1994). Although Freud did not invent psychotherapy, he did launch the first modern exploration of the psychoactive, behavior-modifying, and ultimately brain-altering power of human relationships. The psychoanalytic model of the mind takes into account how relationships are internalized in the course of development to create lasting mental representations of self and other that shape experience and are reactivated in everyday encounters and in all treatments. The focus of psychodynamic psychotherapy always includes the question of how to bring about change by mobilizing these representations in the context of a new relationship.

The Narrative Self

A final point in the convergence between the psychoanalytic model of the mind and cognitive neuroscience is a shared interest in a particular feature of the mind—its innate capacity for narrative expression. Again, Damasio has taken the lead in arguing that consciousness provides an ongoing story about our self-state that serves our need for self-regulation and adaptation to the environment (Damasio 1984; Farber and Churchland 1995). In other words, contemporary brain scientists are beginning to take an interest in the fact that each of us, in the privacy of our own minds, is continually inventing and reinventing a life story as part of an ongoing effort to situate ourselves in the world and to maintain a coherent sense of self. Cognitive psychologists, too, have a strong interest in the narrative structure of the mind, increasingly using the word *script* in their work (Tomkins 1986). In his first book, *Studies on Hysteria*, Freud remarked almost apologetically that he found it "strange that the case histories I write should read like short stories" (Breuer and Freud 1893/1895, p. 160). As we will see, the mind's narrative structure is one of the fundamental aspects of the psychoanalytic model of the mind.

The Psychoanalytic Model of the Mind in the Clinical Setting

A look at developments in contemporary mind science shows that the psychoanalytic model of the mind is ideally suited to help us observe and reveal fundamental aspects of mental life. In the clinical setting, the psychoanalytic model of the mind provides the clinician with a way of making sense of his or her interaction with the patient. It allows the clinician to organize the clinical details—the patient's communication, behavior, modes of relating, and history—so as to construct a picture of the patient's "inner workings" that can be used to understand the current situation, predict responses, and plan interventions. Without such a model, the clinician would quickly become lost in a sea of experiential data. By contrast, the clinician equipped with a sophisticated model of the mind is able to find his or her bearings in the doctor–patient interaction, organize clinical material, and chart a course for potential change.

References

Baron-Cohen S, Leslie AM, Frith U: Does the autistic child have a "theory of mind"? Cognition 21:37–46, 1985

Bartsch K, Wellman H: Children Talk About the Mind. Oxford, UK, Oxford University Press, 1995

Breuer J, Freud S: Studies on hysteria (1893/1895), in The Standard Edition of the Complete Psychological Works of Sigmund Freud, Vol 2. Translated and edited by Strachey J. London, Hogarth Press, 1962, pp 1–335

Chalmers DJ: The Conscious Mind: In Search of a Fundamental Theory. New York, Oxford University Press, 1996

Crick F: The Astonishing Hypothesis: The Scientific Search for the Soul. New York, Simon & Schuster, 1994

Damasio A: Descartes' Error: Emotion, Reason, and the Human Brain. New York, Putnam, 1984

Damasio A: The Feeling of What Happens: Body and Emotion in the Making of Consciousness. New York, Harcourt, Brace, 1999

Dennett DC: Consciousness Explained. Boston, MA, Little, Brown, 1991

Edelman G, Tononi G: A Universe of Consciousness. New York, Basic Books, 2000

Eisenberg L: The social construction of the human brain. Am J Psychiatry 152:1563–1575, 1995

Engel GL: The need for a new medical model: a challenge for biomedicine. Science 196:129–136, 1977

Farber IB, Churchland P: Consciousness and the neurosciences: philosophical and theoretical issues, in The Cognitive Neurosciences. Edited by Gazzaniga MS. Cambridge, MA, Bradford Books/MIT Press, 1995, pp 1295–1306

Freud S: Project for a scientific psychology (1895), in The Standard Edition of the Complete Psychological Works of Sigmund Freud, Vol 1. Translated and edited by Strachey J. London, Hogarth Press, 1962, pp 295–343

Freud S: Letter 52 (Extracts from the Fliess papers) (1896), in The Standard Edition of the Complete Psychological Works of Sigmund Freud, Vol 1. Translated and edited by Strachey J. London, Hogarth Press, 1962, p 233

Freud S: The interpretation of dreams (1900), in The Standard Edition of the Complete Psychological Works of Sigmund Freud, Vol 4/5. Translated and edited by Strachey J. London, Hogarth Press, 1962, pp 1–626

Freud S: Two encyclopaedia articles (1923), in The Standard Edition of the Complete Psychological Works of Sigmund Freud, Vol 19. Translated and edited by Strachey J. London, Hogarth Press, 1962, pp 233–260

Frith C: Making Up the Mind: How the Brain Creates Our Mental World. Malden, MA, Blackwell, 2007

Frith C, Frith U: Interacting minds—a biological basis. Science 286:1692–1695, 1999

Gazzaniga MS, Ivry RB, Mangun GR: The problem of consciousness, in Cognitive Neuroscience: The Biology of the Mind. New York, WW Norton, 1998, pp 527–550

Gopnik A, Aslington JW: Children's understanding of representational change and its relation to the understanding of false belief and the appearance-reality distinction. Child Dev 59:26–37, 1988

Hofer MS: Relationships as regulators: a psychobiologic perspective on bereavement. Psychosom Med 46:183–197, 1984

Kendler KS: A psychiatric dialogue on the mind-body problem. Am J Psychiatry 158:989–1000, 2001

Lakoff G, Johnson M: Metaphors We Live By. Chicago, IL, University of Chicago Press, 1980

Lakoff G, Johnson M: Philosophy of the Flesh: The Embodied Mind and Its Challenge to Western Thought. New York, Basic Books, 1999

Levine J: Purple Haze: The Puzzle of Consciousness. New York, Oxford University Press, 2001

Makari G: Revolution in Mind: The Creation of Psychoanalysis. New York, Harper Collins, 2008

Malle BF: Folk theory of mind: conceptual foundation of human social cognition, in The New Unconscious. Edited by Hassin RR, Uleman JS, Bargh JA. New York, Oxford University Press, 2005, pp 225–255

Mayes L, Cohen D: Children's developing theory of mind. J Am Psychoanal Assoc 44:117–142, 1996

McGinn C: What can your neurons tell you? Review of The Good, True and the Beautiful: A Neuronal Approach, by Jean-Pierre Changeux. New York Review of Books, July 11, 2013, pp 49–50

McHugh PR, Slavney PR: The Perspectives of Psychiatry, 2nd Edition. Baltimore, MD, Johns Hopkins University Press, 1998

Premack DG, Woodruff G: Does the chimpanzee have a theory of mind? Behav Brain Sci 1:515–526, 1978

Rizzolatti G, Craighero L: The mirror-neuron system. Annu Rev Neurosci 27:169–192, 2004

Schore A: Affect Regulation and the Origin of the Self: The Neurobiology of Emotional Development. Hillsdale, NJ, Lawrence Erlbaum, 1994

Sperber D, Premack DG (eds): Causal Cognition: A Multidisciplinary Debate. New York, Oxford University Press, 1995

Thau M: Consciousness and Cognition. New York, Oxford University Press, 2001

Tomkins SS: Script theory, in The Emergence of Personality. Edited by Aranoff J, Rabin AI, Zucker RA. New York, Springer, 1986, pp 147–216

CHAPTER 2

Origins of the Psychoanalytic Model of the Mind

This chapter tells the back story of how the first psychoanalytic model of the mind was formulated, beginning with a lightning tour of the history of scientific psychology, moving from Mesmer, Charcot, and Bernheim, and arriving finally at the case of Anna O., treated by Freud's mentor, Breuer. It will turn to the work of Freud himself, examining how, in the process of abandoning hypnosis, he arrived at the concept of the dynamic unconscious, which forms the basis for the psychoanalytic model of the mind. Vocabulary introduced in this chapter includes the following: *cathartic method, defense, empiricism, free association, fundamental rule, hypnosis, hysteria, materialism, mesmerism, physical determinism, positivism, psychic determinism, psychology, psychotherapy, repression, resistance, suggestion,* and *talking cure.*

Although mental experience has been a subject of fascination since the dawn of consciousness, the history of scientific study of the mind is only about 150 years old. When Freud introduced his first psychoanalytic model of the mind, the term *psychologist* did not even really exist. The word *psychology*—which combines the Greek words *psyche* ("mind/soul") and *–ology* ("the study of")—was introduced into intellectual discourse by a Serbo-Croatian poet (also known as the founder of Serbo-Croatian literature) around 1520 (Krstic 1964), but it did not catch on right away. Poets and philosophers have mused about the nature of the human mind at least since the days of the ancient Greeks. However, psychological reflection did not become organized into a distinct academic or university-based scientific discipline until the end of the nineteenth century, with the birth of two major branches of scientific psychology: the field of experimental psychology (founded by Wundt in Germany in the late 1870s) and the field of psychoanalysis (founded by Freud in Austria in the 1890s).

Birth of Scientific Psychology: The Rise of Psychic Determinism

Modern scientific psychology is the result of the convergence of two major trends in the history of ideas: the Enlightenment (a philosophical movement born in seventeenth-century Europe) and the romantic movement (a trend in culture and the arts beginning in late eighteenth-century Europe). The Enlightenment was characterized by a belief in the power of human reason to triumph over ignorance and superstition. Enlightenment philosophers held to the doctrine of *physical determinism*, which asserts that all events in the natural world obey laws. This attitude led to an explosion of knowledge in the fields of physics and chemistry and in the basic sciences of medicine. In contrast to the Enlightenment, which idealized man's capacity for reason, the romantic movement idealized man's capacity for imagination and feeling. For the romantics, irrationality was not to be overcome, but to be explored as a vital source of creativity. As a result of this idealization, subjectivity became a phenomenon worthy of attention, and introspection became an important route to knowledge about man.

As a result of the combined influence of the Enlightenment and the romantic movement, enthusiasm for successes in the natural sciences had begun to spread to the study of human behavior, so that by the beginning of the nineteenth century in Europe, we see the development of what we now call the social sciences, including anthropology, sociology, economics, political science, and psychology. Much of psychology is based on the principle of *psychic determinism* (analogous to physical determinism), which asserts that psychological life—like physics, biology, physiology, and all other systems in the natural world—is lawfully determined. In other words, psychological events are determined by antecedent psychological events, transformed according to natural laws. Adherence to the principle of psychic determinism does not require abandonment of the idea that mental events result from brain activity; it simply establishes the field of mental activity itself as an appropriate subject for natural science by asserting that mental events obey laws of their own and are not the meaningless epiphenomena of brain processes. The word *psychology* was in use early in the nineteenth century among philosophers, who did much to pave the way for the emergence of psychology as an academic discipline (see Chapter 3, "Evolution of the Dynamic Unconscious"); educators and developmentalists, who studied the best ways to train the minds of children; sexologists, who studied human sexual behavior (e.g., Richard Freiherr von Krafft-Ebing [Krafft-Ebing 1886/1998] and Havelock Ellis [Grosskurth 1985]); proto-psychometricians, who found ways to measure individual differences, such as intelligence (e.g., Alfred Binet [Binet and Simon 1908] and Francis Galton [1869]); neuroanatomists, who discovered areas of the brain responsible for behaviors such as language and motor behavior (e.g., Paul Pierre Broca [1824–1880], Carl Wernicke [1948–1905], and John Hughlings Jackson [1835–1911]) (Stevens 1971); and psychopathologists and psychotherapists, who sought to understand and treat mental illness (e.g., Jean-Martin Charcot, Hippolyte Bernheim, and Josef Breuer) (Ellenberger 1970). Alongside of these scholarly endeavors were dozens of other less intellectually legitimate forays into areas such as phrenology, parapsychology, and even the psychic life of plants (Fancher 1979; Hunt 1993; Robinson 1995).

Franz Anton Mesmer: Early Attempts to Apply Scientific Principles to the Practice of Medicine

The medical historian Henri Ellenberger (1970) has argued that we can trace the origins of scientific psychotherapy to the end of the eighteenth century, when we see a shift in the healing arts from the domain of religion to the domain of science, as doctors and men of science, rather than priests and exorcists, began to dominate the study and treatment of mental suffering. Ellenberger focused on the character of Franz Anton Mesmer (1734–1815), a Viennese physician working more than 100 years before Freud, who was deeply immersed in many aspects of Enlightenment philosophy, particularly the application of science to the practice of medicine. Mesmer believed that he had discovered the existence of a universal, physical fluid, analogous to the forces of gravitation or of electricity. He argued that disturbances of equilibrium in this fluid explain health and disease. Mesmer's theory of cure proposed that the therapist, or "magnetizer," induce in the patient a trance-like state, transmitting his own stronger and better fluid to the patient through the channel of the *rapport*. Although he initially became famous throughout Europe, Mesmer was ultimately discredited by the French Academy of Science (after an investigation carried out by a panel that included America's own Benjamin Franklin). Today, Mesmer's theories of magnetic fluid seem silly to us. His name, while preserved in the English language, is not part of vocabulary of modern medical practice but is memorialized in the word *mesmerize,* which means "to fascinate or enthrall." However, Mesmer's work represents the efforts of a man of science to wrest control of the study of mind from the domain of religion and religious practice (Ellenberger 1970).

By the middle of the nineteenth century, mesmerism had all but disappeared in European medical circles, eclipsed by steady refinements in the techniques of experimental science. However, by the second half of the nineteenth century, we find a new wave of medicalization of the illnesses and the treatments that had been the concern of Mesmer and his followers. This medicalization was fueled by three developments: the widespread prevalence of hysteria, a fascination with hypnosis, and the development of the field of neuroscience.

From Magnetic Illness to Hysteria

Patients with *hysteria* were most often young to middle-aged women who suffered from an odd assortment of sensory and motor symptoms, as well as disorders of thought, emotion, and consciousness, frequently neurological in appearance, that did not fit the pattern of any known neurological condition. Hysteria was a relatively common illness in nineteenth century Europe and the United States, its victims including many famous people (e.g., Alice James, the sister of William and Henry James). However, hysteria was not an illness that was new to the age. The term *hysteria* was coined by the Greek physician Hippocrates (460–370 B.C.E.), who believed that it was caused by irregular movement of blood from the uterus (*hysteros*) to the brain. In the Middle Ages and well into the eighteenth century, people manifesting hysteria were often thought to be suffering from demonic possession and were treated with exorcism. By the middle of the nineteenth century, hysteria had become the focus of healers previously interested in the "magnetic diseases." The illness also drew the attention of the earliest practitioners of our modern field of neurology, who began to offer ideas about disordered functioning within the mind/brain system.[1]

---

[1] These new ideas about the causes of hysteria were presented most systematically in the work of Paul Briquet (1796–1881), a French physician who argued that the ailment was a "neurosis of the brain" caused by the effect of violent emotions on individuals predisposed by heredity factors. For an introduction to the concept of *neurosis,* see Chapter 5, "The Mind's Topography."

From Mesmerism to Hypnosis

As interest in magnetic illnesses was replaced by the study of hysteria, mesmerism was in turn replaced by the practice of *hypnosis*. Like hysteria, hypnotism was an ancient phenomenon that can be traced back to ancient Egypt. However, the term was coined in 1843 by James Braid (1795–1860), a Scottish-born surgeon practicing in Manchester, who named the practice after the Greek word *hypnos*, the god of sleep. Although Braid ultimately recognized that hypnosis and sleep were unrelated, the name nonetheless persisted. Intrigued by the demonstrations of a Swiss mesmerist, Braid began to experiment with inducing trance states in his servants, his friends, and even his own wife. To explain the phenomenon, Braid rejected Mesmer's theory of magnetic fluid and replaced it with his own (somewhat vague) theory of altered brain physiology. His new term *hypnosis* was quickly adopted throughout Europe as the official and newly medicalized name for the practice of inducing a trance for the purpose of treatment.

Emergence of the Fields of Neuroscience, Neurology, and Psychiatry

Both hysteria and hypnotism were of great interest to men whose training was in the new fields of neuroscience and neurology. Whereas the brain had long been understood to be the organ of the mind, described as such in the teaching of both Hippocrates and Galen (129–210 C.E.), human understanding of the specific relationship between the brain and various behaviors, experiences, and symptoms underwent a great leap forward in the second half of the nineteenth century, as scientists began to unlock the secrets of brain structure and function. Scientist-physicians Camillo Golgi (1843–1926) and Santiago Ramon y Cajal (1852–1934) (at the Universities of Pavia and Madrid, respectively) made advances in the microscopic study of brain tissue that led to the development of the *neurone doctrine*, which posits that the basic unit of brain structure is a specialized cell called the *neuron*. In 1906, Golgi and y Cajal shared the Nobel Prize for Medicine for the development of this doctrine, now accepted as the basis for modern neuroscience. Also during the second half of the nineteenth century, the physiologist-physicians Emil du Bois-Reymond (1818–1896) and Hermann von Helmholtz (1821–1894) at the University of Berlin began to elucidate the electrochemical function of the neuron, and neuropathologist-physicians including Paul Pierre Broca (1824–1880), Carl Wernicke (1948–1905), and

John Hughlings Jackson (1835–1911) (at the University of Paris, the University of Breslau, and London Hospital, respectively) began to map the correlations between specific areas of the brain and functions such as speech and language (Broca and Wernicke) and motor function (Hughlings Jackson) (Stevens 1971). Meanwhile, as basic neuroscience is taking off in laboratories throughout Europe, we also see the rise of university-based psychiatry. The neurologist-psychiatrist Wilhelm Griesinger (1817–1869), first director of the university-based Burghölzli mental hospital in Zurich and often called the father of modern academic psychiatry, was famous for having declared that "mental diseases are brain diseases" (Ellenberger 1970, p. 241).

By the end of the nineteenth century, throughout Europe but especially in France, we see an integration between a new fascination with hysteria, the practice of hypnotism, and the new science of the mind/brain system. This integration was brought about largely through the work of two men who, while intensely competitive with each other, did work that made possible the development of modern psychotherapy. These two men were Jean-Martin Charcot, practicing at L'Hôpital Salpêtrière in Paris, and Hippolyte Bernheim, practicing 240 miles away in the city of Nancy. Both of these men exerted a powerful and direct influence on one of their students, the young Sigmund Freud.

Jean-Martin Charcot: Hysteria and Pathogenic Ideas

Jean-Martin Charcot (1825–1893) was one of the most luminous characters in all of nineteenth-century medicine. The son of a middle-class carriage maker, he rose to become one of the most distinguished neurologists of all time, considered by many to be the father of modern neurology. Charcot earned fame through his work at the L'Hôpital Salpêtrière where, in 1862, he was appointed chief physician of one of the hospital's major sections. At the time of his appointment, the Salpêtrière was a vast but decaying complex of 45 buildings that served mainly as a medical poorhouse for thousands of old women and prostitutes. Although famous as the site where Philippe Pinel made medical history by liberating the "insane" from their chains, the mid-nineteenth-century Salpêtrière was not a place where young men of ambition sought appointment. However, Charcot recognized that the Salpêtrière sheltered patients with rare or unknown neurological diseases who could serve as the subjects for clinical research. Within a decade, he had transformed this warehouse for the forgotten into a modern academic medical center with new consulting rooms for treatment, laboratories for research, and a large auditorium. Medical students and scientists from all over the world flocked to the Salpêtrière to hear Charcot's dramatic lectures and to witness his spectacular clinical demonstrations.

Charcot adopted the idea that hysteria was a brain illness that left constitutionally predisposed individuals susceptible to disturbance in the psyche. His work on hysteria began with his effort to distinguish patients with epileptic seizures from those who were having hysterical convulsions. He was also interested in the similarities between hysterical paralyses and traumatic paralyses for which there was no evident organic cause. Traumatic injury had become increasingly common in this era of the railroad, where accidents were frequent and litigation over who could legitimately claim to be paralyzed focused attention on the etiology of syndromes associated with trauma. Charcot and his collaborators developed an elaborate classification system for hysteria, including what he called *traumatic hysteria*.

At the end of the 1870s, Charcot's interest began to include hypnosis, which had gained some acceptance in European medical circles. His experiments quickly revealed that hysterical patients were easy to hypnotize. Using hypnosis, Charcot demonstrated that he could reproduce the same symptoms in patients suffering from hysteria as could be found in those suffering from traumatic paralyses. He also demonstrated that with hypnosis, he was able to remove the same symptoms of paralysis from both groups of patients. On the basis of this work, Charcot concluded that hypnotic, hysterical, and traumatic paralyses were all identical to each another, all the result of *suggestion* (see section "Hippolyte Bernheim and the Nancy School"), and all consisting of lawful, ordered phenomena. He argued that in susceptible individuals with a hereditary predisposition who were exposed to suggestion (either therapist-induced, self-induced, or spontaneous, as in the case of trauma), "a coherent group of associated ideas settle themselves in the mind in the fashion of parasites, remaining isolated from the rest of the mind and expressing themselves outwardly through corresponding motor phenomena" (Ellenberger 1970, p. 149). Charcot introduced the concept that small, sequestered fragments of the mind could follow a course of development separate from the rest of the personality, manifesting themselves through bodily symptoms. These sequestered bits of psychic life became known as *subconscious fixed ideas*, the term given them by Charcot's student Pierre Janet. Charcot's concept marked the first time that ideas were seen as having causal properties in the physical world. His revolutionary concept that ideas outside of awareness can be *pathogenic*, or have the power to cause hysterical and other kinds of neurotic symptoms, would soon be seized upon and modified by another of Charcot's students—the young Sigmund Freud.

Whereas the impressionable young Freud became more than a little enthralled with Charcot, other visitors to the Salpêtrière were more skeptical. Despite his prestige in French medical circles and the excitement created by his dramatic clinical demonstrations, Charcot ultimately ran afoul of the scientific establishment. In the last years of his life, his work in the areas of hypnosis and hysteria fell into disrepute following allegations made by students and patients that many of his famous demonstrations were "faked" by subjects eager to please the master. Charcot's work on hysteria was repudiated by his successors. In 1925, at a celebration of the centennial of Charcot's birth held at the Salpêtrière, the period of Charcot's life devoted to hysteria and hypnosis was dismissed as an unfortunate chapter in an otherwise brilliant career. Only the French surrealists, in their passion for all things at the margins of the acceptable, gave Charcot a posthumous award for his "discovery of hysteria" (Ellenberger 1970, p. 101).

Hippolyte Bernheim and the Nancy School: The Origins of Psychotherapy

Meanwhile, across France in the city of Nancy, Hippolyte Bernheim (1840–1919) was also using hypnosis to treat patients suffering from hysteria. Like Charcot, Bernheim understood hysteria to be a pathogenic effect of *subconscious fixed ideas*. Although decidedly less colorful than Charcot, Bernheim was a distinguished professor of internal medicine at a university hospital in the Alsatian city of Strasbourg. When this province was annexed by Germany in 1871 during the Franco-Prussian War, Bernheim, a fervent French patriot, relocated to Nancy, the old capital of Lorraine, where he rose rapidly in the ranks of the new university hospital.

In Nancy, Bernheim came into contact with Ambroise-Auguste Liébeault (1823–1904), a country physician whom many considered a quack because of his practice of using hypnosis to treat the poor. Bernheim was convinced by Liébeault's assertion (now known to be incorrect) that hypnotic sleep is identical to natural sleep, the sole difference being that the former is induced by the suggestion. In fact, it was Liébeault who made famous the use of the word *suggestion* and Bernheim who defined *suggestibility* (both terms later taken up by Charcot) as "the aptitude to transform an idea into an act" (Garrabé 1999).

In contrast to Charcot, Bernheim and the Nancy School argued that hypnosis was not a pathological brain state that can be induced only in people predisposed through heredity but was itself the result of suggestion, reproducible in everyone to varying degrees. The Nancy School is credited with placing hypnosis (and, by association, hysterical illnesses) on a continuum with normal states of mind, anticipating Freud's assertion that people with hysteria and "normal" people have essentially the same psychological makeup. Finally, and again in contrast with Charcot, Bernheim was interested in developing hypnosis as a therapeutic intervention. In the course of their long collaboration, Liébeault and Bernheim used hypnosis to treat over 30,000 patients suffering from "nervous ailments" including hysteria, but also rheumatism, gastrointestinal diseases, and menstrual disorders. Their method consisted of the use of suggestion to induce hypnosis accompanied by the use of imperative suggestion to remove symptoms. Over time, Bernheim began to dispense with hypnosis altogether, using suggestion alone to influence the expression of the patient's pathogenic ideas. This use of suggestion in the waking state was a treatment procedure that the Nancy School now named *psychotherapy,* the first use of what is now a very common word.

Bernheim introduced his ideas to the medical world in 1882. The same year, Charcot presented a paper on hypnosis and hysteria at the Académie des Sciences. Immediately these two men became bitter rivals, borrowing from and elaborating on each other's ideas. Despite the differences between these two men, their shared insights led to the consolidation of a new theory of hysteria based on a disordered brain/mind system. This new theory explained the bizarre symptoms of hysteria as the result of separate systems of awareness, or consciousness, and/or split fragments of mental life, which in susceptible individuals functioned autonomously. It paved the way for new approaches to treatment based on the goal of reintegrating split-off ideas into ordinary conscious mental life. This new theory and its associated "psychotherapeutics" were disseminated throughout Central Europe by 1885, when we encounter the young neurologist Sigmund Freud on his way to Paris to study with the great Charcot.

Sigmund Freud

Sigmund Freud (1856–1939) was born on May 6, 1856, in Freiburg, a small town in Moravia at the edge of the Austro-Hungarian Empire. He was the oldest son of a wool merchant, Jacob Freud, and Jacob's much younger, third wife, Amalia Nathanson. When Sigmund was 4 years old, the Freud family moved to Leopoldstadt, the predominantly Jewish quarter of Vienna. As was the trend among newly urbanized Jews toward assimilation, Jacob and Amalie Freud raised their children in a German-speaking home with the goals and ideals of the Viennese middle class. It is not known how Jacob Freud supported his family in Vienna, and his financial situation was quite precarious. Nevertheless, he appears to have been able to provide his 10 children with education, music lessons, and even summer vacations at a resort in Moravia. By all accounts, family life revolved around the needs and wishes of the couple's oldest son, whose intelligence inspired awe in his gentle and generous father, and pride in his beautiful and doting mother, who referred to him as "mein guldener Sigi" (Jones 1953/1961, p. 4).

The picture of Freud that emerges from many sources is one of contradiction. By temperament, he was an intense and passionate man who modulated his feelings with hard work, introspection, and a knack for irony. As a suitor, he was affectionate, even ardent, if also possessive, jealous, and self-absorbed. As a friend, he was given to intense, almost desperate and dependent attachments to other men, which were inevitably broken off with hard feelings, mostly on his side. He was at once optimistic, wildly ambitious, and preoccupied with finding a way to become great, even as he was often paralyzed by agonizing self-doubt. Early in his career, he was plagued with neurotic symptoms including palpitations, shortness of breath, indigestion, and extreme moodiness. He saw himself as a loner, isolated in a hostile world, although he greatly exaggerated the extent to which he and his early work were scorned. Although he was thoroughly identified with his Jewishness, through which he claimed to have inherited his comfort with being "in the Opposition" (Freud 1925/1962, p. 9), he had no use for the deity, whom he dismissed as "an illusion" (Freud 1927/1962). His boyhood heroes were not famous philosophers and intellectuals, but "conquistadors" and rebellious heroes of antiquity. The sources from which he drew inspiration were as likely to be great poets as they were to be men of science. However, his own lifestyle was modest, fastidious, and even somewhat ascetic, with long hours spent seeing patients and evenings engaged in writing. Free time was devoted to domestic life or evenings spent playing cards with friends. All of Freud's children described him as an affectionate and devoted father. In other words, his entire appetite for grandeur was given over to the development and promotion of his ideas (Freud 1925/1962; Gay 1988; Jones 1953/1961; Makari 2008).

In his official autobiography, Freud asserts that he was the best student in his class at the gymnasium, and school records support this claim. From the first, he read voraciously in politics, history, literature, art, and the natural sciences. When he entered the University of Vienna at the age of 17, he was already competent in Greek, Latin, Hebrew, English, French, Spanish, and Italian, and thoroughly familiar with the Western canon ranging from the works of Darwin to the classics of Western literature. In a bit of foreshadowing, records from his gymnasium days show that on his final exam, he was asked to translate a passage from Sophocles' *Oedipus Rex* (Freud 1925/1962; Jones 1953/1961).

Freud began at University of Vienna with the plan to study medicine. At first he was in no hurry to make himself independent of his father's financial support. His studies at the university were prolonged by his wide-ranging curiosity and his interest in research. Freud spent most of the first year in the study of the humanities, reading Ludwig Feuerbach, a Hegelian philosopher who argued that man's invention of God leaves him "alienated from himself," and studying with Franz Brentano, the philosopher-priest who proposed a view of the mind as defined by its quality of *intentionality* (or the quality of always "being about" or representing something outside itself). He also found time to translate a volume of the works of British philosopher John Stuart Mill, who viewed mental processes as consisting of the association of related ideas.

After a year of research in comparative anatomy under Carl Claus, Freud published his first paper, on the gonadal structure of the eel. In 1875, he took a position as a research scholar in Ernst Brucke's Institute of Physiology. Brucke was to exert a major influence on the development of Freud's intellectual and professional life.

Freud the Neuropathologist

Brucke's Institute was run according to the principles of a scientific movement called the Helmholtz School of Medicine, which grew out the friendship of four men who worked together at the University of Berlin in the 1840s: Ernst Brucke (1819–1892), Emil du Bois-Reymond (1818–1896), Carl Ludwig (1816–1895), and Hermann von Helmholtz (1821–1894). These four scientists were influenced by the positivist revolution sweeping the German intellectual world in the mid-nineteenth century. *Positivism* was a program for systematizing all knowledge of the world based on "undeniable truths." Since its introduction by Auguste Comte more than 200 years ago,[2] the term *positivism* has come to be used more widely (and more vaguely) to describe any account of the world using

---

[2]Comte introduced the word *positivism* in his multivolume book *The Course in Positive Philosophy* (1830–1842); see http://plato.stanford.edu/entries/comte/ (accessed November 15, 2013).

the language and methods of science. By the middle of the nineteenth century, positivism had become strongly associated with two other important attitudes: *empiricism* (the belief that the only source of true knowledge about the universe comes from the evidence of the senses) and *materialism* (the belief that everything in the universe can be understood in terms of the properties of matter and energy). This triad of positivism, empiricism, and materialism allied itself in opposition to all speculation about the universe based on the power of unseen spiritual forces (Koch 1985, p. 16). In the biological sciences, the positivist revolution fueled the rise of the science of physiology, which attempted to explain organisms in accord with the principles of chemistry and physics. This new physiology played a large role in the development of psychology as an ordered and lawful system that can be studied within the framework of the natural sciences. Both Freud, the father of psychoanalysis, and Wilhelm Wundt (1832–1902), the father of university-based academic/experimental psychology (see Chapter 3), were direct descendants of the Helmholtz School, each having studied under one of its founders (Bernfeld 1944).

Freud's successes as a laboratory scientist were substantial. His investigations of the microscopic neuroanatomy of the lamprey and the crayfish contributed to the revolutionary "neurone doctrine." His training at the Institute of Physiology prepared him for later work on the microanatomy of the human brain stem and the cranial nerves, and in anatomo-clinical neurology in the areas of cerebral palsy and aphasia. His work on the pharmacological effects of cocaine brought him some renown and even some early notoriety. He was appointed to the coveted position of *Privatdozent* at the University of Vienna in 1885 on the basis of his recognized expertise in neuropathology.

Brucke also gave Freud important professional and personal guidance, persuading him that despite his success in research, his future at the Institute was not bright, because pathways for academic advancement were blocked by the presence of talented colleagues several years his senior. Furthermore, the relative penury associated with laboratory life would never be able to provide Freud with the means to marry his fiancée, 21-year-old Martha Bernays (1861–1951), a young woman from a socially prominent German-Jewish family with whom he was passionately in love. In 1882, a year after receiving his medical degree, Freud left Brucke's laboratory and took a position as a house physician at the Viennese Hospital in preparation for beginning the more financially secure life of a clinician. In the next 3 years, he studied internal medicine, surgery, ophthalmology, and dermatology, with the bulk of his time spent in the study of nervous diseases. Finally, it was Brucke who obtained for

Freud the coveted University Jubilee Travel Scholarship, which in 1885 took him to Paris for his life-altering encounter with Charcot.

Freud and Charcot: New Investigations of Psychopathology

At the Salpêtrière, Freud began to think about psychopathology in a new way. His brief 6-month study of psychiatry under Theodor Meynert at the University of Vienna had focused on the study of phenomenology and classification, with no emphasis on the meaning of symptoms. Thrilled by the personal dynamism of Charcot and by the boldness of his ideas about hysteria and hypnosis, Freud returned to Vienna, committed to the study of psychopathology. He quickly devoted himself to the task of translating Charcot's works into German. Freud began clinical practice in 1896, and 6 months later he was earning enough money to marry Martha Bernays. As one of the few specialists in nervous diseases in Vienna at the time, his practice quickly grew, made up largely of women suffering from hysteria whom few wanted to treat. Freud's therapeutic arsenal for the treatment of hysteria included electrotherapy accompanied by deep and whole-body massage, baths for relaxation, and variations on the "rest cure" developed by American physician Silas Weir Mitchell (1829–1914), all of which he used well into the 1890s. He also began to experiment with hypnosis. Because Freud's hero Charcot was not especially enthusiastic about the use of hypnosis for treatment, Freud was most influenced in his technique by Bernheim, whom he visited in Nancy for 2 months in 1889 and whose book on hypnosis he had committed to translate. At the time of this second visit to France, Freud also attended the First International Congress on Hypnotism in Paris (timed to coincide with the opening of the Eifel Tower).

Freud's early technique for the treatment of hysteria included the induction of a hypnotic trance (as described by Bernheim) followed by the use of imperative suggestion for the removal of symptoms. Nevertheless, despite his enthusiastic endorsement of Bernheim's method, Freud quickly became frustrated with the use of suggestion to remove symptoms, complaining of the contrast between the "rosy coloring" of the physician's suggestions and the "cheerless truth" of the patient's suffering (Freud 1891/1962, p. 113). Freud modified Bernheim's technique to include the use of hypnosis not only for therapy but also for "investigation" of the illness. The most immediate influence on this development in his practice came from a Viennese colleague, Josef Breuer, who showed Freud a way by which he might combine clinical work with his passion for a deeper understanding.

Freud and Breuer: *Studies on Hysteria*

Josef Breuer (1842–1925) was a well-known Viennese family physician with an excellent reputation as both a clinician and a researcher. Among other things, he is known today for his description of the Hering-Breuer reflexes governing respiration. Breuer was the leader of a group of prominent Jewish physicians who worked together and helped each other in anti-Semitic Vienna. The older man quickly became Freud's mentor, offering encouragement, friendship, and even financial support. Not only did Breuer send Freud patients for his fledgling practice, but he also shared with Freud his ideas about the treatment of hysteria.

It was Breuer with whom Freud co-authored his first full-length treatise on psychology, *Studies on Hysteria*, published in 1895. This book consists of five case studies (one treated by Breuer and four treated by Freud) and two theoretical chapters—one on the pathogenesis of hysteria (written by Breuer) and one on psychotherapy (written by Freud). The book describes how Breuer and Freud understood the psychopathology of hysteria and how they used what they both referred to as "the cathartic method" to treat patients suffering from this disorder. It also contains several subplots embedded in the text that enliven the story, including the story of how Freud and Breuer broke with each other over their understanding of hysteria; the story of how Freud moved from a trauma theory of hysteria to a theory based on the impact of forbidden, unconscious wishes; and—most relevant here—the story of how Freud gradually moved away from the use of hypnosis, a move that led him to develop a new model of the mind. *Studies on Hysteria* was not a wild success in medical circles, netting its authors about 425 gulden ($85.00) each. However, it launched Freud once and for all on the path of writing about the psychological life of the mind that would ultimately lead him to fill 37 volumes of his collected works (Jones 1953/1961; Makari 2008).

Breuer's Cathartic Method: The Story of Anna O.

As early as 1883, Breuer had shared with Freud the story of his treatment of a woman suffering from hysteria, made famous in the first case report in *Studies on Hysteria* (Breuer and Freud 1893/1895/1962) as "Anna O." Anna O. (whose real name was Bertha Pappenheim) was "a young girl of unusual education and gifts who had fallen ill while nursing her father of whom she was devotedly fond" (Freud 1925/1962, p. 20). When Breuer took over her case in 1882, her symptoms included paralyses of her limbs, paresthesias, disturbances of vision and speech, and states of mental confusion. She had two alternating personalities—one that was normal and the other that she called "naughty" (Breuer and Freud 1893/1895/1962, p. 24). The transition from one to the other was marked by a phase of autohypnosis. Breuer observed that Anna O. could be relieved of her symptoms if, during these self-induced trance states, she were allowed to "express in words the affective phantasy by which she was at the moment dominated" (Freud 1925/1962, p. 20). From this observation, Breuer developed a treatment method in which Anna O. was encouraged to tell stories about her symptoms under the influence of hypnosis. He observed that her stories invariably led to a recounting of her state of mind and her feelings at the time when her symptoms first developed. Careful attention to the details of her stories demonstrated that her symptoms represented symbolic expressions of experiences and memories of which she was not aware in her "normal" state. When she was brought in contact with the emotions connected to these "lost" experiences through storytelling, "the procedure...succeeded, after long and painful efforts, in relieving her...of all her symptoms" (Freud 1925/ 1962, p. 20).

It is clear that Breuer's claim, in *Studies on Hysteria,* to have cured Anna O. of her symptoms was exaggerated. Historians have shown that after her treatment ended, she spent at least a year in a sanatorium before going on to become a prominent social worker whose work with wayward young women earned her commemoration on a German postage stamp in 1954. Nevertheless, Anna O. is generally accepted as the co-inventor with Breuer of a new treatment characterized by introspective investigation, shared narrative, and the expression of feelings. Anna O. called this new procedure "chimney sweeping"; speaking seriously, she named it "the talking cure" (Breuer and Freud 1893/1895, p. 30). Breuer called it "the cathartic method" (Breuer and Freud 1893/ 1895/1962, p. xxix; Freud 1925/1962, p. 22).

At first Freud was enthusiastic about the new treatment, which he referred to as "Breuer's method," applying it to his own patients beginning in 1889. Between 1889 and 1896, Freud hypnotized his patients using the cathartic method with the aim of uncovering dissociated pathogenic ideas and tracing them back through a chain of associations to the point of origin, which was inevitably a traumatic event. In this early phase of his work, traumatic memories (and later, forbidden wishes) were effaced through suggestion (in the manner of Bernheim) or were discharged through words, affective expression, and/or corrective association with the rest of conscious mental life (in the manner of Breuer).

Freud's Abandonment of Hypnosis and Discovery of the Dynamic Unconscious

We now arrive at a crucial episode in our history: the story of how Freud made the transition from the use of Breuer's cathartic method to a new treatment method that led him to develop a new model of the mind. The crucial step in this invention was Freud's abandonment of the use of hypnosis and his substitution of new ways to engage the patient in treatment. Despite his initial enthusiasm for treatments based on hypnosis, Freud gradually became frustrated with the technique, discouraged by the fact that many of his patients were not hypnotizable, or by the fact that their cures often seemed short-lived. Casting about for a treatment method that did not depend on hypnosis, Freud recalled a remark made by Bernheim to the effect that events experienced by patients under hypnosis are only *apparently* forgotten and can be brought to consciousness if the therapist insists that the patient can remember. Freud concluded that this fact might also be true of forgotten ideas in hysteria, and he began to conduct his therapeutic investigations in the waking state. In a technique that he later called *free association,* Freud invited his patients to let thoughts flow freely, with as little conscious control as possible. He also insisted that his patient report to him everything that passed through the mind with as little censorship as possible (Breuer and Freud 1893/1895/1962, p. 56). Freud's insistence that the patient report to the analyst everything in his or her mind with as little censorship as possible would later come to be known as the *fundamental rule* of psychoanalysis (Freud 1901/1962, p. 39). Fortified by the principle of psychic determinism, Freud was confident that every thought or feeling that came to the patient's mind would be a link in a determined chain of associations, leading back ultimately to the original pathogenic idea or memory. In other words, while relatively free of conscious censorship, the patient's thoughts would not be guided by chance at all, but would lead the investigation in the right direction. The net effect of the modifications Freud made in Breuer's method was that his patients were now fully "awake" and as a result were more actively engaged in the treatment process. His own role, by contrast, became less intrusive and controlling.

With these changes, Freud had inadvertently discovered a treatment method that afforded him a view of the patient's mind at work that had not been apparent before. When Freud encouraged his patients to become active participants in the treatment investigation, he was rewarded with his first glimpse of a world of psychological activity that lay behind the patient's symptoms, a world more vast than previously imagined. His first observation was that despite his patients' best attempts to adhere to the demands of the new treatment, they were not always able to bring themselves to report all of their thoughts and feelings or even to allow themselves to be fully aware of their own mental activity. The patients' efforts at free association inevitably produced gaps and discontinuities in the train of thought and incoherence in the story. Freud used the word *resistance* to describe discontinuity in the flow of association. His next observation was that he and his patients had to work hard to overcome this resistance. He had to admonish his patients repeatedly to say whatever came to mind, and they, in turn, had to struggle to cooperate with his demand. Freud concluded that his patients' conscious motivation to adhere to the technique of free association was opposed by another, less conscious motivation to conceal aspects of mental life, not only from the doctor but also from the patient him- or herself. Finally, Freud observed that all of the bits of mental life that his patients were reluctant to reveal turned out to be of a "distressing nature, calculated to arouse the affects of shame and of self-reproach...they were all of a kind that one would prefer not to have experienced, that one would rather forget" (Breuer and Freud 1893/1895/1962, p. 269; Makari 2008).

By combining all of these observations, Freud concluded that his patients wanted to keep certain ideas, feelings, memories, and wishes out of consciousness because they needed to defend themselves from associated feelings of shame and self-reproach. Freud used the word *repression* to refer to the defensive process of removing unacceptable thoughts and feelings from consciousness. In other words, for the first time, Freud was able to see a psychological battle going on in his patient's mind that had previously been obscured by the use of hypnosis.

It was around these observations of resistance to self-awareness, and of the work needed to overcome it, that Freud organized his new theory of hysteria. Whereas Breuer, Charcot, Bernheim, Janet (Charcot's student), and others understood that hysteria was the result of pathogenic ideas becoming walled off from ordinary conscious mental life, they all believed that these splits in consciousness were the result of pathological brain processes, such as "hypnoid states" (Breuer), innate weaknesses in the capacity for synthesis (Janet), or familial "mental degeneration" (Charcot). Freud introduced the revolutionary idea that in hysteria, thoughts and feelings are separated from consciousness not because of diseased brain processes but rather because of the emotional needs of the patient—or from "the motive of defense" (Breuer and Freud 1893/1895/1962, p. 285). In contrast to Charcot's "traumatic hysteria" or Breuer's "hypnoid hysteria," Freud described what he called "defense hysteria," asserting that individuals with hysteria do not suffer from brain disease, but are essentially normal people struggling with thoughts and feelings that they find unacceptable (Breuer and Freud 1893/1895/1962, p. 285). In his view, hysteria is the result of a battle over unacceptable thoughts, memories, and wishes that are barred from consciousness but that continue to seek expression in the form of symptoms. Initially, Freud saw what he called *resistance* as a barrier to exploration of inner life. However, over time, he learned to be as curious about the patient's reasons for keeping secrets as he was about the secrets themselves. In other words, Freud became increasingly interested in observing resistance as the most important clue to areas of conflict in the patient's emotional life. When his patients were able to overcome their resistance and to accept these warded-off aspects of psychological lives, their symptoms disappeared.

A "New Psychology" of the Unconscious: Psychoanalysis

By 1896, Freud had given up use of hypnosis almost entirely as a method for the treatment of hysteria and had devoted himself fully to the practice of what he initially called "psychical analysis" but by the end of the year had named *psychoanalysis* (Freud 1896b/1962, p. 151). As his practice grew, Freud applied his new treatment method to many new patients and even to himself. The years between 1895 and 1900 were exciting as Freud mined the possibilities afforded him by his novel treatment method. However, although his concept of defense hysteria was a revolution in thinking about the cause of hysteria, the greatest revolution was yet to come. Not content with the clinician's job of understanding and treating patients, Freud was a highly ambitious man who sought to leave a lasting mark in the world. He was drawn to large questions, the answers to which might shed light on the "nature of man" (Jones 1953/1961, p. 175). Even while engaging in the treatment of his growing caseload of patients, collaborating with Breuer to write *Studies on Hysteria*, and working to extend his theory of defense hysteria to include other illnesses, Freud was already beginning to explore how the processes of defense and repression operate not just in psychopathology but in psychological health as well.

   In the years between the publication of *Studies on Hysteria* in 1895 and the turn of the century in 1900, Freud worked feverishly to expand his theory of hysteria into a general theory of mind. As early as 1896, in a letter to a friend, Freud remarked that he was well on his way to inventing a "new psychology" that would apply not just to people suffering from neuroses but to everyone (Freud 1896a/1962, 1901/1962, 1933/1962). From the first, Freud's new psychology, known now as psychoanalysis, was founded on his ideas about parts of the mind that in everyone are unconscious. As we will see in Chapter 3, the concept of the unconscious is at the core of all psychoanalytic models of the mind.

References

Bernfeld S: Freud's earliest theories and the school of Helmholtz. Psychoanal Q 13:341–362, 1944

Binet A, Simon R: Le developpement de l'intelligence chez les enfants. L'Année Psychologique 14:1–94, 1908

Breuer J, Freud S: Studies on hysteria (1893/1895), in The Standard Edition of the Complete Psychological Works of Sigmund Freud, Vol 2. Translated and edited by Strachey J. London, Hogarth Press, 1962, pp 1–335

Ellenberger H: The Discovery of the Unconscious: The History and Evolution of Dynamic Psychiatry. New York, Basic Books, 1970

Fancher RE: Pioneers of Psychology. New York, WW Norton, 1979

Freud S: Hypnosis (1891), in The Standard Edition of the Complete Psychological Works of Sigmund Freud, Vol 1. Translated and edited by Strachey J. London, Hogarth Press, 1962, pp 233

Freud S: Letter 52 (Extracts from the Fliess papers) (1896a), in The Standard Edition of the Complete Psychological Works of Sigmund Freud, Vol 1. Translated and edited by Strachey J. London, Hogarth Press, 1962, p 233

Freud S: Heredity and the aetiology of the neuroses (1896b), in The Standard Edition of the Complete Psychological Works of Sigmund Freud, Vol 3. Translated and edited by Strachey J. London, Hogarth Press, 1962, pp 141–156

Freud S: The psychopathology of everyday life (1901), in The Standard Edition of the Complete Psychological Works of Sigmund Freud, Vol 6. Translated and edited by Strachey J. London, Hogarth Press, 1962, pp 1–310

Freud S: An autobiographical study (1925), in The Standard Edition of the Complete Psychological Works of Sigmund Freud, Vol 20. Translated and edited by Strachey J. London, Hogarth Press, 1962, pp 1–74

Freud S: The future of an illusion (1927), in The Standard Edition of the Complete Psychological Works of Sigmund Freud, Vol 21. Translated and edited by Strachey J. London, Hogarth Press, 1962, pp 1–56

Freud S: The question of a Weltanschauung (Lecture XXXV), New introductory lectures on psychoanalysis (1933), in The Standard Edition of the Complete Psychological Works of Sigmund Freud, Vol 22. Translated and edited by Strachey J. London, Hogarth Press, 1962, pp 158–182

Galton F: Hereditary genius: an inquiry into its laws and consequences. London, Macmillan/Fontana, 1869

Garrabé J: Hippolyte Bernheim (1840–1919), in Anthology of French Language Psychiatric Texts. Edited by Ousin FR, Garrabé J, Morozov D. Paris, Empecheurs Penser en Rond; Psychoanalyse et psychiatrie edition, 1999

Gay P: Freud: A Life for Our Time. New York, WW Norton, 1988

Grosskurth P: Havelock Ellis: A Biography. New York, New York University Press, 1985

Hunt MH: The Story of Psychology. New York, Random House, 1993

Jones E: The Life and Work of Sigmund Freud (1953). Edited by Trilling L, Marcus S. New York, Basic Books, Harper, 1961

Koch S: Foreword: Wundt's creature at age zero—and as centenarian: some aspects of the institutionalization of the "new psychology," in A Century of Psychology as Science. Edited by Koch S, Leary DE. New York, McGraw-Hill, 1985, pp 7–39

Krafft-Ebing R: Psychopathia Sexualis (1886). New York, Arcade Publishing, 1998

Krstic K: Marulic M—the author of the term "psychology." Acta Instituti Psychologici Universitatis Zagrabiensis 36:7–13, 1964. Available at: http://psychclassics.yorku.ca/Krstic/marulic.htm. Accessed October 12, 2013.

Makari G: Revolution in Mind: The Creation of Psychoanalysis. New York, Harper Collins, 2008

Robinson DN: An Intellectual History of Psychology. Madison, University of Wisconsin Press, 1995

Stevens LA: Explorers of the Brain. New York, Knopf, 1971

CHAPTER 3

Evolution of the Dynamic Unconscious

This chapter explores the concept of the unconscious in greater depth. It explains what it means when we say that the psychoanalytic unconscious is *dynamic*. It will review the history of the concept of the unconscious in Western philosophy and compare the concept of the psychoanalytic unconscious to related concepts from neighboring disciplines. In the face of overwhelming evidence, why do so many people deny the existence of the unconscious? Vocabulary introduced in this chapter includes the following: *automatic thoughts, behaviorism, cognitive psychology, cognitive unconscious, dynamic, dynamic unconscious, functionalism, introspectionism, mind–body dualism, structuralism,* and *unconscious.*

The unconscious is a core feature of every psychoanalytic model of the mind. Although psychoanalytic models of the mind may vary, the idea that feelings, thoughts, memories, wishes, fears, fantasies, and patterns of personal meaning outside of our awareness influence experience and behavior is a core feature of all of them. The theory that symptoms, troublesome personality traits, or problems in living represent efforts to solve unconscious conflict is central to the psychodynamic understanding of human suffering. The observation that shared investigation into unconscious mental life can lead to relief from suffering is one of the cornerstones of psychodynamic psychotherapy. Although ideas about unconscious mental life have been modified continuously since their introduction more than a century ago, the basic idea that unconscious factors influence mental life remains the most important shared feature of the psychoanalytic model of the mind. The goal of this chapter is to explain more about the psychoanalytic view of the unconscious and to explore how this view differs from other approaches.

The Unconscious in the Psychoanalytic Model of the Mind

As we have seen in Chapter 2, Freud invented the psychoanalytic model of the mind when he applied the principle of psychic determinism to data derived from waking therapy, arriving at the concept of a dynamic unconscious. At the moment when he abandoned the use of hypnosis in favor of a new treatment strategy based on the use of free association, Freud was able to observe forces at work in the mind that no one had ever seen before. He observed that his patients struggled with conflict between revealing what was on their minds and concealing it from themselves and from the doctor. Freud's exploration of this conflict led to the first description of how the mind is divided by inner strife. From the concept of defense hysteria, it was a short step to a view that all minds are divided by a struggle between conscious acceptable thoughts/feelings and unconscious unacceptable thoughts/feelings. In contrast to other theoreticians working at the time, Freud saw the mind as split not because of brain disease or degeneration but because of motivations, or dynamic forces. For this reason, in the psychoanalytic model of the mind, we often refer to the unconscious as the *dynamic unconscious* to distinguish it from other kinds of nonconscious aspects of mind. Let's explain what we mean.

What Does the Word *Dynamic* Mean in the Context of the Unconscious?

The word *dynamic,* familiar to readers as part of the word *psychodynamic,* is an old word in the language of psychoanalysis, borrowed from the language of physics, where it describes a state of continuous interplay of multiple forces. In psychoanalysis, because we are talking about the mind, *dynamic* refers to psychological forces—or, more precisely, to motivational forces. In other words, as described by psychoanalysts, the unconscious consists of a world of hidden motivational forces—including wishes, needs, hopes, and fears—that influence all aspects of mental life and behavior.

In the psychoanalytic model of the mind, unconscious mental life is dynamic in two senses. First, it is dynamic in the sense that it makes its influence felt in everything we do, not just in some states of mind some of the time. Second, the unconscious is dynamic in the sense that its contents are actively denied access to consciousness by a psychological force called *repression*. Repression, as we already know, is the term Freud used to describe a purposeful—or, again, motivated—unconscious process in which thoughts or feelings judged to be irrational, immoral, distressing, or otherwise unacceptable are excluded from awareness. In other words, thoughts and feelings become part of the dynamic unconscious when they are kept out of awareness by other dynamic mental forces, which oppose our efforts to know our minds.

What Can We Learn From Ordinary Introspection?

What can ordinary introspection tell us about our mental life outside of consciousness? The fact is, all human beings, even those with no knowledge of the details of any psychological theory, operate with some notion of an unconscious. Everyday experiences point to the idea that the mind is at work outside of awareness. For example, we all have the experience of suddenly remembering something we had forgotten, which must have been stored somewhere in the mind in the meantime. Most of us have had the experience of waking up in the morning to discover that we have found the answer to a lingering problem we were not aware of working on while asleep. It is easy to demonstrate that responses to subliminal stimulation occur daily. For example, we find images in our dreams that we have borrowed from waking experience, but which we did not register consciously during the day. In addition, we know that our minds can process information in ways that make it possible for us to do all kinds of things—from reading a book to hitting a golf ball to driving a car—even though we are not able to describe exactly what it is that we know or what we are doing. Ordinary experience prepares us, at least somewhat, for the idea that the mind is at work outside of awareness.

The psychoanalytic model of the mind, with its particular concept of the unconscious, includes the idea that the mind can store information, work on intellectual problems, and register stimuli outside of consciousness. It also includes the idea that lots of information processing occurs outside of awareness. However, the real significance of the psychoanalytic concept of the unconscious lies not in its storage function, its capacity for subliminal perception, or its capacity for information processing. The idea specific to the psychoanalytic view of the mind is that thoughts and feelings outside of awareness are not just stored in some unseen compartment in the mind waiting to be noticed or called upon but are alive, powerful, and ever-present, influencing all of our experiences and life choices, both large and small. Also, in contrast to mental activity kept from awareness in the interest of speed and efficiency (as in information processing that allows for judging distance while walking upstairs or for decoding letters and words while reading), the contents of the dynamic unconscious are kept from awareness because we do not *want* to know about them.

Even the fact that we do not want to know all of our own thoughts is not entirely beyond our capacity for ordinary introspection. We all know that from time to time we react to situations in ways that do not make sense, or do things for reasons that we cannot explain. We are certainly able to spot these moments in other people, often with the conviction that we know the "real" motives behind what others do. We fear, often correctly, that others can see things about us that we do not see about ourselves (Vazire and Mehl 2008). Even the implication of self-deception, embedded in the concept of repression, is not entirely beyond the reach of self-reflection. From time to time we have all had to admit, often in the face of vehement protest to the contrary, that we have not been honest with ourselves about our reasons for a response or an action, or that we did something for reasons of which we are not particularly proud—a bit of self-interest, a competitive or vengeful impulse, or a secret longing? Again, such instances of self-deception are easy to spot in other people. As it turns out, the capacity to understand how and why people hide their real feelings and motives from themselves is part of the psychological equipment of every normal child. Research shows that children as young as 6 or 7 years old are aware that people often go to elaborate lengths to obscure their true motives and/or feelings from themselves, so as to avoid feelings of shame and guilt (Chandler et al. 1978). In other words, there is a lot that introspection can tell us about the unconscious, even the dynamic unconscious.

Early Investigations of the Conscious Mind

Although many people imagine that Freud was the first person to write about unconscious mental life, or even that he somehow "discovered" it, he was not the first to argue for the possibility of mental life outside of awareness.[1] However, it is true that when Freud began explicating his "new psychology," he was at odds with the rest of the new field of

---

[1]Fritz Perls, the founder of Gestalt Psychology in America, referred to Freud as the "Livingstone of the unconscious," thus comparing the father of psychoanalysis with the British explorer who "discovered" the source of the Nile (Perls 1947/1969, p. 86). See also Charles Van Doren (1992), *A History of Knowledge: Past, Present, and Future.*

academic/experimental psychology, which took as its aim "an exact description of consciousness."[2]

The Theories of Wilhelm Wundt and His Followers: Introspectionism and Functionalism

The founder of this new field was the physician Wilhelm Wundt (1832–1902). In contrast to Freud, Wundt was the son of a Lutheran pastor in southwest Germany and came from a long line of scholars and university presidents. In 1857, a year after Freud's birth, Wundt took a position as a research assistant in the newly established Berlin Physiological Institute under the direction of Freud's hero, Hermann von Helmholtz. In 1879, just as Freud was hitting his stride as a neuropathologist in Ernst Brucke's Institute in Vienna, Wundt took possession of an abandoned storage closet at the University of Leipzig to set up his first laboratory at what he called the "Institute of Psychology." Wundt's research program was based on an investigative technique called *introspection*, which involved controlled attention to minute bits of conscious experience such as sound, light, and color. Indeed, in later years, the psychology with which Wundt is associated came to be called *introspectionism*. Wundt's mission was to elucidate the basic elements of conscious psychic life (which he identified as sensation and feeling), and to discover how these basic elements interact to form conscious experience. Therefore, when we compare psychoanalysis with the official discipline of university-based psychology, we find considerable overlap in their origins in the Helmholtzian tradition. However, we also find that Freud was at odds with this growing branch of "the establishment" in his interest in unconscious mental states.

Wundt's student Edward Bradford Titchener (1867–1927), the English-born psychologist who founded the psychology laboratories at Cornell University in 1892, continued the tradition of equating mind with consciousness. Titchener developed a branch of psychology known as *structuralism*, which carried on Wundt's project of delineating the structures of the conscious mind. William James (1842–1910), the physician-philosopher-turned-psychologist who offered the first university-based instruction on physiological psychology at Harvard University in 1875, was the chief proponent of a school of psychology known as *functionalism*. In contrast to the introspectionism and/or structuralism of Wundt and Titchener, James' functionalism argued that

---

[2]See http://plato.stanford.edu/entries/wilhelm-wundt/ (accessed November 25, 2013).

the goal of psychology was to elucidate the function, or purpose, of mental life. Wundt and Titchener's structuralism and James' functionalism vied for supremacy in American psychology for three decades between 1890 and 1920, together dominating the field of psychology until the rise of *behaviorism* (about which we will have more to say in a moment). In spite of their rivalry, these men had in common the view that mental life can be equated with consciousness. James, like most psychologists of his day, understood that mental events are connected to brain processes; however, in contrast to Freud, he argued that "consciousness…'corresponds' to the entire activity of the brain…at the moment" (James 1890, p. 177; see also Edwards and Jacobs 2003, p. 25; Fancher 1979; Hunt 1993; Reiber 1980; Robinson 1995).

The Legacy of René Descartes: Mind as Consciousness

Wundt, Titchener, James, and many others in the early years of academic psychology took for granted the idea that mind and consciousness can be equated. In one way or another, all were intellectual descendants of the French mathematician and philosopher René Descartes (1596–1650). A giant in Western intellectual history, Descartes was a major force in the movement from medieval science and philosophy to the modern era and has been heralded as the father of modern psychology. In 1639, he began work on his most famous work, *Meditations*,[3] which consists of a series of reflections concerning the possibility of knowledge (*scientia*). Rejecting the authority of Church-sanctioned scholasticism (the integration of the works of Aristotle and the teachings of the church offered by Thomas Aquinas), Descartes began his reflections from a position of radical doubt, wondering what, if anything, one could be certain of. As Descartes famously argued, the only thing that cannot be doubted is doubt itself—or more to the point, one's own experience of doubt. This is the essence of his famous sentence *cogito, ergo sum* ("I think, therefore I am"). We would be going far afield were we to fully examine how Descartes used this first "truth" to arrive at certainty as to the existence of a nondeceiving God, and then, at certainty with regard to the existence of an external world that can be investigated using the methods of mathematics. What is important for our purpose is to understand how, in the process of developing his epis-

---

[3]The full title of Descartes' book was *Meditations on the First Philosophy: In Which the Existence of God and the Distinction Between Mind and Body Are Demonstrated*.

temology, Descartes arrived at both a novel foundation for seeking knowledge and a view of the mind itself.[4]

Some historians of psychology venerate Descartes as an important ancestor of the field of cognitive psychology (more about this in a moment), reminding us that he posited a thinking mind (referred to often as his *cogito*) at the center of knowledge (Gardner 1985). However, there are other features of Descartes' view of the mind that are less admired today. The first of these—and perhaps the best known to students of mind science—is what has been called Cartesian *mind–body dualism*, or the view that the mind and the body are two entirely and essentially different things. For Descartes, the essential feature of physical reality (including the body) is that it occupies space or is extended (*res extensa*). This means that everything in physical reality is susceptible to mathematical measurement and description. In contrast to physical reality, the essence of mind is to think (*res cogitans*). As mind does not occupy space, it is not susceptible to mathematical description. In Descartes' view, the mind is equivalent to the soul and belongs not to the domain of science but to that of religion. Although Descartes did consider the question of how mind and body interact, his basic mind–body dualism influenced all subsequent discourse on the nature of mind.

A second feature of Descartes' view of the mind was his equation of mental life with thinking. Descartes considered feelings and emotions to be generated by the body, and he considered ideas and thoughts to be generated by the mind, which could therefore be understood as distinct from emotion. As we explore the psychoanalytic model of the mind in greater depth, we will consider the shortcomings of this view (see also Damasio 1984).

A final feature of Descartes' view of the mind, and the one most relevant to the subject of the unconscious, was his view that the mind and consciousness are the same thing. Because Descartes' epistemology depends on the idea that thinking is the only thing of which we can be certain, it also requires a denial of the possibility that thinking can take place without one's being aware of it (Rosenzweig 1985, p. 29). Descartes' view that the mind is transparent to itself—that we have "clear and direct," privileged, automatic, and accurate access to our minds (a viewpoint referred to by contemporary philosophers of mind as "the concept of first-person knowledge" [Gopnik 1993])—was part of the legacy of Cartesian psychology inherited by many of Descartes' followers, including Wundt and other early university-based students of psychology (Fancher 1979; Hunt 1993).

---

[4]See http://plato.stanford.edu/entries/descartes/ (accessed October 12, 2012).

The Unconscious From Descartes to Freud

Outside of university-based academic psychology, however, there were many who felt that important mental events do occur outside of awareness (Edwards and Jacobs 2003, p. 16). Indeed, it would be easy to fill a book full of pithy aphorisms dating all the way back to ancient times about the mind's hidden aspects. For example, Plato's (428–348 B.C.E.) view that knowledge is the rediscovery of forgotten ideas points to the possibility of unconscious mental life. The Christian philosopher Augustine (354–430 C.E.), influenced by Plato, wrote that his own mind was hard to grasp in that much of it was beyond awareness. St. Thomas Aquinas, the father of medieval scholasticism, proposed a theory of mind that emphasized mind–body unity and the importance of unconscious factors (Whyte 1962, p. 80). Although Descartes profoundly influenced the founders of formal academic psychology, there are other traditions in modern European thought that did not assume that mental life is the same as consciousness (Ellenberger 1970; Klein 1997; Tallis 2002; Talvitie 2009; Whyte 1962).

Enlightenment Philosophy and the Unconscious

For example, Gottfried Wilhelm Leibniz (1646–1716), the German polymath whose works included treatises on law, philosophy, mathematics (calculus and binary systems), logic, mechanics, and physics, has often been cited as the first post-Cartesian European scientist to argue for the idea of unconscious mental activity (Whyte 1962, p. 99). In his 1704 book *New Essays Concerning Human Understanding*, Leibniz asserted that there are many small perceptions (*petites perceptions*) below the threshold of what he called "apperception" that have a profound impact on conscious experience. In contrast to Descartes, who had confidence in his "clear and direct" experience, Leibniz asserted that these "clear concepts are like islands which arise above the ocean of obscure ones" (Whyte 1962, p. 99).[5]

Johann Friedrich Herbart (1776–1841), a German philosopher, psychologist, and educator, expanded the idea of unconscious mental processes into a complete theory of mind. Building on Leibniz's idea of a threshold of perception, Herbart added a dynamic component, conceiving of ideas as forces. Herbart borrowed the term *dynamic* from Leibniz, who first used it (in opposition to the word *static*) in discussions of mechanics (Ellenberger 1970, p. 289). Indeed, Herbart defined psychology as "the mechanics of the mind" (Jahoda 2009). He argued that all mental phenomena result from the interaction of multiple perceptions, representations, and ideas that compete with each other at the threshold of consciousness. In Herbart's view, stronger ideas push weaker ideas below this threshold in a process that he called *verdrängt*—the same word Freud used for his concept of repression. In Herbart's view, "repressed" ideas strive to reemerge, reinforcing themselves through association with other ideas (Ellenberger 1970, p. 312; Edwards and Jacobs 2003; Whyte 1962, pp. 143–144).

Gustav Theodor Fechner (1801–1887), a professor of physics, philosophy, and medicine at the University of Leipzig, introduced an experimental approach to the study of the unconscious. Fechner is probably best known today for his metaphor (borrowed by Freud, and perhaps itself borrowed from Leibniz's "islands in the ocean") comparing the mind to an iceberg floating on the sea (Jones 1953/1961, p. 374). Less well known to us but more important historically was the fact that in 1850, Fechner began a series of experiments testing the relationship between the intensities of stimulation and perception (Ellenberger 1970, p. 217) that are considered by many to be the starting point of experimental psychology and were influential on Wilhelm Wundt (Ellenberger 1970, p. 217).[6]

The German Romantic Movement and the Unconscious

In contrast to the philosophers of the Enlightenment, with their "cult of reason," philosophers of the German romantic movement were fascinated by the irrational and the individual. Prominent in the first third of the nineteenth century, German romantic philosophers took a special interest in phenomena such as creativity, genius, dreams, and mental illness, all of which were seen as having sources in the unconscious. However, in contrast to the Leibnizian "cognitivists," romantic philosophers were interested in unconscious motivation. They were all influenced by one the first romantic philosophers, the Swiss-born Jean-Jacques Rousseau (1712–1778), who left an account of his life in the form of *Confessions* (1782), arguably the first autobiography based on the author's

---

[5]Leibniz's views had widespread influence on many fields and many writers. Scottish judge and philosopher Henry Home, Lord Kames (1696–1781), influenced by Leibniz, was the first person who used the English word *unconscious* (in 1751) to refer to a particular mental function—again, the function of perception. Twenty-five years later, the German philosopher and physician Ernst Platner (1744–1818) was the first person to use the German word *Unbewusstsein* (unconsciousness)—the same word used by Freud—in 1776 to describe ideas outside of consciousness. Thus, by the end off the eighteenth century, the concept and the word *unconscious* had developed a strong foothold in discussion about the mind. See http://plato.stanford.edu/entries/leibniz/ (accessed September 24, 2012).

personal feelings. Rousseau's reflections on his actions and motives, including those "not so clear to me as I have for a long time imagined," rival the *Meditations* of Descartes in their influence on subsequent European thought. Romantic poets including Goethe (1749–1832), Schiller (1759–1851), and Coleridge (1772–1834) argued that the unconscious was the storehouse of hidden treasures of the mind and the source of all creativity (Ellenberger 1970, pp. 200–202; Whyte 1962, pp. 126–129).

A particular brand of German romanticism that had a profound influence on all aspects of German culture, including the development of psychology, was the Philosophy of Nature (*Naturphilosophie*), founded by Friedrich Wilhelm Joseph von Schelling (1775–1854) at the University of Munich. In Schelling's philosophy, the visible world emerged from a common spiritual principle, the "world soul" (*Weltseele*), which over successive generations produced matter, nature, and consciousness (Ellenberger 1970, pp. 203–205). The unconscious was rooted in the

---

[6]While Fechner was hard at work on his experiments on Leipzig, another group of thinkers interested in psychology—including the psychology of unconscious mental processes—was forming across the sea in England. The founder of this group was Sir William Hamilton (1788–1856), a Scottish-born professor of medicine, law, and metaphysics at the Royal Institute who was one of the first British philosophers to take note of the important developments in German philosophy and science in the mid-nineteenth century. Hamilton began to include German ideas in his own lectures at the University of Edinburgh. In his view of the mind, Hamilton argued that "the sphere of our conscious modifications [by which he meant mental *activities*] is only a small circle in the centre of a far wider sphere of action and passion, of which we are only conscious through its effects" (Hamilton 1860, p. 242).

Hamilton's most important students in the world of psychology were other British physicians, including Thomas Laycock (1812–1876), a British-born, German-educated physiologist at the University of London who first posited "the reflex action of the brain," by which he meant "an unconsciously acting principle of organization" (Whyte 1962, p. 162), and William Benjamin Carpenter (1813–1885), an English physician and naturalist who in 1853 coined the term *unconscious cerebration*, which soon became widely used in the English-speaking world (Jones 1953/1961, p. 378). Carpenter's *Principles of Mental Physiology* (1874) was devoted to a discussion of the evidence for this unconscious cerebration gleaned from its downstream effects on consciousness and behavior (Whyte 1962, p.155). For Laycock, Carpenter, and the other medically oriented students of Hamilton, it mattered little whether the concept of unconscious cerebration was formulated in terms of metaphysics or of brain physiology. Their goal was to understand the patient as part of a body-mind unit (Whyte 1962, p. 162). In contrast to Descartes, their assumption was that brain and mind are not different at all but are made of exactly the same stuff (Whyte 1962).

invisible life of the universe, forming the link between man and nature. Although this philosophy sounds odd and mystical to our modern ears, it was highly influential among European philosophers and writers of the time.[7]

Arthur Schopenhauer (1788–1860), born in Poland but educated in Germany, worked largely outside of the German university. His work *The World as Will and Representation* was first published in 1819 but did not become widely read until the second half of the nineteenth century, when Schopenhauer became fashionable as part of a neo-romantic revival in Europe. Although Schopenhauer's philosophy is impossible to classify, his ideas are important to our story because of his emphasis on the concept of "will to live" (*Wille zum Leben*), a blind, unconscious force driving the entire universe, including the mind of man. In Schopenhauer's view, man in a self-deceiving, irrational creature motivated by internal instincts serving the larger universal will (Ellenberger 1970, p. 208).

The work of Schopenhauer profoundly influenced Friedrich Nietzsche (1844–1900), another giant in Western philosophy. Endowed with a brooding and stormy temperament, the young Nietzsche quickly became disillusioned with religion, finding inspiration instead in the works of Schopenhauer and the music of Richard Wagner. Preoccupied with man's capacity for self-deception, Nietzsche tried to demonstrate that every emotion, attitude, opinion, behavior, and apparent virtue is rooted in an unconscious lie (Ellenberger 1970, p. 273). In Nietzsche's view, the unconscious is the essential part of every individual and consists of a turbulent cauldron of thoughts, emotions, and instincts, including needs for pleasure and struggle, sexual and herd instincts, instincts for knowledge and truth, and ultimately the one basic instinct, the "will to power" (Ellenberger 1970, p. 274). Nietzsche's work describes the vicissitudes of these instincts, their inhibitions, and their multiple disguises. The most shocking of Nietzsche's ideas, presented in his book *On the Genealogy of Morality* (1887), was his view that professions of Christian morality are nothing more than a disguised form of

---

[7]Gustav Theodor Fechner reenters our story at this point, for although we have noted his role in the founding of experimental psychology, Fechner was also a midlife convert to the school of *Naturphilosophie* (Ellenberger 1970, p. 216). In our previous discussion of Fechner, we neglected to mention that the tens of thousands of experiments published in his multivolume *Psychophysics* were largely an effort to provide proof for his highly speculative universal principles of nature, which included the principle of tending to stability (or constancy), the pleasure/unpleasure principle (especially as it related to the principle of constancy), the principle of repetition, and the concept of psychic energy.

inhibited, unconscious "resentment." Unsparing even of himself, Nietzsche argued, in a dark refrain of Rousseau, that every religion and every philosophy (presumably including his own) is no more than a disguised confession.

Late-nineteenth-century speculation about unconscious mental life culminated in the work of Karl Robert Eduard von Hartmann (1842–1906), whose book *The Philosophy of the Unconscious* was first published in 1869. In this massive 1,200-page treatise, von Hartmann discussed the subject of the unconscious in relation to 26 topics, including neural physiology, movements, reflexes, will, instinct, idea, curative processes, energy, sexual love, feeling, morality, language, history, and ultimate principles, to mention a few (Whyte 1962, p. 164). Claiming to present the unconscious as a systematic philosophy, von Hartmann's work is largely unread and forgotten today, dismissed by most historians as "neither good philosophy nor good science" (Whyte 1962, p.165). However, *The Philosophy of the Unconscious* was wildly popular in its day, printed nine times between 1869 and 1881 and translated into both French and English.

The popularity of von Hartmann's book belies any notion that the idea of unconscious mental life was not considered before Freud. Although Freud acknowledged only "the great Fechner" as having been important to him (Freud 1900/1962, p. 536; Freud 1925/1962, p. 59), there is plenty of evidence that Freud was familiar with all of the major psychological treatises of his day. For example, although Freud never cited Herbart, we know that he was familiar with Herbart's work through its central place in Gustav Adolf Lindner's (1828–1887) textbook of psychology, which he read in his gymnasium days (Ellenberger 1970, p. 536; Jones 1953/1961, p. 372). Most interesting, perhaps, are Freud's attitudes toward Schopenhauer and Nietzsche, whose ideas are strikingly similar to his own. Freud denied having been influenced by either man, claiming that he avoided the works of both Schopenhauer and Nietzsche until later life "with the deliberate object of not being hampered in working out the impressions received in psychoanalysis by any anticipatory ideas" (Freud 1914/1962, pp. 15–16; Freud 1925/1962, pp. 59–60). Clearly, Freud had a special interest in protecting the originality of his theory of repression, which he saw as the cornerstone of psychoanalysis, arguing that it "quite certainly came to me independently of any sources" (Freud 1914/1962, p. 15). As Ellenberger points out, regardless of whether Freud had read Schopenhauer or Nietzsche while he was at work on his own ideas, he was certainly part of a tradition that Ellenberger (following Klages) likes to call "the great unmasking trend" in the literature and philosophy of mid- to late-nineteenth-century Europe, which consisted of a "systematic search for deception and self-deception and the uncovering of truth" (Ellenberger 1970, p. 537). The unmasking trend included not only Schopenhauer and Nietzsche but also Karl Marx and writers such as Henrik Ibsen, whose plays exposing life's lies were cited by Freud with great admiration (see also Ricoeur [1977] on "the hermeneutics of suspicion").

Unconscious Mental Processes and Contemporary Academic Psychology

We have learned how Freud proposed the concept of a dynamic unconscious. We have also learned that the concept of the unconscious was not new in Western philosophy. However, it was at odds with prevailing ideas in Wundt's new academic psychology. Much has changed in academic psychology since its founding in 1879, so that psychoanalysts are no longer alone among psychologists in their efforts to chart unconscious mental life. However, this change did not happen right away. Although various forms of Wundt's introspectionism dominated American psychology for the three decades between 1890 and 1920, the 1930s and 1940s saw the rise of behaviorism as the dominant paradigm in the field of academic psychology.

The Emergence of Behaviorism

Behaviorism is a branch of psychology that seeks to explain human (and animal) activity as a chain of stimulus-response connections linked together by reinforcement. The founding members of this new psychology included Ivan Pavlov (1849–1936), who invented the concept of *conditioned reflexes;* Edward Lee Thorndike (1874–1947), who invented the concept of *reinforcement;* and James B. Watson (1878–1958), who coined the term *behaviorism* itself. Strict behaviorists argued that the data of introspection are not only unreliable but unnecessary for the study of human activity, which can best be explained as a series of conditioned reflexes. In pursuit of scientific objectivity, behaviorism argued that it should restrict itself exclusively to the study of overt actions, turning away not only from the idea of the unconscious but also from the idea of the mind itself. In this view, the mind is an illusion created by brain activity, a meaningless by-product of the nervous system with no causal role in human behavior. While behaviorism argued that human behavior is based on "nonconscious" activity, it rejected the idea of unconscious mind. Behaviorism created the image of psychology as the study of rats scurrying through mazes and across electric grids in pursuit of rewards or of cheerful children (from B.F. Skinner's [1948] best-selling novel *Walden Two*) behaviorally engineered to create a perfect society. Despite the heroic efforts of Dollard and Miller (1950) in the 1950s to link social learning theory to psychoanalysis, for the most part these fields remained far apart (Fancher 1979; Hunt 1993; Watson 1924).

The Rise of Cognitive Psychology

Around the middle of the twentieth century, however, the field of academic psychology began to move away from behaviorism toward the study of *cognition* (Gardner 1985, p. 6). This new psychology is referred to as *cognitive psychology, cognitive science,* or *cognitive neuroscience.* Each name includes the word *cognitive,* which refers to the question of how human beings know things. Cognitive science is a multidisciplinary approach to psychology that grew out of the fields of computer science, artificial intelligence, psycholinguistics, ethology, anthropology, neuroscience, and philosophy of mind.

Beginning in the 1940s, theorists from these disciplines became increasingly dissatisfied with explanations of behavior as sequences of conditioned reflexes. They argued that many human capacities—such as language, problem solving, planning, remembering, creating, and imagining (as well as some complex animal behaviors such as nest building and mating)—cannot be explained on the basis of reflex chains, however elaborate. These theorists began to posit the existence of stable, autonomous cognitive structures, or *representations,* operating within the organism (and analogous to the software programs in a computer) that account for its behavior (or output). Depending on the field of inquiry, these representational structures included symbols, rules, images, programs, schema, mental maps, expectations, plans, and goals, to name a few. Linguists posited the existence of *deep structures* of language that matured without having been learned; computer scientists programmed machines capable of computation based on algorithms; personality theorists described stable and patterned traits, some of which appeared to be innate; and mathematicians established a new discipline, *information theory,* all replacing chains of conditioned reflexes. In other words, cognitive scientists argued that it is impossible to understand the human organism without speaking about a mind (Gardner 1985; Hunt 1993).

In the second half of the twentieth century, cognitive science had become so popular that it became common to speak of "the cognitive revolution" (Baars 1986; Neisser 1967). As we noted in Chapter 1, cognitive psychology has created a parallel track for the study of unconscious mental processes, exploring capacities related to *information processing*. The *cognitive unconscious* (Kihlstrom 1987, 1995) includes *implicit knowledge, tacit knowledge, procedural knowledge, implicit learning, implicit memory, nondeclarative memory, nonconscious construals, the adaptive unconscious, subliminal perception,* and *pre-attentive processing*, to mention only a few important concepts (Bargh and Barndollar 1996; Edwards and Jacobs 2003; Gazzaniga 1967, 1992; Greenwald 1992; Hassin et al. 2005; Kahneman 2011; Kihlstrom 1987, 1995; Schacter et al. 2011; Stein 1997; Weinberger and Weiss 1997; Westen 1998; Wilson 2002; Zellner 2012a). In the world of cognitive-behavioral therapy, which is based somewhat on cognitive psychology, unconscious mental processes are referred to as *automatic thoughts* (Bargh and Chartrand 1999; Beck 1976; Edwards and Jacobs 2003; Hassin et al. 2009; Weinberger and Weiss 1997). The term *nonconscious processing* can be confusing because it has been used to refer both to aspects of the cognitive unconscious and to aspects of the neural underpinnings of all mental functioning. Indeed, the neural underpinnings of nonconscious processing have been explored in areas such as split-brain experiments (Gazzaniga 1967, 1992), pathways by which the brain processes anxiety (LeDoux 1996), and the phenomenon of "blindsight" (Weiskrantz 1997; Weiskrantz et al. 1974), to mention only a few.

There is some overlap between these aspects of the cognitive unconscious and Freud's *descriptive unconscious* (see Chapter 5, "The Mind's Topography"). There is also much overlap between the cognitive unconscious and ideas posited 300 years ago by Leibniz and his followers. However, the types of unconscious mental functioning of interest to cognitive scientists are different from those of most interest to psychoanalysts. The cognitive unconscious mostly includes phenomena related to information processing outside of awareness. This unconscious processing is thought to be necessary because it affords greater efficiency and speed. The writer Malcolm Gladwell (2005), in his book *Blink: The Power of Thinking Without Thinking*, intrigued readers of popular science with descriptions of phenomena related to unconscious information processing. Gladwell's *Blink* pays special attention to our capacity to process complex information from many sources quickly—or "in the blink of an eye"—at a subliminal level. Most of this unconscious information processing cannot become conscious, even with close attention.

However, the dynamic unconscious of interest to psychoanalysts includes unconscious motivations and/or feelings that are kept from awareness not for greater efficiency but because they have been judged to be unacceptable. More recently, we have seen increasing overlap between the psychoanalytic dynamic unconscious and the cognitive unconscious in the emergence of new ideas from cognitive psychology, including *unconscious affect, nonconscious goal pursuit,* and *unconscious motivation* (Bargh and Barndollar 1996). Conflict mediation is made possible by *unconscious scanning operations,* or *metacognition*—terms by which cognitive psychologists describe the capacity to monitor one's own mind so that compromises can be forged among priorities. As we will see, the psychoanalytic model of the mind has much to say about how the mind forges compromise in the midst of conflict (Bargh and Barndollar 1996; Metcalfe and Shimamura 1994).

When approaching the literature about unconscious mental processing, it is important to remember that efforts to correlate aspects of the psychoanalytic unconscious with concepts derived from cognitive psychology are complicated by the "discourse politics" that have prevailed in the world of mind science, because war between points of view has ensured that no common language has been adopted by the scientific community to describe any aspect of mind (Edwards and Jacobs 2003). Important comparisons between the cognitive unconscious and the dynamic unconscious, as well as much empirical evidence for both, can be found in the work of Erdelyi (1995), Hassin et al. (2005), Wakefield (1992), Weinberger and Weiss (1997), Westen (1998), and many others. Evidence of the neuronal pathways that might be involved is summarized in the work of Panksepp (1998), Solms and Turnbull (2002), and Zellner (2012b). To make matters even more interesting, we find concepts pertaining to unconscious mental functioning emerging from fields such as in economics (Ariely 2008; Kahneman 2011), evolutionary psychology (Smith 2004), political science (Covington 2002; Jameson 1982), and cultural theory (Saul 1997), among others.

Controversy Surrounding the Unconscious: Self-Knowledge and Self-Deception

It is a paradox that although the concept of unconscious mental functioning is accepted by most people as a matter of common sense, its existence is highly controversial. Despite the fact that the concept of mental life outside of awareness has a long history and is recognized by most contemporary psychologists and philosophers of mind, it is still widespread, even common, to hear educated, otherwise knowledgeable people assert that they "do not believe in the unconscious." How can we understand this widespread skepticism with regard to the concept of mental life outside of awareness?

The fact is, human beings are powerfully attached to the idea that we have immediate, privileged, and complete access to our own psychological life—or, in other words, to the idea that through the act of introspection, we can know our own minds. When Descartes argued that he had "clear and direct" access to his own inner life, this confidence formed the basis of his philosophy. Although we know that Descartes had many critics, his claim to what philosophers of mind call "first-person knowledge" has powerful resonance with what we would like to believe—that we do indeed know what we are thinking (Gopnik 1993). Some historians have argued that Western philosophy in particular has a long history of valorizing man's capacity for self-awareness, beginning in the Renaissance, when words for "awareness" and "self-consciousness" first began to enter philosophical discourse, and peaking during the European Enlightenment with its "cult of reason" (Whyte 1962). In this view, Descartes was only the strongest voice in a philosophical tradition that venerated conscious awareness, rationality, and self-determination.

Some have also argued that our conviction that we have "first-person knowledge" is not just a cultural value but also an innate, or "hardwired," feature of the human species (Carruthers and Smith 1996; Wegner 2002, 2005). Indeed, the annals of neuroscience and psychology are full of observations of our human tendency to claim understanding of our behavior in ways that are clearly at odds with the facts. For example, subjects who do strange things under the influence of posthypnotic suggestion—such as crawling under the table to "look for a chicken"— are compelled to offer all kinds of post hoc explanations for their behavior, all the while unaware that they are acting out the command of the hypnotist. In the split-brain experiments referred to earlier (see section "The Rise of Cognitive Psychology"), patients who have undergone a surgical procedure to disconnect the hemispheres of the brain from each other (a rarely used treatment for intractable epilepsy) respond with complex behavior to stimuli presented to the nonconscious/nonverbal half of the brain even though they have no conscious awareness of those stimuli. When asked what they are doing and why (e.g., laughing in response to a cartoon presented to the nonconscious/nonverbal half of the brain), subjects will invariably give an explanation that bears no relationship to the stimulus presented (Gazzaniga 1967, 1992).[8] It is astonishing how rarely these patients express puzzlement or astonish-

---

[8]See also *New York Times*, November 6, 2007, on "rationalization" (Tierney 2007).

ment at their own behavior. It seems that it is almost impossible for human beings to admit, or probably more accurately even to recognize, that when it comes to understanding our own minds, we often simply do not know what we are thinking.

When Freud was in an especially devilish mood, he enjoyed provoking his readers by reflecting on just how disturbing his idea about the unconscious might be. Never modest, he declared his ideas to be as shocking as those of Copernicus and Darwin, asserting that along with those two great pioneers of Western science, he shared the honor of having caused one of the three great "narcissistic injuries" to mankind. It was Copernicus who, in a "cosmological blow" to our self-love, first proposed that the Earth is not the center of the universe. It was Darwin who, in a "biological blow," first suggested that man is not the special creation of a divine being. In the most wounding blow of all, Freud asserted that the concept of the unconscious demands that we accept that we do not even know what we are thinking (Freud 1917/1962, pp. 140–141). Despite our best efforts to heed the ancient maxim "Know thyself," it seems that we are fated to be unable—indeed, unwilling—to fully know even our own selves.

References

Ariely D: Predictably Irrational: The Hidden Forces That Shape Our Decisions. New York, HarperCollins, 2008

Baars BJ: The Cognitive Revolution in Psychology. New York, Guilford, 1986

Bargh JA, Barndollar K: Automaticity in action: the unconscious as repository of chronic goals and motives, in The Psychology of Action: Linking Cognition and Motivation to Behavior. Edited by Gollwitzer PM, Bargh JA. New York, Guilford, 1996, pp 457–481

Bargh JA, Chartrand TL: The unbearable automaticity of being. Am Psychol 54:462–479, 1999

Beck AT: Cognitive Therapy and Emotional Disorders. New York, International Universities Press, 1976

Carpenter WB: Principles of Mental Physiology: With Their Applications to the Training and Discipline of the Mind, and the Study of Its Morbid Conditions. London, H.S. King & Company, 1874

Carruthers P, Smith PK (eds): Theories of Theories of Mind. New York, Cambridge University Press, 1996

Chandler MJ, Paget KF, Koch DA: The child's demystification of psychological defense mechanisms: a structural and developmental analysis. Developmental Psychology 14:197–205, 1978

Covington C: Terrorism and War: The Unconscious Dynamics of Political Violence. London, Karnac, 2002

Damasio A: Descartes' Error: Emotion, Reason, and the Human Brain. New York, Putnam, 1984

Dollard J, Miller N: Personality and Psychotherapy: An Analysis in Terms of Learning, Thinking and Culture. New York, McGraw, 1950

Edwards D, Jacobs M: Conscious and Unconscious. Berkshire, UK, Open University Press, 2003

Ellenberger H: The Discovery of the Unconscious: The History and Evolution of Dynamic Psychiatry. New York, Basic Books, 1970

Erdelyi M: Psychoanalysis: Freud's Cognitive Psychology. New York, WH Freeman, 1985

Fancher RE: Pioneers of Psychology. New York, WW Norton, 1979

Freud S: The interpretation of dreams (1900), in The Standard Edition of the Complete Psychological Works of Sigmund Freud, Vol 4/5. Translated and edited by Strachey J. London, Hogarth Press, 1962, pp 1–626

Freud S: On the history of the psycho-analytic movement (1914), in The Standard Edition of the Complete Psychological Works of Sigmund Freud, Vol 14. Translated and edited by Strachey J. London, Hogarth Press, 1962, pp 1–66

Freud S: A difficulty in the path of psycho-analysis (1917), in The Standard Edition of the Complete Psychological Works of Sigmund Freud, Vol 17. Translated and edited by Strachey J. London, Hogarth Press, 1962, pp 135–144

Freud S: An autobiographical study (1925), in The Standard Edition of the Complete Psychological Works of Sigmund Freud, Vol 20. Translated and edited by Strachey J. London, Hogarth Press, 1962, pp 1–74

Gardner H: The Mind's New Science: A History of the Cognitive Revolution. New York, Basic Books, 1985

Gazzaniga MS: The split brain in man. Scientific American 217:24–29, 1967

Gazzaniga MS: Nature's Mind. New York, Basic Books, 1992

Gladwell M: Blink: The Power of Thinking Without Thinking. New York, Back Bay Books, Little, Brown, 2005

Gopnik A: How we know our minds: the illusion of first-person knowledge. Behavioral and Brain Sciences 16:1–14, 1993

Greenwald AG: New look 3: unconscious cognition reclaimed. Am Psychol 47:766–779, 1992

Hassin RR, Uleman JS, Bargh JA (eds): The New Unconscious. New York, Oxford University Press, 2005

Hassin RR, Bargh JA, Zimerman S: Automatic and flexible: the case of nonconscious goal pursuit. Soc Cogn 27:20–26, 2009

Hunt MH: The Story of Psychology. New York, Random House, 1993

Jahoda G: The metaphysical mechanics of the mind: Johann Friedrich Herbart. Psychologist 22:558–559, 2009

James W: The Principles of Psychology, Vol 1. New York, Henry Holt, 1890

Jameson F: The Political Unconscious: Narrative as a Socially Symbolic Act. Ithaca, NY, Cornell University Press, 1982

Jones E: The Life and Work of Sigmund Freud (1953). Edited by Trilling L, Marcus S. New York, Basic Books, Harper, 1961

Kahneman D: Thinking Fast and Slow. New York, Farrar, Straus & Giroux, 2011

Kihlstrom J: The cognitive unconscious. Science 237:1445–1452, 1987

Kihlstrom J: The rediscovery of the unconscious, in The Mind, the Brain, and Complex Adaptive Systems, Vol 22. Edited by Morowitz H, Singer J. Reading, MA, Addison-Wesley, 1995, pp 123–143

Klein DB: The Unconscious: Invention or Discovery? Santa Monica, CA, Goodyear, 1977

LeDoux J: The Emotional Brain: The Mysterious Underpinnings of Emotional Life. New York, Simon & Schuster, 1996

Metcalfe J, Shimamura AP (eds): Metacognition: Knowing About Knowing. Cambridge, MA, MIT Press, 1994

Neisser U: Cognitive Psychology. New York, Appleton-Century-Crofts, 1967

Panksepp J: Affective Neuroscience: The Foundations of Human and Animal Emotions. Oxford, UK, Oxford University Press, 1998

Perls FS: Ego, Hunger, and Aggression (1947). New York, Vintage Books, 1969

Reiber RW (ed): Wilhelm Wundt and the Making of Scientific Psychology. New York, Plenum, 1980

Ricoeur P: Freud and Philosophy: An Essay on Interpretation. New Haven, CT, Yale University Press, 1977

Robinson DN: An Intellectual History of Psychology. Madison, University of Wisconsin Press, 1995

Rosenzweig S: Freud and experimental psychology: the emergence of idiodynamics, in A Century of Psychology as Science. Edited by Koch S, Leary DE. New York, McGraw-Hill, 1985, pp 135–207

Saul JR: The Unconscious Civilization. New York, Free Press, 1997

Schacter DL, Gilbert DT, Wegner DM (eds): Psychology, 2nd Edition. New York, Worth, 2011

Smith DL: Why We Lie: The Evolutionary Roots of Deception and the Unconscious Mind. New York, St. Martin's Press, 2004

Solms M, Turnbull O: The Brain and the Inner World: An Introduction to the Neuroscience of Subjective Experience. New York, Other Press, 2002

Stein DJ (ed): Cognitive Science and the Unconscious. Washington, DC, American Psychiatric Press, 1997

Tallis F: Hidden Minds: A History of the Unconscious. New York, Arcade, 2002

Talvitie V: Freudian Unconscious and Cognitive Neuroscience: From Unconscious Fantasies to Neural Algorithms. London, Karnac, 2009

Tierney J: Go ahead, rationalize. Monkeys do it, too. New York Times, November 6, 2007

Van Doren C: A History of Knowledge: Past, Present, and Future. New York, Random House, 1992

Vazire S, Mehl MR: Knowing me, knowing you: the relative accuracy and unique predictive validity of self-ratings and other ratings of daily behavior. J Pers Soc Psychol 95:1202–1216, 2008

Wakefield JC: Freud and cognitive psychology: the conceptual interface, in The Interface of Psychoanalysis and Psychology. Edited by Barron JW, Eagle MN, Wolitzky DL. Washington, DC, American Psychiatric Publishing, 1992, pp 77–98

Watson JB: Behaviorism. New York, People's Institute, 1924

Wegner DM: The Illusion of Conscious Will. Cambridge, MA, MIT Press, 2002

Wegner DM: Who is the controller of controlled processes? in The New Unconscious. Edited by Hassin RR, Uleman JS, Bargh JA. New York, Oxford University Press, 2005, pp 19–36

Weinberger J, Weiss J: Psychoanalytic and cognitive conceptions of the unconscious, in Cognitive Science and the Unconscious. Edited by Stein DJ. Washington, DC, American Psychiatry Publishing, 1997, pp 23–54

Weiskrantz L: Consciousness Lost and Found: A Neuropsychological Exploration. Oxford, UK, Oxford University Press, 1997

Weiskrantz L, Warrington EK, Sanders MD, et al: Visual capacity in the hemianopic field following a restricted occipital ablation. Brain 97:709–728, 1974

Westen D: The scientific legacy of Sigmund Freud: toward a psychodynamically informed psychological science. Psychol Bull 124:333–371, 1998

Whyte LL: The Unconscious Before Freud. London, Tavistock, 1962

Wilson T: Strangers to Ourselves: Discovering the Adaptive Unconscious. Cambridge, MA, Harvard University Press, 2002

Zellner MR: The cognitive unconscious seems related to the dynamic unconscious—but it's not the whole story. Neuropsychoanalysis 13:59–63, 2012a

Zellner MR: Toward a materialist metapsychology: major operating principles of the brain provide a blueprint for a fundamentally psychodynamic infrastructure. Psychoanal Rev 99:563–588, 2012b

Core Dimensions of
Psychoanalytic Models
of the Mind

This chapter defines five core dimensions emphasized in all psychoanalytic models of the mind: topography, motivation, structure/process, development, and psychopathology/treatment. It also provides a quick tour of four leading psychoanalytic models of mental functioning: the Topographic Model, the Structural Model, Object Relations Theory, and Self Psychology. The reader is introduced to the basic outline of the book, which is organized around a chart showing how each psychoanalytic model conceptualizes each of the core dimensions of mental functioning and psychopathology/treatment. The goal of the book is to work toward a unified psychoanalytic model of the mind. Vocabulary introduced in this chapter includes the following: *adaptational perspective, developmental lines, developmental point of view, epigenesis, genetic perspective, hedonic principle, motivational/dynamic point of view, nature and nurture, pleasure/unpleasure principle, reality principle, structural point of view,* and *topographic point of view.*

In Chapter 2, we described how Freud arrived at the concept of the dynamic unconscious, the foundation for the psychoanalytic model of the mind. In Chapter 3, we discussed the concept of the unconscious in greater depth, exploring how we experience aspects of unconscious mental functioning in moments of ordinary introspection, how philosophers and psychologist throughout history thought about the unconscious, how contemporary psychologists think about it, and finally why, in the face of so much evidence, many continue to deny the possibility of unconscious mental functioning. The idea that hidden motivational forces—feelings, thoughts, memories, wishes, fears, fantasies, and patterns of personal meaning that are kept out of awareness because they are unacceptable—continuously influence our experience and behavior is a basic feature of the psychoanalytic model of the mind that, as we will see, is central to the topographic point of view. At the same time, there are four other basic features of all psychoanalytic attempts to model the mind, bringing the total to five. We begin this chapter by delineating these five key domains of the mind.

Key Domains of Mental Functioning

All psychoanalytic models of the mind will have much to say about the domains of topography, motivation, structure/process, development, and psychopathology/treatment. The first four of these are fundamental dimensions that any model of the mind must take into account. The last is a dual category that each model must formulate in depth in order to be useful to patients. On some occasions, these basic aspects of mental life are referred to as *points of view* (Rapaport and Gill 1959). By providing a strategy for reframing observations about mental life in terms of general principles, these five key domains allow the clinician to turn information about the patient into knowledge about the patient's mind and, ultimately, about his or her suffering. Delineating the core dimensions of the mind makes the psychoanalytic model of the mind easier to understand, easier to integrate, and easier to use in the task of helping patients.

Topography

The notion that the mind, whether normal or pathological, is always divided into conscious and unconscious parts is often called the *topographic point of view*. Descriptions of the mind's topography—or what is conscious and what is unconscious—are part of every psychoanalytic model of the mind. Because the topographic point of view is so fundamental, we list it first among the basic features of the psychoanalytic model of the mind. As we will see, the earliest psychoanalytic model of the mind was itself called the Topographic Model (Freud 1900/1962). This early model relied heavily on the topographic point of view of mental functioning but included the other four points of view as well.

Motivation

Motivation is the second feature shared by all psychoanalytic models of the mind. *Motivation* is another word for the impetus for mental and/or physical activity. It may take the form of needs, fears, wishes, purposes, and intentions. In the psychoanalytic model of the mind, the search to understand motivation is called the *dynamic* or *motivational point of view*. Put simply, the motivational point of view addresses the question "Why do people do what they do?" or "What makes people tick?" The motivational point of view is almost as important as the topographic point of view in the evolution of the psychoanalytic model of the mind. As we have seen, inherent in the concept of dynamic unconscious is the idea that behavior results from an interaction of two motivational forces—a wish to express unconscious mental content and a wish to keep this content hidden. In other words, mental content can be unconscious because we do not want to know about it, or "from the motive of defense" (Breuer and Freud 1893/1895/1962, p. 285).

There is ongoing debate within psychoanalysis about the basic nature of human motivation. We will explore this debate further in each successive chapter of the book. Nevertheless, despite differences, there are several aspects of the theory of motivation about which most psychoanalysts agree. First, in contrast to the case in behaviorism or social learning theory, in the psychoanalytic model, **experience and action are understood as being motivated from within the mind.** In other words, behavior is not simply a collection of responses to stimuli from the external world. The mind is viewed as capable of spontaneous activity and is not merely reactive to the environment. Indeed, as we shall see, when Freud abandoned his *seduction hypothesis* in favor of a view of motivation as arising from within the mind of the child, psychoanalysis became increasingly committed to the study of internal mental life (see Chapter 7, "The Oedipus Complex"). In any case, whether motivation is seen as originating from biological imperatives or from the internalization of cultural mandates, in the psychoanalytic model, motivation always has a mental component that plays a causal role in determining behavior.

Second, in addition to seeing motivation as originating in the mind, **the psychoanalytic model sees motivation as guided by the** *pleasure/ unpleasure principle.* This principle asserts that behavior and mental activity always seek to maximize feelings of pleasure and to escape from feelings of unpleasure or pain. In general psychology, this principle is known as the *hedonic principle* (Schacter et al. 2011, p. 326). The history of psychoanalysis can be told as a long argument about the nature of the basic pleasures that guide human mental life. For example, Freud emphasized the pleasure that accompanies the satisfaction of sexual and aggressive drives, and he saw all other pleasures as transformations of these more basic pleasures (see Chapter 9, "The Id and the Superego," for an exploration of drive theory). Other theorists have pointed to the pleasures inherent in attachment, dependency, and feelings of safety, arguing that these satisfactions cannot be reduced to those already mentioned (see Chapter 11, "Object Relations Theory"). Still other theorists have emphasized the pleasures that accompany autonomy, mastery, and self-actualization (see Chapter 12, "Self Psychology"). Despite this ongoing debate, most psychodynamic psychiatrists agree that the pleasure/unpleasure principle provides the basic compass that guides human behavior. The pleasure principle is not unique to the psychoanalytic model; it forms the basis of many kinds of psychology. However, by keeping this principle in awareness, clinicians can understand even the most painful behavior as serving a hidden pleasure, or as defending against even worse pain.

Third, **the psychoanalytic model of the mind takes into account the fact that motivation develops in an interaction between the mind and the external environment.** In other words, the mind operates according to the *reality principle* in addition to the pleasure principle. The search within the psychoanalytic model to understand those aspects of individual human behavior and mental life that represent efforts to cope with the reality of the external world is called the *adaptational perspective.* Because the psychoanalytic model of the mind understands motivation as both originating within the organism and adapted to the environment, it is able to consider both internal and external factors in the development of human desire. Much debate within psychoanalysis focuses on the relative emphasis placed on internal versus external contributors to motivation. For example, Freud conceptualized basic motivations as derivatives of biologically rooted drives that unfold in a largely predetermined maturational sequence. Other theorists have emphasized wishes, fears, and desires that are socially and culturally determined. Most contemporary psychodynamic psychiatrists see motivation as resulting from a complex interplay of *nature* and *nurture,* wherein inborn preferences are shaped by interactions with the environment, especially by the social matrix.

Finally, **the psychoanalytic model of the mind includes the idea that the mind is always working to reconcile conflicting motivations.** It is impossible for any given behavior or mental experience to satisfy both the pleasure principle and the reality principle. Indeed, there are even many competing imperatives for various kinds of pleasure, not to mention many competing imperatives created by fears and moral constraints. As a result, the psychoanalytic model of the mind includes the concept of *conflict* (also called *psychic conflict*). In this view, the mind seeks to reconcile its conflicting wishes, fears, and moral constraints with the demands imposed by reality through *compromise formation*. Every conscious experience and/or behavior represents a compromise among competing demands. In psychodynamic psychotherapy, the clinician seeks to explore the wide variety of compromises made by people as they seek to reconcile these competing demands. Psychological health can be assessed by evaluating compromises in terms of adaptation to reality and yield of pleasure. Psychodynamic psychotherapy seeks to expand the range of compromises available to the patient.

Structure and/or Process

Structure is the third feature of the psychoanalytic model of the mind. A mental structure can be defined as a relatively stable mental configuration with a slow rate of change (Rapaport and Gill 1959). The *structural point of view* arises from the observation that the motivational forces controlling mental life, along with the processes by which they are modulated, are not fleeting or erratic, but instead represent enduring patterns that are stable over time. Although, again, there is considerable argument about the best description of psychic structure, all psychoanalytic models of the mind draw on this important concept, with different schools of thought defined in part by what each sees as the basic structure of the mind. The term *structure* has been used to refer to mental events and processes at varying levels of abstraction, ranging from fantasies, memories, ideals, moral standards, character traits, and representations of self and other to more abstract and/or complex concepts such as mental agency or modes of function such as defense. Freud's well-known tripartite model of the mind, which divides mental life into *id, ego,* and *superego,* is only one example of how the broader concept of psychic structure has been used to create a model of the mind (Freud 1923/1962).

An important aspect of the concept of structure is its built-in historical component. For example, whereas the concept of wish can be conceived of as existing only in the present, the concept of structure allows us to talk more easily about the history and development of the inner world. By talking about development, we can talk about the possibility of change. If we can understand how stable configurations in the mind are formed, how they are threatened, and what makes them change, we can build a theory that encompasses both psychopathology and psychological change. This needed theory of change provides a rational basis for all approaches to psychotherapy.

Another important aspect of the concept of structure is that every structure has certain capacities, or processes. It is often hard to separate these processes—for example, primary process, secondary process, defense, reality testing, and so forth—from the structure itself. Indeed, sometimes we see a process that is itself defined as a structure. For this reason, we include process with structure and discuss both concepts together.

Development

The *developmental point of view* is the fourth important feature of the psychoanalytic model of the mind. It seeks to understand behavior and mental life as part of a meaningful progression from infancy to adulthood. It assumes that an adult can be understood as a psychological being only by exploring his or her history. The developmental point of view seeks to understand the origins of the patient's wishes, fears, ideals, values, attitudes, and adaptive strategies. It also explores how all of these change over time. The developmental aspects of the psychoanalytic model of the mind borrow extensively from developmental psychology, given that these overlapping fields share an interest in the mental life of the child (Gilmore and Meersand 2013).

Unique to psychoanalysis, the *genetic perspective* takes as its focus the patient's subjective story of his or her past as told to the therapist in treatment. The word *genetic* here refers not to the molecular basis of heredity but rather to the idea of *genesis*, or "the story of origins" (Hartmann and Kris 1945). By contrast, the developmental point of view is not unique to psychoanalysis. The developmental dimension seeks to understand the history of psychological life from the point of view of an objective observer, often through use of empirical methodology.

Initially Freud's developmental theory focused on describing *wishes,* which are organized into *drives* and which emerge according to an inborn, biologically determined plan consisting of oral, anal, phallic, and oedipal/genital phases (see Chapter 9, "The Id and the Superego"). However, most contemporary psychodynamic psychiatrists prefer the notion of *developmental lines* along which one can trace the history of any number of aspects of mental life, including wishes, fears, morality, the self, the quality of object relatedness, and all dimensions of ego functioning, to mention only a few (A. Freud 1981).

In addition, for the most part, psychodynamic psychiatrists adopt an epigenetic perspective of development. The concept of *epigenesis* views the formation of structure as the result of successive transactions between the individual and the environment. The outcome of each phase depends on the outcomes of all previous phases, as each new phase integrates previous phases and each has a new level of organization. The concept of epigenesis allows for a tension between the fact that wishes, fears, and conflicts from earlier years are preserved in the mind and that they are also, to some extent, transformed and superseded. The concept of epigenesis also allows for *regression,* by which certain phenomena represent a return to earlier states of development. Indeed, many aspects of psychopathology can be understood as representing a regression to strategies that were adaptive at earlier stages of development but now appear inappropriate.

The developmental point of view adds depth to the adaptational perspective by asserting that what may be been adaptive for a child at one phase of development may be maladaptive in the same person as an older child or as an adult. Finally, the developmental point of view allows us to understand how the mind of a child may be preserved in the mind of an adult, so that we are forever influenced by our childhood wishes, fears, and ways of thinking.

Theory of Psychopathology and Treatment (Therapeutic Action)

Every psychoanalytic model of the mind includes both a theory of psychopathology and an associated theory of therapeutic action. The theory of psychopathology attempts to account for how and why the mind of the patient causes suffering. The theory of treatment attempts to explain how psychodynamic psychotherapy might help the patient find relief. Freud's famous statements that psychodynamic psychotherapy seeks to "make conscious everything that is pathogenically unconscious" (Freud 1901/1962, p. 238; Freud 1916–1917/1962, p. 282) and that "where id was, there ego shall be" (Freud 1923/1962, p. 56; Freud 1933/1962, p. 80) are examples of how he conceptualized psychopathology and treatment within the model of the mind he was using at the time. Although theories of psychopathology and treatment have grown vastly more complex than they were in Freud's day, all clinicians must use these theories in their work in order for their aims and strategies to be coherent.

For a detailed review of the psychoanalytic approach to psychopathology, readers are referred to *Psychodynamic Psychiatry in Clinical Practice,* 4th Edition (Gabbard 2005), and *Psychodynamic Diagnostic Manual* (Psychodynamic Diagnostic Manual Task Force 2006). There are also several good textbooks about psychodynamic psychotherapy (Cabaniss et al. 2011; Caligor et al. 2007; Dewald 1964; Gabbard 2004; Summers and Barber 2009).

Four Foundational Psychoanalytic Models of the Mind

The four psychoanalytic models of the mind examined in this book are the Topographic Model, the Structural Model, Object Relations Theory, and Self Psychology. These four models have emerged over the past 120 years of psychoanalytic thought and represent major ways of thinking about mental functioning. Soon after Freud elaborated his first model of the mind, he became dissatisfied with it; he subjected both this early model and all subsequent models to continuous revision. In doing so, he established a tradition in which models of the mind are questioned and changed in response to new data (Arlow and Brenner 1964). Evolving clinical experience demands modification of each existing model, leading to the development of new models. As mentioned in the Introduction, the result is that the contemporary psychoanalytic model of the mind is a composite of several models, each of which attempts to address the insufficiencies of the others. As we will see, each of the four psychoanalytic models of the mind has much to say about the five core dimensions of mental functioning. Each of these models looks at the core dimensions slightly differently, and each emphasizes different aspects. Throughout this book, these four models will be explained in relation to each other, with the ultimate goal of integrating them into a single contemporary model of the mind.

Topographic Model

The Topographic Model was Freud's first model of the mind, introduced in 1900. It posited a basic structure of *conscious, preconscious,* and *unconscious* domains separated by a barrier of defense, or repression. Although this model contained rudimentary ideas about motivation, structure, development, and psychopathology/treatment, its main focus was the topography of the mind. The basic features of the Topographic Model, as well as its lasting impact on theories of psychopathology and treatment, will be explored in Part II (Chapters 5, 6, and 7) of this book.

Structural Model

Increasingly dissatisfied with his Topographic Model, Freud introduced his Structural Model in 1923. In this model, the mind is divided into three parts, *ego, id,* and *superego,* each differing in structure and motivational aims and each having unconscious features. As Freud and his followers became increasingly interested in the functioning of the ego, the Structural Model came to be known as Ego Psychology. The basic features of the Structural Model, in addition to the work of well-known ego psychology theorists such as Anna Freud, Heinz Hartmann, and Erik Erikson, will be explored in Part III (Chapters 8, 9, and 10) of this book.

Object Relations Theory

Object Relations Theory was developed in the 1940s, after the death of Freud. In contrast to previous models, Object Relations Theory views the mind as organized by internal *object relations*—self and object representations linked by an interaction between self and object. Object Relations Theory seeks to understand basic motivations such as attachment and separation, positing that infants are object seeking from the beginning of life. It explores how object relations develop over time under the influence of various pressures and how different configurations in these object relations can lead to psychopathology and can suggest associated treatment strategies. The basic features of Object Relations Theory, in addition to the work of well-known object relations theorists such as Melanie Klein, Wilfred Bion, D. W. Winnicott, Margaret Mahler, John Bowlby, and Otto Kernberg, will be explored in Part IV (Chapter 11) of this book.

Self Psychology

Introduced by Heinz Kohut in the 1960s, Self Psychology looks at mental functioning as representing the functioning of a basic structure called the *self*. Kohut explored basic inborn *narcissistic* needs in all of us, positing that we all seek recognition and encouragement from caregivers, whom he described as *selfobjects*. Self Psychology proposes that during childhood, in interactions with *empathic* caregivers, each of us developed a self that was more or less robust in terms of agency, energy, and ability to form ideals. It also describes a treatment strategy based on an understanding of the selfobject function of the therapist. The basic features of Self Psychology, in addition to the work of well-known self psychology theorists such as Kohut and his followers, will be explored in Part IV (Chapter 12) of this book.

Core Dimensions Across the Four Models

In Part II ("The Topographic Model") of this book, readers will be introduced to a chart that will help them with the task of understanding the psychoanalytic models of the mind. In this chart, the core dimensions emphasized by all psychoanalytic models of mental functioning—Topography, Motivation, Structure/Process, Development, and Psychopathology/Treatment—are plotted for each of the four foundational models of the mind examined in this book—the Topographic Model, the Structural Model, Object Relations Theory, and Self Psychology. Table 4–1 shows the form that the master chart will take.

As each model of the mind is introduced, the chart will become filled in. In the process of watching the chart grow, the reader will learn how concepts that are familiar but may be difficult to grasp or to integrate—for example, libido or separation-individuation—can be understood as an approach to motivation, structure/process, development, and/or psychopathology/treatment. In addition, aspects of the four component models of the mind can be understood in relation to one other, pointing the way to useful integration. The ultimate goal is for the reader to arrive at a usable composite psychoanalytic model of the mind. How to do this will be discussed in Chapter 13, "Toward an Integrated Psychoanalytic Model of the Mind."

References

Arlow J, Brenner C: Psychoanalytic Concepts and the Structural Theory. New York, International Universities Press, 1964

Breuer J, Freud S: Studies on hysteria (1893/1895), in The Standard Edition of the Complete Psychological Works of Sigmund Freud, Vol 2. Translated and edited by Strachey J. London, Hogarth Press, 1962, pp 1–335

Cabaniss D, Cherry S, Douglas CJ, et al: Psychodynamic Psychotherapy: A Clinical Manual. Oxford, UK, Wiley-Blackwell, 2011

Caligor E, Kernberg OF, Yeomans FE: Handbook for Dynamic Psychotherapy for Higher Level Personality Pathology, Washington, DC, American Psychiatric Publishing, 2007

Dewald P: Psychotherapy: A Dynamic Approach. New York, Basic Books, 1964

Freud A: The concept of developmental lines–their diagnostic significance. Psychoanal Study Child 36:129–136, 1981

Freud S: The interpretation of dreams (1900), in The Standard Edition of the Complete Psychological Works of Sigmund Freud, Vol 4/5. Translated and edited by Strachey J. London, Hogarth Press, 1962, pp 1–626

Freud S: The psychopathology of everyday life (1901), in The Standard Edition of the Complete Psychological Works of Sigmund Freud, Vol 6. Translated and edited by Strachey J. London, Hogarth Press, 1962, pp vii–296

Freud S: Introductory lectures on psycho-analysis (1916–1917), in The Standard Edition of the Complete Psychological Works of Sigmund Freud, Vol 16. Translated and edited by Strachey J. London, Hogarth Press, 1962, pp 241–463

TABLE 4–1. Core Dimensions of Psychoanalytic Models of the Mind

	Topography	Motivation	Structure/ Process	Development	Psychopathology	Treatment
Topographic Model Addressed in Part II (Chapters 5, 6, and 7)						
Structural Model Addressed in Part III (Chapters 8, 9, and 10)						
Object Relations Theory Addressed in Part IV (Chapter 11)						
Self Psychology Addressed in Part IV (Chapter 12)						

Freud S: The ego and the id (1923), in The Standard Edition of the Complete Psychological Works of Sigmund Freud, Vol 19. Translated and edited by Strachey J. London, Hogarth Press, 1962, pp 1–66

Freud S: New introductory lectures on psycho-analysis (1933), in The Standard Edition of the Complete Psychological Works of Sigmund Freud, Vol 22. Translated and edited by Strachey J. London, Hogarth Press, 1962, pp 1–182

Gabbard GO: Long-Term Psychodynamic Psychotherapy: A Basic Text. Washington, DC, American Psychiatric Publishing, 2004

Gabbard GO: Psychodynamic Psychiatry in Clinical Practice, 4th Edition. Washington, DC, American Psychiatric Publishing, 2005

Gilmore KJ, Meersand P: Normal Child and Adolescent Development: A Psychodynamic Primer. Arlington, VA, American Psychiatric Publishing, 2013

Hartmann H, Kris E: The genetic approach in psychoanalysis. Psychoanal Study Child 1:11–30, 1945

Psychodynamic Diagnostic Manual Task Force: Psychodynamic Diagnostic Manual. Silver Spring, MD, Alliance of Psychoanalytic Organizations, 2006

Rapaport D, Gill M: The points of view and assumptions of metapsychology. Int J Psychoanal 40:153–162, 1959

Schacter DL, Gilbert DT, Wegner DM (eds): Psychology, 2nd Edition. New York, Worth, 2011

Summers RF, Barber JP: Psychodynamic Psychotherapy: A Guide to Evidence-Based Practice. New York, Guilford, 2009

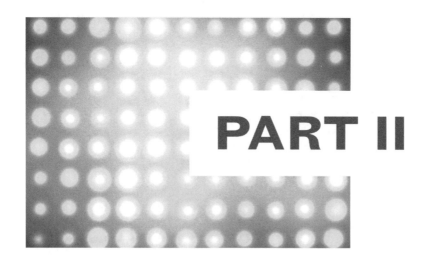

PART II

The Topographic Model

CHAPTER 5

The Mind's Topography

This chapter describes the Topographic Model of the mind. In this model, the mind consists of conscious, preconscious, and unconscious domains separated by a barrier of repression. All psychodynamic approaches to psychopathology and treatment draw upon aspects of the Topographic Model, with the aim of bringing pathogenic unconscious wishes, fears, and feelings into awareness. Vocabulary introduced in this chapter includes the following: *censor, condensation, conscious, descriptive unconscious, displacement, insight, interpretation, neurosis, overdetermination, parapraxis, preconscious, primary process, psychic reality, reconstruction, repetition compulsion, resistance, return of the repressed, secondary process, symbolization, transference,* and *wish.*

The Topographic Model was Freud's first fully developed psychoanalytic model of the normal mind. As discussed earlier, after introducing the concept of the dynamic unconscious in his work on hysteria, Freud immediately began work on a model of the mind that would apply to everyone, not just those suffering from psychopathology. Introduced more than 100 years ago, the Topographic Model of the mind seems primitive or antiquated to us when judged by the standards of contemporary psychology. Nevertheless, it continues to exert a profound influence on the contemporary psychoanalytic model of mind and treatment.

Freud first introduced this Topographic Model of the mind in Chapter 7 of *The Interpretation of Dreams* (Freud 1900/1962), but he did not formally designate it as reflecting a *topographic point of view* until 15 years later (Freud 1915/1962). The word *topographic* is derived from the Greek word *topo,* meaning "place." The choice of this word represents Freud's conception of the mind as consisting of structures, each of which occupies a particular psychical locality and functions in a particular spatial relation to the others (Freud 1900/1962, p. 536). Having abandoned his earlier efforts to establish a brain-based psychology, Freud made it clear that he did not intend for these "places" in the mind to refer to any existing brain anatomy. The idea of a psychic locality was intended to serve as a metaphor for an imaginary mapping of the mental terrain in which the unconscious is conceived of as lying "beneath" the domain of consciousness as a kind of psychic underworld.

As we can see by its name and by our brief introductory description, the Topographic Model of the mind looks at the mind largely from the *topographic* point of view, emphasizing which mental contents are allowed access to consciousness. However, the Topographic Model also includes a description of the ongoing *motivational* (or dynamic) interactions among the three regions of the mind, which work both together and in conflict, each influencing the others. In addition, the Topographic Model also includes a description of the *structural* properties of each part of the mind, including the characteristics and modes of functioning of each. Finally, the Topographic Model of the mind is tied to a *developmental* point of view that accounts for how the psychological life of the child lives on in the adult.

Mental Topography: The Mind's Three Layers

In the Topographic Model, the mind is divided into three regions, conceptualized on a vertical axis from the surface of the mind to its depth, differentiated from one another by their relationship to consciousness. These three regions of the mind are the *conscious* mind, the *preconscious* mind, and the *unconscious* mind. Consciousness lies on the surface of the mind and includes mental experience that is within awareness at any given moment. Just beneath consciousness is the preconscious, which includes mental contents that are in the *descriptive unconscious,* meaning that although they are not within awareness at any given moment, they can easily be brought to awareness if attention is applied to them. Beneath the preconscious lies the unconscious, buried in the deepest region of the mind. In contrast to the preconscious, which is only descriptively unconscious, the unconscious is *dynamically unconscious,* meaning that its contents cannot be brought to awareness by a simple act of attention but are actively denied access to consciousness by the force of repression.

Motivation

The most significant feature of the Topographic Model of the mind is the dynamic interaction among the unconscious, preconscious, and conscious regions of the mind. Indeed, as we explored in Part I of this book, the Topographic Model of the mind grew directly out of the concept of the *dynamic unconscious,* which is made up of wishes. A *wish* is defined by Merriam-Webster as an act of desire.[1] In the psychoanalytic model of the mind, a wish is a striving to experience some kind of satisfaction. According to the Topographic Model, the most important interaction in the mind is the ongoing struggle between the preconscious and the unconscious, which are separated by a *censor* with the authority to decide which wishes are socially or morally acceptable. During this early period, Freud became increasingly convinced that wishes of a sexual nature are the most important wishes in the mind. He also believed that sexual wishes are the most unacceptable. In Chapter 9, when we explore the Structural Model of the mind and the concept of the id, we will see how Freud organized wishes into libidinal and aggressive drives, developing drive theory to explain how these different types of motivations worked.

As we discussed in our description of the dynamic unconscious, in this model, the unconscious is dynamic in two senses. First, it is dynamic in that unconscious wishes seek to express themselves all of the time, affecting all that we experience and do. Second, it is dynamic in that unconscious wishes are repressed, or held outside of awareness, because we do not want to know about them, having judged them to be unacceptable. An example of unacceptable content might be a young woman's wish to have the love, sexual attention, and admiration of everyone, and/or her wish to do away with all rivals. The censor may judge these wishes to be unacceptable in terms of social norms. Such a judgment may lead this young woman to repress these unacceptable wishes or to banish them from consciousness. However, repressed wishes are not destroyed; instead, they are preserved in the unconscious and continue to exert an active effect on all of mental life and

---

[1] See http://www.merriam-webster.com/dictionary/wish (accessed January 9, 2012).

behavior. In other words, this young woman may have repressed her unacceptable wishes, but these wishes are still active in that she feels extremely anxious to the point of panic whenever the unacceptable wishes are stirred up. Furthermore, she avoids all efforts to make herself more attractive, such as dressing up or getting her hair and nails done. Despite being decidedly dowdy, she is preoccupied with how other women express their femininity. In the sections below, we will learn more about how a therapist, by bringing her patient's unacceptable wishes into awareness, can help relieve this young woman of suffering.

In the Topographic Model, there is little dynamic interaction between consciousness and the preconscious. Indeed, as we mentioned earlier, the contents of the preconscious are not within awareness at the moment but can easily be brought to consciousness if attention is paid to them. For example, the preconscious might include the answers to questions such as the following: "How many windows are in your bedroom?" or, more relevant here, "Where is your local nail salon or beauty parlor?" If the young woman mentioned above attends to these questions, she can access the information to answer them correctly, by turning attention to what had been preconscious. However, she does not know the answer to the question of why she is so anxious when she thinks about having a manicure. The thoughts, feelings, and/or wishes associated with her anxiety are unconscious, or repressed.

Structure/Process

In the Topographic Model of the mind, the unconscious, preconscious, and conscious regions of the mind each have a characteristic structure, and each operates in a characteristic way. As we have seen, the unconscious consists exclusively of unacceptable wishes that have been separated from the rest of the mind by repression. In addition, according to the Topographic Model, the unconscious operates according to what has been called *primary process*, in which wishes strive for immediate expression or satisfaction through whatever means possible, obeying the pleasure principle without regard for consequences. As a result, the unconscious is incapable of social judgment or moral concern. Freud believed at this point that primary process also accounts for the peculiar form that thoughts take in the unconscious, which is unperturbed by logical contradictions and operates without a sense of time. Primary process is also responsible for the fact that unconscious ideas are often represented by highly personal and idiosyncratic concrete symbols rather than words (*symbolization*). *Visual symbolism* is especially pronounced in dreams, which reflect the predominance of the primary process. The specific organizing mechanisms of primary process include *condensation* (wherein a single idea is capable of representing many related ideas, linked by private, idiosyncratic associations) and *displacement* (wherein an idea is capable of representing another idea, again linked by personal, often *symbolic* association). An example of unacceptable wishes represented in primary process form might be a dream image recounted by our same young woman (dreamer) in which, as she is getting a manicure, "the bottle of nail polish is suddenly filled with blood." Through exploration of this young woman's associations, the nail polish and the manicure appear to represent both a wish to be "the most glamorous of all women" and a wish to "polish off" all rivals in a bloody attack (see Chapter 6, "The World of Dreams," for a more in-depth discussion of dreaming and dream theory). As we can see here, primary process is responsible for the phenomenon of *overdetermination,* often seen in dreams and symptoms, in which a single idea or symbol may represent many ideas.

The preconscious is the seat of reason. In other words, the preconscious operates according to *secondary process,* which obeys the reality principle. It includes the capacity to judge mental contents and censor those judged to be unacceptable according to conventional mores. It includes the capacities for assessment of external reality, delayed gratification, and planned action for the purpose of solving problems. Preconscious thoughts, organized by the secondary process, are logical, goal directed, and language based. They rely on the stable, conventional, or culturally shared meaning of words, as opposed to the highly personal and idiosyncratic symbolic language of primary process.

Freud theorized that primary process was the original, or earliest mode of mental functioning, with secondary process developing only after the child learns through experience that wishing alone does not bring satisfaction and that more advanced forms of thought and action are necessary for gratification. Indeed, the word *primary* here refers to what comes first in the development of the mind. However, contemporary psychodynamic theorists no longer adhere to this view, arguing instead that both kinds of mental organization develop simultaneously in the mind and that primary process should not be confused with immature cognition. Contemporary theorists also understand that there are probably multiple ways of encoding experience, which are best studied by cognitive psychologists (Bucci 1997).

The conscious mind is the same as the preconscious mind in terms of structure. Consciousness also functions according to secondary process, using the logical processes with which we are all familiar. Indeed, most of the time we are aware only of secondary process, and we are used to conscious, purposeful thought. However, under conditions in which censorship is relaxed, or when mental life is especially dominated by unconscious wishes, feelings, and thoughts (as in dreams, daydreams, slips of the tongue, the play of children, art, poetry, neurotic symptoms, or any highly emotional state), it becomes possible to observe the penetration of primary process into conscious mental life. For example, we see this in the dream recounted above by the young woman with extreme anxiety who avoids going to a nail salon. When awake, this young woman had no realization of her unacceptable wishes but was aware only of her own anxiety at the thought of doing anything to improve her appearance, including getting a manicure, going shopping, or fixing her hair.

Development

Finally, the Topographic Model of the mind is attached to a view of development. We have seen how the unconscious consists of unacceptable wishes. We have seen how Freud came to believe that the most important of these wishes were sexual. He also came to understand that many of them date from infancy and childhood. Again, we will explore what is called *infantile sexuality* more thoroughly in Chapter 7 ("The Oedipus Complex") and Chapter 9 ("The Id and the Superego"). In any case, as the child grows older, his or her childhood wishes become increasingly unacceptable in terms of conventional morality and the surrounding society, and these wishes are repressed. Indeed, the self-centered and competitive wishes of our young woman are appropriate for a very little girl but not for a young adult. However, despite repression, this young woman's childhood wishes have not gone away but continue to be active in her mind.

At the same time as the censoring capacities of the child develop, other mental processes develop as well (see Chapter 7, "The Oedipus Complex," and Chapter 8, "A New Configuration and a New Concept: The Ego"). However, contemporary psychodynamic practitioners know that everyone possesses an unconscious mind, ruled in part by primary process, which continues to be active even in adulthood. In other words, the Topographic Model describes a mind that is divided, from the earliest days of life, forever and permanently into two domains of psychological life—one layered on top of the other—that are separated by a censor. The upper layer of the mind constitutes a reality oriented, rational, and morally constrained domain of reason, responsive to the constraints of society. The lower layer is in part a pleasure-seeking, illogical, and amoral domain of childhood wishes, subject to highly idiosyncratic forms of symbolic representation. The upper layer partially obscures the lower layer but is not able to control it completely. Indeed, the two domains of the psyche coexist in dynamic relationship with one other, each making its own unique contribution to psychological life.[2]

What Can the Topographic Model Help Us to Understand?

Psychic Reality and Subjective Experience

Although the Topographic Model of the mind is flawed in ways (see Chapter 8, "A New Configuration and a New Concept: The Ego"), it is useful in understanding many aspects of human mental life and behavior, both normal and pathological. According to this model, all experience is the result of the continuous interaction of unconscious and preconscious/conscious regions of the mind, as our experience of inner wishes and fears interacts with our experience of external social reality. Indeed, Freud described the unconscious as a *psychic reality* with importance equal to—if not greater than—external reality in terms of influence on our experience (Freud 1916, p. 444). The Topographic Model of the mind helps us to understand the idiosyncratic, personal, and often not-so-rational private world of personal meaning that constitutes each

---

[2]In the early days of the Topographic Model of the mind, Freud was uncertain about what was included in the unconscious. He talked about repressed memories (*reminiscences*), unacceptable thoughts/feelings, and wishes (Breuer and Freud 1893/1895/1962; Freud 1900/1962). Over time, he came to see that repressed wishes are forged in childhood and often involve an element of sexuality. The oedipus complex, one of the most famous scenarios imagined by Freud, which many readers may have already detected in the clinical material mentioned above, involves Freud's ideas about the oedipus complex. Indeed, the oedipus complex is so well known that we will devote the whole of Chapter 7 to exploring this idea, both how it developed alongside the early Topographic Model of the mind and how it is used by psychodynamic clinicians today. In later chapters of this book, we will also see how elements other than wishfulness are included in unconscious mental functioning. We will explore these elements, examining what contemporary psychodynamic practitioners think about how the mind functions, with particular attention to what we now think might be included in the unconscious.

individual's ongoing subjective experience. As each of us develops, inner experience interacts with the experience of external reality, and unconscious interacts with conscious, in a matrix of subjectivity, as past and present desires, feelings, fears, hopes, expectations, prejudices, and attitudes shape every new experience, even as they are in turn being shaped by new experience. Some aspects of subjective experience are universal, in that we are all human beings who have many things in common. Other aspects of subjective experience are highly idiosyncratic, as each of us develops in a unique way, under unique circumstances.

Transference

In the formation of subjective experience, unconscious wishes, hopes, and fears evade the censor by assuming many forms of disguise, so that every aspect of mental life represents a mixture of unconscious wish and disguise. In describing how this mixture of wish and disguise comes about, Freud proposed the concept of *transference,* first introduced as part of the Topographic Model. In any mental state, an unconscious wish may transfer, or displace, some of its intensity to an unobjectionable preconscious thought with which it might have some symbolic or associative connection (Freud 1900/1962). Returning again to the young woman described earlier, we find an example of this phenomenon in her intense interest in helping her best friend "look great" whenever she goes to a party. In this instance, the young woman's interest in "looking glamorous" is displaced onto her investment in her friend's appearance, which is more acceptable to her than interest in her own. This transference of intensity is the mechanism behind the well-known clinical phenomenon in which a patient transfers strong feelings from a person of emotional importance (often from the patient's childhood) to the therapist (Freud 1905a/1962). For example, in psychotherapy, this same young woman monitors her female therapist carefully for evidence that the therapist is trying to look beautiful. Throughout this book, we will see how transference phenomena are useful in all kinds of psychodynamic psychotherapy as a way to understand the unconscious mind of the patient. For now, we see that in the Topographic Model of the mind, transference is an ongoing process connecting the wishes of the unconscious system to the language-based thoughts of the preconscious/conscious system, explaining how all experience comes to represent a blend of unconscious and conscious influences.

Slips of the Tongue, Jokes, and Dreams

As noted earlier in our discussion of primary and secondary process, in any situation in which censorship is relatively relaxed, we can see the influence of the unconscious on aspects of mental life. Indeed, excited by the possibilities presented by his new theories, Freud enjoyed entertaining himself and his readers by demonstrating the contribution of his Topographic Model to our understanding of all kinds of phenomena. In *The Psychopathology of Everyday Life* (Freud 1901/1962), he wrote about how slips of the tongue and bungled actions, or *parapraxes*, reveal unconscious life when the mind is relatively relaxed by intense feeling or fatigue. For example, when a committee chairman announces at a public meeting that Mr. X will make a "stupor" (rather than "super") new member of the committee, he is revealing a hidden and forbidden opinion that the man in question is both boring and stupid. In the same vein, when a political candidate declares himself to be "on the side of anti-bias, anti-hatred, and anti-Semitism," he cannot expect to win the endorsement of the Anti-Defamation League (Motley and Baars 1979). In addition, we can see the contribution of the dynamic unconscious when a young woman heading out for dinner in a flashy, revealing dress mishears her doorman yelling "Sexy! Sexy!" as he hails her a taxi cab. In another example, a young man, angry in the aftermath of an argument with his boss, misreads a street sign as saying *murder* when it really says *Maeder* (Arlow 1969, p. 9).

A collector of humorous puns and jokes, Freud also enjoyed demonstrating that jokes achieve their desired effect by introducing forbidden, unconscious ideation into previously innocuous situations. For example, to quote from one of Freud's favorites, "A wife is like an umbrella; sooner or later one takes a cab." Freud analyzed this joke as drawing a laugh because we all know, but do not "venture to declare aloud and openly, that marriage is not an arrangement calculated to satisfy a man's sexuality" (Freud 1905b/1962, p. 77).

Finally, as we have seen earlier, in the world of dreams we are also able to observe the interactions of the unconscious and preconscious mind under circumstances in which the censor is a bit more relaxed, or "asleep at the switch." Dreams are so central to the development of the Topographic Model and so important to the work of psychodynamic psychotherapy that we will devote the whole of Chapter 6 to exploring the purpose and meaning of these phenomena.

Theory of Psychopathology in the Topographic Model: The Concept of Neurosis

The Topographic Model of the mind has made a lasting contribution to the study of psychopathology. As discussed above, the Topographic Model posits that all experience is the result of a mixture of unconscious and preconscious elements, as inner unconscious experience combines with the experience of external and social reality to form subjectivity. This formula applies to pathological as well as normal mental phenomena. Indeed, it is important to remember that the concept of the dynamic unconscious was first invented for the purpose of understanding human mental suffering, allowing Freud and his followers to talk about the role of unconscious mental forces in the formation of the symptoms of hysteria, and soon, of other kinds of psychopathology.

Pathological phenomena best accounted for by the psychoanalytic model of the mind are described with the concept of neurosis. *Neurosis* is defined as any inflexible, maladaptive behavior that represents a solution to unconscious conflict. In all human experience there is ongoing conflict between efforts to satisfy unconscious wishes and efforts to repress these same wishes when they are judged to be unacceptable. Therefore, in neurosis also, wishes are always both partially expressed and partially hidden. However, in neurosis, unlike more ordinary experience, there is a cost to the solution in terms of the suffering that accompanies symptoms. In the field of psychiatry, the term *neurosis* has been decried as being vague, overinclusive, and impossible to verify empirically, and in 1980 it was dropped from the official psychiatric nomenclature in favor of the word *disorder,* a term more easily defined with the purely descriptive approach favored by the DSM system (American Psychiatric Association 1984). However, despite its relative disuse as a formal nosological category in psychiatry, neurosis remains one of the most important concepts in psychodynamic psychiatry, because all psychodynamic treatment seeks to help patients gain freedom from neurotic suffering. As we progress through this book, we will see how our developing model of the mind adds to the theory of psychopathology and/or neurosis.

The word *neurosis* did not originate with psychoanalysis or with Freud. It was coined by the Scottish physician William Cullen in the 1770s to designate functional disturbances of the nervous system for which there was no demonstrable structural lesion in the afflicted organ. In the nineteenth century, the neuroses included a wide variety of diverse ailments, including many that are now considered neurological, such as epilepsy and Parkinson's disease. The term also included hysteria. Writing extensively as he did about hysteria, Freud co-opted the word *neurosis* so that nowadays this word has little meaning outside the context of psychodynamic psychiatry. Although Freud first used the term as a purely nosological category, he soon expanded and redefined the concept in his discussion of what he called *the neuropsychoses of defense* (which included hysteria, obsessional neurosis, phobias, and some kinds of paranoia) (Freud 1894/1962). Freud explained these ailments as representing *the return of the repressed*—that is, the reappearance of unacceptable ideas, disguised in the form of symptoms (Freud 1896/1962, p. 161). In other words, in a view that was radical at the time, neurotic symptoms do not differ from aspects of ordinary experience, in that both represent the mixed impact of unconscious wishes and social reality. However, in neurosis we find unacceptable wishes "returning" disguised as symptoms, whereas in nonpathological experience, the mixture causes less distress.

Let us turn to some examples of how the Topographic Model helps us to understand various kinds of neurotic psychopathology. A young woman with hysterical conversion disorder may suffer from the symptom of a paralyzed arm, evincing no neurological disorder upon exam. We will say that her symptoms comprise a neurosis if they represent her fear of the emergence of forbidden unconscious wishes to strike out at her mother, or to masturbate to satisfy forbidden sexual wishes. In this young woman's case, the symptom of the paralyzed arm represents the solution to a conflict between wishing to attack her mother, or to masturbate, and feeling that this wish is unacceptable.

Unconscious conflict may be expressed not only in the form of neurotic symptoms but also in the form of troubling neurotic personality traits, such as difficulties in work, troubles in love relationships, crippling life patterns, or disturbances in mood and/or self-esteem. For example, a self-effacing young man may exhibit the character traits of timidity and deference. In his case, these character traits may be understood to represent the young man's fear of his own unconscious wish to strike out at authority figures, so that he always "pulls his punches." We will return to this same young man to learn a great deal about the expression of conflict in character when we explore the Structural Model (see Chapter 10, "Conflict and Compromise"). In the young woman who felt anxious, especially whenever she thought of a nail salon, we see both symptoms (anxiety and avoidance) and character traits (excessive goodness and asexuality) caused by disguised unacceptable unconscious wishes.

The Topographic Model of the mind enables us to understand not only the content but also the peculiar form in which symptoms often appear. All symptoms are symbolic communications that, like dreams, make use of primary process mechanisms such as condensation, displacement, and symbolization to represent personal and idiosyncratic hidden thoughts and feelings. Indeed, the similarity between the organization of symptoms and the organization of dreams was one of Freud's first brilliant observations. His contribution included the ability to read symptoms and character traits as texts in which we can see the partial expression of a patient's forbidden unconscious wishes and his or her fears. In the example of the young woman with the paralyzed arm, we see how some patients make use of body parts to express more complex thoughts. Even the strange and fragmented thoughts of many psychotic patients can be better understood if we understand the "logic" of primary process. Although psychotic symptoms are caused mainly by disordered brain processes, we see in them the exposure of primary processes in a situation where secondary processes are destroyed or severely fragmented. For example, a psychotically depressed young man who is struggling with unacceptable anger may feel that his body is filled with "poison" or that his brain is being taken over by "malignancy." Another psychotic schizophrenic young woman may spend hours collecting and eating "teeny pieces of tin" so as to feel closer to her mother, whose name is Christina.

Finally, a last important contribution made by the concept of the dynamic unconscious to the understanding of neurotic psychopathology is that it allows us to understand not only the hidden content and complex form of symptoms, character traits, and problematic patterns but also their striking inflexibility. Indeed, neurosis is characterized, and even defined, by its failure to respond to the demands of common sense or current reality. For the person suffering from neurotic problems, the advice of friends and family, the reading of self-help books, and even the most determined efforts of willpower fail to provide relief or bring about change. Our understanding of the nature of the dynamic unconscious helps us to understand this rigidity by suggesting that repressed ideas are not just hidden but take on new qualities by virtue of having been repressed. In other words, repressed ideas, feelings, and motivation have become sequestered from the rest of the personality. As we have seen, in describing this sequestered aspect of the repressed unconscious, Freud was fond of using metaphors from archeology. He suggested that when unconscious ideas/wishes/feelings become separated from the rest of the mind by repression, they are not "worn away" by exposure to the reality of new experience. Instead, they continue to exist, timeless and unchangeable, maintaining their childish, timeless, and irrational qualities in the same way the artifacts from ancient civilizations are preserved from erosion by their burial in the depths of the earth (Freud 1909b/1962).

In contrast to ancient artifacts, however, repressed wishes and fantasies do not remain inert but continue to be active in mental life. They contribute to the *repetition compulsion* of neurotic patients, who repeatedly enact specific scenarios during the course of their lives without ever recognizing the relationship of these scenarios to unconscious memories or wishes. For example, a young woman whose sister died from traumatic brain injury during their childhood came to treatment with a chief complaint of feeling "brain dead." Despite unusually high intelligence, she had long been unable to fully use her mind. She also proved to be highly accident prone, especially with regard to accidents endangering the cranium. In treatment, this young woman endangered herself by failing to follow the low-tyramine diet appropriate for those on monoamine oxidase inhibitors. Although none of her neurotic patterns was connected consciously with memories or feelings about her sister's death, the exposure of this link led ultimately to a resolution of her self-destructive feelings and behaviors.

Theory of Therapeutic Action in the Topographic Model: Psychodynamic Psychotherapy

The Topographic Model of the mind is central to our understanding not only of how people develop symptoms or fixed ways of feeling/acting that lead to suffering but also of how psychodynamic psychotherapy can bring about relief. Although modern conceptions of the therapeutic action of psychodynamic psychotherapy no longer view exploration of the unconscious as the only aim of treatment, the goal of making the unconscious conscious is part of most treatments (Freud 1901/1962, p. 238; Freud 1916–1917/1962, p. 282). Many of the clinical techniques used in psychodynamic psychotherapy were developed with the aim of bringing unconscious mental contents into conscious awareness. As we have seen, Freud developed free association in the hope that if the patient abandons conscious control of his or her thought processes, it will be easier to observe the unconscious determinants of his or her subjective experience. In psychodynamic psychotherapy, the patient is still asked to "say whatever comes to mind," speaking as candidly as possible. The patient and the therapist work together to infer the nature of unconscious determinants in the sequencing, patterning, and content of the patient's flow of ideas and feelings, the nature of his or her avoidance of engaging in exploration, and the transferences he or she experiences or enacts in the process. *Resistance* is the word that psychodynamic psychiatrists use to describe the clinical phenomenon of a patient's active but unconsciously motivated avoidance of knowing his or her own mind. Exploration of resistance leads patient and therapist directly to the heart of the patient's most intense struggles between the unconscious wishes and feelings seeking expression and the effort to avoid awareness of these unconscious wishes and feelings. As we have also seen, *transference* is the word Freud used to describe the automatic, unconsciously determined repetition within the therapist-patient relationship of unconscious feelings/thoughts involving other people, often important caretakers from childhood. Exploration of transference allows for examination of emotionally intense feelings about the patient's experience in relation to important others. Exploration of both resistance and transference takes place in the controlled setting of psychotherapy, where both phenomena are emotionally alive, yet subject to a degree of detached observation on the part of both the patient and the therapist.

In the language of psychodynamic psychotherapy, an explicit inference about the working of the dynamic unconscious is called an *interpretation.* An interpretation that makes inferences about the forgotten or repressed past is called a *reconstruction.* Knowledge about the unconscious gained through interpretation is called *insight.* The Topographic Model of the mind proposes that insight is useful to patients because when wishes, feelings, thoughts, and memories are made conscious, they become subject to secondary process thinking rather than to primary process thinking. In other works, when conscious, they become subject to rational assessment and judgment. Patients become more able to choose how to act in the face of inner demands and less at the mercy of a rigid, stereotyped tendency to act out unconscious scenarios. Although psychodynamic psychiatrists no longer see insight as the only—or even at times the most important—element in treatment, it is still a central part of all psychodynamic psychotherapy, as the patient gains increased awareness of and mastery over the unconscious factors that affect his experiences or his choices, or about unconscious barriers to becoming the person he wants to be. (We provide a more extensive discussion of the value of consciousness in the next section, "The Nature and Function of Consciousness.")

In the case of the young woman whose sister died from traumatic brain injury, exploration of her complaints of not being able to use her brain, her communications during her session, her dreams, and her various moments of avoidance all contributed to understanding her unconscious memories and feelings about her sister's death. Originally, although the patient had recounted the fact of her sister's illness and death, her feelings about these events were not within her awareness. She complained about feeling "brain dead" herself but did not connect these feelings with the facts of her sister's brain injury. At the same time, she talked often about both angry and guilty feelings in reaction to friends who sought or needed help. Her dreams contained images of someone who was injured and/or dying. Exploration of all of these feelings, memories, and dreams led to deepening understanding. However, in this young woman's psychotherapy, the most important insight came from the exploration of transference. Patient and therapist were able to understand frightening interactions in which the patient misused medication in ways that might damage her brain, as a powerful window into her unconscious feeling of connection with her dead sister and her unconscious feelings of guilt and anger about her sister's injury and death. When her feelings were brought into awareness, she no longer needed to express them in the form of self-destructive symptoms and character traits.

In the same way, the anxious young woman who avoided the nail salon and who was anxious to the point of panic at the thought of any efforts to make herself beautiful, learned in her psychodynamic psychotherapy that her anxiety was connected to her repressed and unacceptable wishes to attack other beautiful women, beginning with her mother. When this young woman was able to consciously reflect on her wishes and fears and to integrate them with the rest of her mental life, she no longer felt severe anxiety in the face of her wishes to look more attractive.

The Nature and Function of Consciousness

Although neuroscientists and psychologists do not agree about the precise definition of consciousness, most include a quality of mental awareness in their definition (Hirst 1995). As used by neurologists, definitions of consciousness emphasize levels of arousal of brain centers. In contrast, as used by psychodynamic psychiatrists, definitions of consciousness emphasize the subjective aspect of experience, or self-awareness. In contemporary psychodynamic psychotherapy, we continue to use the technique of bringing unconscious mental contents into awareness, with the aim of increasing the patient's ability to choose a course of action in the face of conflicting imperatives. According to this practice, when patients are conscious or aware of their inner life, they are better able to regulate and control themselves and to make choices and judgments about how to feel and act. How does this idea fit with what is going on in the rest of mind science?

As noted earlier, in contrast to earlier branches of psychology that equated mind with consciousness, the field of cognitive neuroscience is rapidly charting the unseen realms of unconscious mental life. This map-making endeavor began with exploration of information process- ing that takes place in the *cognitive unconscious* (Kihlstrom 1987, 1995) and has moved on to include processes of motivation and intention. Most recently, it has included processes of self-regulation such as atten- tion, metacognition (self-monitoring), working memory, and other pro- cesses previously thought to be under conscious control (Uleman 2005). Indeed, this rapidly expanding map of unconscious mental function has left many wondering what the role of consciousness is. This ques- tion has plagued thoughtful scientists for many years, including Freud himself, who referred to "the long-looked-for evidence that conscious- ness has a biological function" (Freud 1909a/1962, p. 145).

Freud saw consciousness as part of "the superiority of humans over animals" (Freud 1900/1962, p. 617), strongly rejecting any idea that consciousness is a mere epiphenomenon or only "a superfluous re- flected picture of the completed psychical process" (Freud 1900/1962, p. 616). He suggested that consciousness makes higher-order mental processes possible, contributing to self-regulation by playing a role in the capacity for reality testing, judgment, and "temperate and purpose- ful control" (Freud 1900/1962; Freud 1909a/1962, p. 145; Freud 1911/ 1962). In Freud's view, the reason for making the unconscious conscious is so that repression can be replaced by "condemning judgment carried out along the best lines" (Freud 1910/1962).

In contemporary psychodynamic psychiatry, questions about the re- lationship between consciousness, attention, language, integration, and higher-order mental functions such as self-reflection, self-monitoring, judgment, self-control, and volition are the subject of ongoing investi- gation (Klein 1959, 1970). For example, Shevrin (Shevrin et al. 1996), supported by Brakel (1997), argued that the role of consciousness is to categorize experience, deciding whether a mental event should be clas- sified as perception, sensation, dream, thought, or memory. Conscious- ness thereby distinguishes experiences from one another and helps to organize the mind. Olds (1992) emphasized the feedback functions of consciousness, in which sense data are re-represented symbolically and thereby made independent of their sources. According to Olds, in self- reflective consciousness, the self and its interactions can be represented, making introspection possible. Levin (1997) and Rosenblatt and Thick- stun (1977) also emphasized similar "re-entrant mechanisms" of consciousness that make possible many complex functions, such as empathy, insight, object relatedness, and psychological mindedness, allowing for flexibility in the ways human beings conceptualize themselves and make decisions (Auchincloss and Samberg 2012, p. 43–45).

As noted, in the rest of cognitive neuroscience we also see expanding research into the function of consciousness. In recent years, Posner and Rothbart (1998) have argued that aspects of self-regulation, such as volition, are dependent on elements of consciousness, including awareness, self-monitoring, and executive attention. Bargh (2005, p. 53), who otherwise argued for the recognition of unconscious self-regulation, asserted that consciousness serves the purpose of greater integration and coordination through its "assemblage" of various kinds of experience. Other aspects of consciousness emphasized by researchers include self-control offered by language (Bucci 1997), reconsolidation of memory (Nader and Hardt 2009; Sara 2000), modulation of emotion (Phelps 2005), access to a common narrative (Damasio 1984; Farber and Churchland 1996), and many other aspects of self-control (Hirst 1995; Pally 2000; Pally and Olds 1998; Payne et al. 2005).

In short, we see that psychodynamic psychiatry holds a view of the importance of conscious awareness that is in accord with what is going on in the rest of mind science. When clinicians discovered ways to enhance the self-regulation of patients by increasing their self-awareness, they discovered what many researchers are finding in the laboratory—that enhanced consciousness does indeed improve one's ability to choose how to live, even if unconscious factors are also seen to be increasingly powerful.

Chapter Summary and Chart of Core Dimensions

Table 5–1 introduces our Topographic Model chart of core dimensions, in which we have placed the following key concepts:

- **Topographic point of view:** The mind is divided into conscious, preconscious, and unconscious domains. The preconscious mind can be made conscious when attention is paid to its contents; the unconscious mind cannot by made conscious by the simple act of attention, but is denied consciousness by the forces of repression.
- **Motivational point of view:** The unconscious mind consists of wishes that continually strive for expression. The conscious/preconscious mind has the capacity for repression of these wishes when they are judged to be unacceptable.

- **Structural point of view:** The unconscious mind is characterized by *primary process;* the conscious/preconscious mind is characterized by *secondary process.* The unconscious mind and the conscious/preconscious mind are separated by a *censor* that has the task of judging wishes to be either acceptable or unacceptable.
- **Developmental point of view:** Primary process develops before secondary process. Wishes come from childhood and form the basis of *infantile sexuality.* Over time, they are judged to be increasingly unacceptable. Meanwhile, the capacity for repression (i.e., the *censoring capacity*) grows. The end result is an adult mind that is forever split between conscious/preconscious and unconscious domains.
- **Theory of psychopathology:** Neurosis—inflexible, maladaptive patterns of thought, emotion, or behavior—results from unconscious conflict between the conscious/preconscious domains and the unconscious domain. Neurosis is characterized by the *return of the repressed* (in which unacceptable wishes that have been repressed reappear in the form of symptoms) and often by the *repetition compulsion* (a tendency to reenact specific scenarios without awareness of their relationship to early repressed wishes or fantasies).
- **Theory of therapeutic action:** The goal of psychodynamic psychotherapy is for the patient to acquire more *insight* into the unconscious mind—to "make the unconscious conscious." Through the technique of *free association* (which operates according to the *fundamental rule* that the patient will say whatever comes to mind as candidly as possible to the therapist), the unconscious determinants of the patient's subjective experience gradually come to light. The therapist and patient then observe *transference* and *resistance,* using both to piece together a picture of the unconscious mind. The therapist also makes use of *interpretation,* defined as a statement about the unconscious mind. Interpretations about childhood are called *reconstructions.*

TABLE 5–1. Topographic Model Part 1: The Mind's Topography

Topography	Motivation	Structure/Process	Development	Psychopathology	Treatment
The mind is divided into three regions: Conscious Preconscious Unconscious	The unconscious mind consists of wishes always striving for expression	The unconscious operates according to primary process; the preconscious/conscious operates according to secondary process	Primary process is the earliest mode of mental functioning; secondary process develops later	Neurosis arises from conflict between the conscious/preconscious domains and the unconscious domain	Free association ("fundamental rule")
	Unacceptable wishes are kept in check by forces of repression from the preconscious/conscious mind	A censor separates the unconscious and the conscious/preconscious mind	Wishes come from childhood and form the basis of infantile sexuality	Return of the repressed	Examination of transference and resistance
			Wishes become increasingly unacceptable	Repetition compulsion	Therapeutic interpretation and reconstruction
			Censoring capacity grows		Insight ("Make the unconscious conscious")

References

American Psychiatric Association: Diagnostic and Statistical Manual of Mental Disorders, 3rd Edition, Text Revision. Washington, DC, American Psychiatric Association, 1984

Arlow J: Unconscious fantasy and disturbances of mental experience. Psychoanal Q 38:1–27, 1969

Auchincloss EL, Samberg E: Psychoanalytic Terms and Concepts. New Haven, CT, Yale University Press, 2012

Bargh JA: Bypassing the will: toward demystifying the nonconscious control of social behavior, in The New Unconscious. Edited by Hassin RR, Uleman JS, Bargh JA. New York, Oxford University Press, 2005, pp 37–58

Brakel L: Commentary on Solms' What Is Consciousness? J Am Psychoanal Assoc 45:714–720–703, 1997

Breuer J, Freud S: Studies on hysteria (1893/1895), in The Standard Edition of the Complete Psychological Works of Sigmund Freud, Vol 2. Translated and edited by Strachey J. London, Hogarth Press, 1962, pp 1–335

Bucci W: Psychoanalysis and Cognitive Science: A Multiple Code Theory. New York, Guilford, 1997

Damasio A: Descartes' Error: Emotion, Reason, and the Human Brain. New York, Putnam, 1984

Farber IB, Churchland P: Consciousness and the neurosciences, in Consciousness and the Brain. Produced by Lawrence Bauman. Audio Scholar, 1996

Freud S: The neuro-psychoses of defense (1894), in The Standard Edition of the Complete Psychological Works of Sigmund Freud, Vol 3. Translated and edited by Strachey J. London, Hogarth Press, 1962, pp 41–61

Freud S: Further remarks on the neuro-psychoses of defense (1896), in The Standard Edition of the Complete Psychological Works of Sigmund Freud, Vol 3. Translated and edited by Strachey J. London, Hogarth Press, 1962, pp 157–185

Freud S: The interpretation of dreams (1900), in The Standard Edition of the Complete Psychological Works of Sigmund Freud, Vol 4/5. Translated and edited by Strachey J. London, Hogarth Press, 1962, pp 1–626

Freud S: The psychopathology of everyday life (1901), in The Standard Edition of the Complete Psychological Works of Sigmund Freud, Vol 6. Translated and edited by Strachey J. London, Hogarth Press, 1962, pp 1–310

Freud S: Fragment of an analysis of a case of hysteria (1905a), in The Standard Edition of the Complete Psychological Works of Sigmund Freud, Vol 7, London, Hogarth Press, 1962, pp 3–124

Freud S: Jokes and their relation to the unconscious (1905b), in The Standard Edition of the Complete Psychological Works of Sigmund Freud, Vol 8. Translated and edited by Strachey J. London, Hogarth Press, 1962, pp 1–247

Freud S: Analysis of a phobia in a five-year-old boy (1909a), in The Standard Edition of the Complete Psychological Works of Sigmund Freud, Vol 10. Translated and edited by Strachey J. London, Hogarth Press, 1962, pp 1–150

Freud S: Notes upon a case of obsessional neurosis (1909b), in The Standard Edition of the Complete Psychological Works of Sigmund Freud, Vol 10. Translated and edited by Strachey J. London, Hogarth Press, 1962, pp 151–318

Freud S: Five lectures on psycho-analysis (1910), in The Standard Edition of the Complete Psychological Works of Sigmund Freud, Vol 11. Translated and edited by Strachey J. London, Hogarth Press, 1962, pp 1–56

Freud S: Formulations on the two principles of mental functioning (1911), in The Standard Edition of the Complete Psychological Works of Sigmund Freud, Vol 12. Translated and edited by Strachey J. London, Hogarth Press, 1962, pp 213–226

Freud S: The unconscious (1915), in The Standard Edition of the Complete Psychological Works of Sigmund Freud, Vole 14. Translated and edited by Strachey J. London, Hogarth Press, 1962, pp 166–204

Freud S: The history of the psychoanalytic movement. Psychoanalytic Review 3:406–454, 1916

Freud S: Introductory lectures on psycho-analysis (1916–1917), in The Standard Edition of the Complete Psychological Works of Sigmund Freud, Vol 16. Translated and edited by Strachey J. London, Hogarth Press, 1962, pp 241–463

Hirst W: Cognitive aspects of consciousness, in The Cognitive Neurosciences. Edited by Gazzaniga M. Cambridge, MA, MIT Press, 1995, pp 1307–1319

Kihlstrom J: The cognitive unconscious. Science 237:1445–1452, 1987

Kihlstrom J: The rediscovery of the unconscious, in The Mind, the Brain, and Complex Adaptive Systems, Vol 22. Edited by Morowitz H, Singer J. Reading, MA, Addison-Wesley, 1995, pp 123–143

Klein GS: Consciousness in psychoanalytic theory: some implications for current research in perception. J Am Psychoanal Assoc 7:5–34, 1959

Klein GS: Perception, Motives and Personality. New York, Knopf, 1970

Levin F: Commentary on Solms' What Is Consciousness? J Am Psychoanal Assoc 45:714–720–703, 1997

Motley MT, Baars BJ: Effects of cognitive set upon laboratory induced verbal (Freudian) slips. J Speech Hear Res 22:421–432, 1979

Nader K, Hardt O: A single standard for memory: the case for reconsolidation. Nat Rev Neurosci 10:224–234, 2009

Olds D: Consciousness: a brain-centered informational approach. Psychoanalytic Inquiry 12:419–444, 1992

Pally R: The Mind-Brain Relationship. London, Karnac, 2000

Pally R, Olds D: Consciousness: a neuroscience perspective. Int J Psychoanal 79:971–98, 1998

Payne BK, Jacoby LL, Lambert AJ: Attitudes as accessibility bias: dissociating automatic and controlled processes, in The New Unconscious. Edited by Hassin RR, Uleman JS, Bargh JA. New York, Oxford University Press, 2005, pp 393–420

Phelps EA: The interaction of emotion and cognition: the relation between the human amygdala and cognitive awareness, in The New Unconscious. Edited by Hassin RR, Uleman JS, Bargh JA. New York, Oxford University Press, 2005, pp 61–76

Posner MI, Rothbart MK: Attention, self-regulation and consciousness. Philos Trans R Soc Lond B Biol Sci 353:1915–1927, 1998

Rosenblatt A, Thickstun J: A study of the concept of psychic energy. Int J Psychoanal 51:265–278, 1970

Sara SJ: Retrieval and reconsolidation: toward a neurobiology of remembering. Learn Mem 7:73–84, 2000

Shevrin H, Bond J, Brakel L, et al: Conscious and Unconscious Processes: Psychodynamic, Cognitive, and Neurophysiological Convergences. New York, Guilford, 1996

Uleman JS: Introduction: becoming aware of the new unconscious, in The New Unconscious. Edited by Hassin RR, Uleman JS, Bargh JA. New York, Oxford University Press, 2005, pp 3–18

CHAPTER 6

The World of Dreams

This chapter explains how dreams are understood and used in contemporary psychodynamic psychiatry. It also examines how dream theory has been updated and discusses dream theory from neighboring disciplines. Vocabulary introduced in this chapter includes the following: *activation-synthesis hypothesis, day residue, dream, dream work, latent dream thoughts, manifest dream,* and *self-state dreams.*

A *dream* is defined as a mental experience that occurs when the dreamer is asleep. It includes images, thoughts, and feelings that the dreamer remembers when he or she awakens. Dreams are reported by people living in every corner of the world. Since the beginning of time, people have wondered about the meaning of dreams, often using them to foretell the future or for religious ritual. Literature and poetry from all parts of history and all parts of the world are replete with stories about the importance of dreams. More recently, scientists have used empirical methods to understand how dreams are created and what they might mean.

Meanwhile, many patients in psychotherapy, and certainly many patients in psychodynamic psychotherapy, report their dreams to their therapists. Psychodynamic psychotherapists work with patients to explore their dreams as part of a shared search for better understanding of the patient's psychological life. There are many approaches to understanding dreams, including approaches from anthropology, sociology, and other branches of psychology. For example, we know that dream states are produced by the brain, primarily during rapid eye movement (REM) sleep but also during other stages of sleep (Dement and Wolpert 1958). In their work with patients, psychodynamic psychotherapists may use many models from many disciplines to understand dreams, but when doing therapy, they call upon the psychoanalytic model of the mind to help them understand what the patient's dreams mean and how those dreams can help them to learn about the patient's inner life.

The Topographic Model, the Dynamic Unconscious, and the Psychoanalytic Theory of Dreams

Freud introduced the Topographic Model of the mind in 1900 at the same time that he offered the first psychoanalytic theory of dreams. We have seen how Freud turned from exploration of hysteria to development of the first model of the normal mind. In the process of doing this, he also turned from exploration of neurotic symptoms to the study of the normal phenomenon of dreaming. In *The Interpretation of Dreams*, Freud related how he became interested in dreams after observing that his patients invariably inserted dreams into their free associations (Freud 1900/1962). As he became increasingly immersed in dream interpretation (exploring his own dreams as well as those of his patients, children, family, friends, and colleagues), Freud found support for his concept of the dynamic unconscious. Indeed, Freud is well known for having written that "The interpretation of dreams is the royal road to knowledge of the unconscious activities of the mind" (Freud 1900/1962, p. 608). Although aspects of psychoanalytic dream theory have changed since it was first introduced in *The Interpretation of Dreams* in 1900, much of the theory, vocabulary, and practice of dream interpretation remains similar to Freud's first efforts.

Freud's theory of dreams addresses two issues: the purpose of dreams and the meaning of dreams. The second of these issues is most important to contemporary practitioners. Freud argued that the purpose of dreams is to protect sleep in the face of disturbing sensations, such as noise and thirst, or from mental preoccupations, including both current concerns (such as getting to work on time) and unacceptable unconscious wishes. Freud proposed that dreams manage these disturbing stimuli in ways that protect sleep. For example, a person who is late to work may dream that he is already at his desk, or a thirsty person may dream of drinking water. Freud also argued that both mental preoccupations and unconscious wishes are represented as being fulfilled in the dream, albeit in a disguised form. He went on to say that if unconscious wishes are not sufficiently disguised, they will arouse anxiety, so that the dream fails to protect sleep, and the dreamer awakens. Nowadays, psychodynamic psychiatrists do not attempt to account for the purpose of dreams, understanding that data from the clinical situation does not lend itself to the exploration of this important question. In fact, debate rages throughout mind science about how best to understand the purpose served by dreaming and dream states for human beings and other animals (Crick and Mitchison 1983).

In contrast to his ideas about the purpose of dreams, Freud's efforts to understand the meaning of dreams have persisted and are still in use today. Here's how the psychoanalytic theory explaining the meaning of dreams works. Freud used the term *manifest dream* to describe the dream as recalled and narrated by the dreamer on awakening. He understood that the manifest content of dreams often changes, because we remember different versions of the dream at different times. Freud distinguished the manifest dream from what he called *latent dream thoughts,* or underlying thoughts expressed by the dream. Finally, he used the term *dream work* to describe the process (within the dreamer) of transforming the latent dream thoughts into the manifest dream.

According to Freud, in the process of making a dream, the latent dream thoughts attach themselves through association to unconscious wishes from childhood. The latent thoughts and the childhood wishes, both of which are unacceptable to the censor, then attach themselves, again by association, to a bit of *day residue,* or an innocuous image and/ or event from current experience, which then appears in the manifest dream. In other words, the power of forbidden unconscious wishes is transferred to unobjectionable day residues, or bits of conscious experiences from everyday life that serve as symbols for the formation of the dream. In this way, latent dream thoughts are altered or disguised for the purpose of evading the censor, which is charged with the task of keeping unacceptable thoughts out of awareness. As we can see, Freud argued that the structure of dreams resembles the structure of neurotic symptoms, which he understood as resulting from a struggle between the unacceptable thoughts seeking expression in consciousness and the forces of repression.

Dreams can be interpreted by the therapist by breaking them down into component parts, images, or phrases and asking the patient to associate to each component. As with exploration of a symptom, the patient's associations to parts of a dream provide both therapist and patient with a method for unraveling the dream work and finding the latent dream thoughts hidden beneath the manifest content. In this process (or in some variant of this process), therapist and patient uncover unacceptable thoughts from present life, as well as thoughts from many stages of childhood. Indeed, if they work long enough on any dream, patient and therapist will discover very early childhood wishes.

In the example introduced in Chapter 5 ("The MInd's Topography"), the young woman with panic attacks who avoided the nail salon reported a manifest dream in which she was getting a manicure when the bottle of nail polish suddenly filled with blood. Through exploration of her associations to images in the dream, she and her therapist found latent dream thoughts of murdering other women. In another example, an unmarried young woman in psychotherapy reported a manifest dream that included the image of a plastic doll sitting on the uppermost shelf of a bookcase, which she "could not reach." The patient's associations to the dream led to her recounting that she had been "playing dolls" with her niece on the previous day and had wondered to herself what had become of the dolls of her own childhood. Further associations led to concerns that her need to feel "above it all" (on the uppermost shelf) would lead to her remaining unmarried. Her deepest concern, not previously conscious during the first telling of the dream, was that she too might be "left on the shelf" and, unlike her sister, never get married or have children of her own. There was also resonance between the image of the plastic doll and the patient's feelings about how her father had treated her during childhood. Finally, there was resonance between the patient's feeling that the doll was "out of reach" and her feeling that she could not recapture feelings from childhood that dated from before her mother's death when she was 4 years old. In Chapter 7 ("The Oedipus Complex"), we will see how this dream might reveal aspects of early childhood wishes and conflicts.

As we see in this example, this patient's dream of the plastic doll on the shelf involved harmless material, or day residue, from her everyday life (her bookshelves and her niece's dolls), which symbolized many layers of experience and thought from various stages of her life. When the patient (and her censor!) was awake, inhibitory and defensive mechanisms prevented unacceptable thoughts from gaining access to consciousness, in this case because they were too painful. When the patient was asleep, the censor relaxed a bit, and we see greater penetration of these painful (latent dream) thoughts into consciousness, albeit still disguised in the form of a dream.

We can also see that when the logical processes of mental life are relatively inactive during dream sleep, primary processes can be more easily observed in the unusual thought processes that characterize dreams.

As we have seen in Chapter 5, primary process includes condensation, displacement, and symbolism. For example, in the dream about the nail polish, we see the wish to be glamorous and the wish to "polish off" rivals represented in the symbol of the bottle of polish. In the dream of the doll on the shelf, we can also see many thoughts and wishes represented in just a few images (*condensation*). We see the patient's fear of not getting married represented in a doll "left on the shelf" (*displacement*), and we see the feeling of being superior or being "above it all" also represented by the doll on the shelf. In both cases, the representation makes use of the concrete, pictorial image of a doll (*symbolization*).

The Use of Dreams in Contemporary Psychodynamic Psychiatry

Most psychodynamic psychiatrists since Freud continue to see dreams as an important source of information about unconscious mental life. However, our focus on dreams is based on a newer understanding of the mind. Freud's early theory of dreams was based on the Topographic Model and was never updated when he improved on this model. For example, the idea of a censor that sits between the unconscious and the preconscious/conscious is an idea that has been discarded (see Part III). In addition, much of early dream theory is based on Freud's ideas about "psychic energy," which most contemporary psychodynamic psychiatrists think of as highly flawed. For example, in Freud's energy-based theory, only wishes have enough "energy" to cause a dream to be created, so that latent dream thoughts must attach themselves to wishes to gain enough energy to create a dream—hence Freud's famous assertion that "dreams are the fulfillment of a wish" (Freud 1900/1962, p. 121). Contemporary work with dreams has broadened to include exploration not only of unacceptable latent thoughts but also of the defensive modes of functioning that are revealed in dreams (see also Part III). Contemporary clinicians also use dreams to gather information about the state of the transference. Finally, as we will see when we examine Self Psychology in Chapter 12, Heinz Kohut (1977) proposed that certain *self-state dreams* are not founded on unconscious infantile wishes but rather are attempts to master threats to the self. However, diverse points of view share an understanding that sleeping patients are less vigilant about preventing themselves from becoming aware of aspects of psychological life. For that reason, dreams can be very useful in psychodynamic psychotherapy.

An example of another patient dream illustrates how a dream can be useful in psychodynamic psychotherapy. A young woman came to therapy for help with "excessive sexual restraint" and trouble finding a romantic partner. She was very successful as a high-level administrator in her life at work, but she had never had a boyfriend. She reported having had a very traumatic childhood, filled with physical abuse at the hands of her father and brother. In the second session of psychodynamic psychotherapy, this young woman reported the following dream: "A huge grizzly bear, a ferocious tiger, and many snakes" threatened to come into the patient's house while she was "stirring her dinner on the stove." She had been "trying to relax," and yet she awoke in "terrible fear." Over time, as the patient and her therapist explored this dream, they understood that the wild animals who interrupt and threaten the patient represented her frightening memories and feelings, her father and brother who abused her when she was a child, and her therapist who threatened to "stir up trouble" by exploring these feelings. The dream, to which patient and therapist referred throughout the therapy, helped them both to better understand these important issues.

Freud's *The Interpretation of Dreams:* Why Is It Important?

Let us pause for a moment to explore a question that many readers have asked: Why is Freud's book *The Interpretation of Dreams* considered one of the most important works of the modern age? Most students have been told that it is, but few know why. *The Interpretation of Dreams* was written between 1895 and 1899 and was published in 1900. In Freud's estimation, it was his greatest book. Indeed, writing about this book many years later, Freud said, "Insight such as this falls to one's lot but once in a lifetime" (Freud 1900/1962, p. xx). What is *The Interpretation of Dreams* about, and what are the insights of which Freud was so proud?

The Interpretation of Dreams, as the title suggests and as we have explored in this chapter, is a treatise on the subject of dreams—their structure, function, and meaning. But it is also much more. From its very first page, Freud engages his readers with the promise of something both intriguing and potentially shocking. In his selection of a title, the German word *Traumdeutung,* meaning "dream interpretation," Freud chose a word familiar to readers that referred to the dream interpretations offered by Gypsy fortune tellers living at the fringes of society. In other words, Freud's choice of the title *Traumdeutung* was guaranteed to challenge, even provoke, a scientific audience and intrigue others (Ellenberger 1970, p. 452). Then, in his choice of a verse for his epigraph, Freud borrowed the lines from Virgil's *Aeneid* (Book VII, 312), again familiar to his readers and again guaranteed to ignite their curiosity:

> *Flectere si nequeo Superos, Acheronta movebo.*
> ("If I cannot sway the Higher Powers, I will move the Underworld.")

These words are the battle cry of the goddess Juno, who, frustrated by her failure to enlist the help of Jupiter in her plan to destroy the Trojan warrior Aeneas, summons the Furia Alecto and her band of enraged women from Hades to assist in her attack on the young hero as he makes his way to found the city of Rome. At the end of *The Interpretation of Dreams*, Freud elegantly weaves these famous lines of ancient poetry into the intellectual plot of the book to represent the "fate of repressed ideas," which even when banished to the underworld by the "Higher Powers" of consciousness, are far from vanquished but instead find renewed power to influence—and, by implication, even to destroy—our lives (Freud 1900/1962, p. 608). By using these words, Freud offers his readers a dramatic and stirring bit of foreshadowing of the story he plans to tell. He promises his readers that he will in fact "raise hell."

The plot of *The Interpretation of Dreams* unfolds through the interplay of at least three subplots, which interact with and inform each other throughout the course of the book's seven chapters. As we have seen, the first subplot of the book is Freud's theory of dreams—what dreams mean, what they are for, and how they work. The second subplot is the presentation of Freud's first fully developed theory of the unconscious in the workings of the normal human mind—the Topographic Model of the mind. The third subplot is the story of Freud's own coming of age and his struggles with insecurity, self-doubt, and competition on the way to becoming a man, told through the recounting of his own dreams. The genius of *The Interpretation of Dreams* lies in the way Freud moves back and forth from one subplot to the others, developing each in relation to the others in a brilliant fugue, at once highly personal and vast in scope. The style of the book is both literary and scientific, the subject matter is both highly intimate and universal, and the preoccupations of the author are both mundane and existential, predicting the great tensions that enliven psychodynamic psychiatry to this day. It is no wonder that *The Interpretation of Dreams* is considered Freud's masterpiece.

Psychodynamic Dream Theory and Neuroscience

For a long time, Charles Fisher (1954, 1965; Fisher and Paul 1959) was one of the few psychoanalysts who applied empirical techniques from neuroscience to investigate the psychoanalytic approach to dreams. However, several important critiques of psychoanalytic dream theory have emerged from neuroscience and cognitive neuroscience. Among the most important of these is the work of John Allan Hobson and Robert W. McCarley, Harvard University sleep researchers who published a series of articles about dreaming (Hobson 1988; Hobson and McCarley 1977). Hobson and McCarley posited that REM sleep is instigated by the periodic firing of pontine reticular neurons, especially gigantocellular tegmental field cells. Discharges from these cells provide sensorimotor information, which activates the forebrain. The forebrain then constructs a dream by synthesizing random sensorimotor information from the pons with information stored in memory. Hobson and McCarley called their theory the *activation-synthesis hypothesis* of dream formation.

In many of his writings, Hobson points out that the activation-synthesis theory accounts for the instigation and the formal properties of dreams but has few, if any, implications for understanding the meaning of dreams. However, in other statements, Hobson has challenged theories about what dreams might mean, especially those derived from psychoanalysis (Hobson 1988; Hock 2009). At the same time, Hobson and McCarley have critiqued other aspects of dream theory, including the idea that dreams may be "forgotten" by patients because they reveal feelings that are upsetting, thereby instigating motivated forgetting, or repression. In contrast to this view, Hobson and McCarley argue that the forgetting of dreams results from changes in the ratio of neurotransmitters during REM sleep that affect forebrain neurons involved in memory. These changes impair long-term memory while leaving short-term memory intact. Therefore, a subject is more likely to have good recall—even of affectively charged dream material—on awakening from REM sleep in a laboratory than on awakening at home the following morning. In other words, Hobson and McCarley (1977; McCarley 1981) view the poor recall of dreams as being due to neuronal changes rather than to repression.

Some neuroscience research findings contradict Hobson's conclusions by suggesting that dreaming is generated by forebrain structures and/or that forebrain structures are involved with motivational circuitry, offering support to Freud's views of dreaming as connected to wish fulfillment (Braun 1999; Solms 1997, 2000). Other researchers review empirical evidence about dreams from both neuroscience and cognitive psychology, as well as from the clinical situation, discussing the many complex implications for Freudian and other psychoanalytic theories, exploring issues such as the dreams of different kinds of patients, including those with trauma, and how dreams are used in—and change with—treatment (Ellman 1992; Fonagy et al. 2012).

Many authors who support Hobson's findings have also pointed out that there need be no contradiction between his findings and those of psychoanalysis with regard to understanding the meaning of dreams. These authors argue that Hobson's theory and the theories of psychoanalysis represent two separate sets of findings that originate from different methods of study and emphasize different aspects of dream states, dreaming, and dreams. Hobson's theory explores the neural correlates of the dream state, and psychoanalytic theory explores the meaning of dreams. Findings in one theory should strive to be consistent with the other, but neither theory can be translated into the terms of the other. In other words, although Hobson's neuroscientific findings are very important to the project of developing a complete theory of dreaming, they shed no light on the question of whether meaning is present in dreams, or what that meaning might be. And likewise, although Hobson and McCarley's understanding of how memory functions in relation to dreams is very important, this understanding sheds no light on aspects of memory that are influenced by psychological factors. As many have argued, until we have a framework that connects brain and mind, we must be careful about making explanatory or causal statements that link these two realms. For now, brain and mind must be treated "as two distinct orders, each having its own peculiar language, conceptualizations, and levels of abstraction" (Labruzza 1978, p. 1537; Mancia 1999; Wasserman 1984).

As an example of how to usefully integrate findings from very different fields, we can link theories from neuroscience to those from psychoanalysis by understanding that the neurophysiological processes that occur during dreaming, such as motor paralysis or penile erection, are sometimes utilized by the dreamer as symbolic elements that can assist in representing important thoughts. As one theorist has written in an effort to link theories from neuroscience to those from psychoanalysis,

> a loose analogy can be made with the relatively random inkblots of a Rorschach test. The patient projects onto these the meanings that reflect his particular psychology. Since the pontine discharges would presumably be even more random than the inkblots of the Rorschach, there

would be even more room within the frame for the dreamer to project his psychological conflicts. (Wasserman 1984, p. 842)

Exploring the Meaning of Dreams

Exploration of the meaning of dreams and/or of motivated forgetting requires use of the correct methods. These methods must be in the domain of psychology, not neuroscience. Data from the clinical situation is an important source of such psychological data. Other psychological methods appropriate for the study of the meanings of dreams include those using computers and "data mining" techniques. For example, according to Kelly Bulkeley of the International Association for the Study of Dreams (of which Hobson is also a member), researchers have been using quantitative methods of analysis for many years to study the content of dreams. In collaboration with psychologist G. William Domhoff at the University of California, Santa Cruz, Bulkeley describes a technique he calls "blind analysis," which exploits advances in digital technology to explore recurring patterns in dreams. As Bulkeley writes, the findings from several studies "provide compelling evidence that dreaming is not meaningless 'noise' but rather a coherent and sophisticated mode of psychological functioning" (Bulkeley 2013, p. SR 14).

Bulkeley and others publish often in the journal *Dreaming*. This journal explores dreams from many points of view, including the neuroscience of dream states, the meaning of dreams and nightmares, and the relationship of dreams to trauma, coping, and stress, to mention a few important topics.[1] Indeed, as Bulkeley goes on to write, "From the American Indian ritual of the vision quest to the Muslim prayer and dream-incubation practice of *istikhara*, there have been cultural traditions of enhancing people's awareness of their dreams and deriving insights from them. Modern researchers can learn from such practices and combine them with today's technologies, using new tools to fulfill an ancient pursuit" (Bulkeley 2013, p. SR 14). Bulkeley's techniques, and those of many others, support the understanding of psychodynamic psychiatry that dreams have meaning and that investigation of this meaning can be very useful in the exploration of psychological life.

---

[1]For an index of topics, see the website of the International Association for the Study of Dreams (http://www.asdreams.org) and the journal *Dreaming*, published by the American Psychological Association (http://www.apa.org/pubs/journals/drm/index.aspx).

Chapter Summary and Chart of Core Dimensions

Table 6–1 shows our Topographic Model chart of core dimensions with the addition of key concepts for Structure/Process and Treatment.

- **Topographic point of view:** Dreams are both conscious/preconscious and unconscious. The manifest dream is conscious; the latent dream thoughts are unconscious.
- **Motivational point of view:** In dream sleep, latent dream thoughts combine with wishes from childhood to seek expression. The forces of repression are at work even during sleep.
- **Structural point of view:** In the dream-making process, latent dream thoughts linked with wishes from childhood attach themselves, by association, to *day residue* (an innocuous image and/or event from current experience), which then appears in the manifest dream. In this way, latent dream thoughts are altered or disguised for the purpose of evading the censor, which is charged with the task of keeping unacceptable thoughts out of awareness.
- **Theory of therapeutic action:** The exploration of dreams is part of almost all psychodynamic psychotherapies.

TABLE 6–1.   Topographic Model Part 2: The World of Dreams

Topography	Motivation	Structure/Process	Development	Psychopathology	Treatment
The mind is divided into three regions: Conscious Preconscious Unconscious	The unconscious mind consists of wishes always striving for expression	The unconscious operates according to primary process; the preconscious/ conscious operates according to secondary process	Primary process is the earliest mode of mental functioning; secondary process develops later	Neurosis arises from conflict between the conscious/ preconscious domains and the unconscious domain	Free association ("fundamental rule")
	Unacceptable wishes are kept in check by forces of repression from the preconscious/ conscious mind	A censor separates the unconscious and the conscious/ preconscious mind	Wishes come from childhood and form the basis of infantile sexuality	Return of the repressed Repetition compulsion	Examination of transference and resistance
			Wishes become increasingly unacceptable		Therapeutic interpretation and reconstruction
		Dreams	Censoring capacity grows		Insight ("Make the unconscious conscious")
					Dream exploration

References

Braun A: The New Neuropsychology of Sleep: Commentary by Allen Braun (Bethesda, MD). Neuropsychoanalysis 1(2):196–201, 1999

Bulkeley K: Data-mining our dreams. New York Times, October 18, 2013

Crick F, Mitchison G: The function of dream sleep. Nature 304:111–114, 1983

Dement W, Wolpert E: The relation of eye movements, bodily motility, and external stimuli to dream content. Journal of Experimental Psychology 55:543–553, 1958

Ellenberger H: The Discovery of the Unconscious: The History and Evolution of Dynamic Psychiatry. New York, Basic Books, 1970

Ellman SJ: Psychoanalytic theory, dream formation, and REM sleep, in The Interface of Psychoanalysis and Psychology. Edited by Barron JW, Eagle MN, Wolitzky DL. Washington, DC, American Psychological Association, 1992, pp 357–374

Fisher C: Dreams and perception: the role of preconscious and primary modes of perception in dream formation. J Am Psychoanal Assoc 2:389–445, 1954

Fisher C: Psychoanalytic implications of recent research on sleep and dreaming. J Am Psychoanal Assoc 13:197–303, 1965

Fisher C, Paul IH: The effect of subliminal visual stimulation on images and dreams: a validation study. J Am Psychoanal Assoc 7:35–83, 1959

Fonagy P, Kächele H, Leuzinger-Bohleher M, et al (eds): The Significance of Dreams: Bridging Clinical and Extraclinical Research in Psychoanalysis. London, Karnac, 2012

Freud S: The interpretation of dreams (1900), in The Standard Edition of the Complete Psychological Works of Sigmund Freud, Vol 4/5. Translated and edited by Strachey J. London, Hogarth Press, 1962, pp 1–626

Hobson JA: The Dreaming Brain. New York, Basic Books, 1988

Hobson JA, McCarley RW: The brain as a dream state generator: an activation-synthesis hypothesis of the dream process. Am J Psychiatry 134:1335–1348, 1977

Hock RR: Forty Studies That Changed Psychology: Explorations Into the History of Psychological Research, 6th Edition. Upper Saddle River, NJ, Prentice Hall, 2009

Kohut H: The Restoration of the Self. New York, International Universities Press, 1977

Labruzza AL: The activation-synthesis hypothesis of dreams: a theoretical note. Am J Psychiatry 135 1536–1538, 1978

Mancia M: Psychoanalysis and the neurosciences: a topical debate on dreams. Int J Psychoanal 80:1205–1213, 1999

McCarley RW: Mind-body isomorphism and the study of dreams, in Sleep, Dreams, and Memory. Edited by Fishbein W. New York, Spectrum, pp 205–237, 1981

Solms M: The Neuropsychology of Dreams: A Clinico-Anatomical Study. Mahwah, NJ, Lawrence Erlbaum, 1997

Solms M: Dreaming and REM sleep are controlled by different brain mechanisms. Behav Brain Sci 23:843–850, 2000

Wasserman MD: Psychoanalytic dream theory and recent neurobiological findings about REM sleep. J Am Psychoanal Assoc 32:831–846, 1984

CHAPTER 7

The Oedipus Complex

This chapter explains what is meant by the oedipus complex. It explores concepts related to the oedipus complex, both historically and in contemporary theory. Finally, it delineates research in support of the concept from developmental psychology and other neighboring disciplines. Vocabulary introduced in this chapter includes the following: *castration anxiety, complex, fantasy, internalized homophobia, narrative structure of the mind, negative oedipus complex, oedipal victor, oedipus complex, penis envy, positive oedipus complex, preoedipal stage, primal scene, primary femininity,* and *seduction hypothesis.*

The *oedipus complex* consists of a set of feelings and thoughts that we all have about our role in a three-way relationship between ourselves and our parents. The oedipus complex emerges when we are children between the ages of 3 and 6 years. It includes the wish for romantic union with one parent, along with a wish to be rid of the other, competing parent. The oedipal child wishes to be the primary recipient of the love from the desired parent, and fears retaliation from the rival parent. The result is a complex network of feelings, including love and hate, desire and jealousy, disappointment and hope, and competition and fear. This network of feelings forms a template in the mind that lasts for the rest of our lives and influences everything we do. Because the oedipus complex is founded in childhood experience, it is affected by the cognitive immaturity of the child. In other words, it contains many illogical and fantastical thoughts and feelings. As the child grows older and repression sets in, the oedipus complex becomes increasingly unconscious. However, it is universal and has a lasting effect on the psychological life of all of us, whether male or female, young or old.

Freud first formulated the oedipus complex as he was developing his earliest theories on hysteria and the Topographic Model of the mind. He discovered the oedipus complex in his own self-analysis, inspired by the death of his father (in 1896), and in his work with patients. His first published account of the importance of this set of feelings appeared in the book *The Interpretation of Dreams* (Freud 1900/1962).

The oedipus complex represents Freud's foray into several important areas in the development of the psychoanalytic model of the mind. In Chapter 1 ("Overview: Modeling the Life of the Mind"), we mentioned several of these areas as being very important also in contemporary mind science:

1. The oedipus complex represents Freud's first fully developed idea about the contents of the unconscious. We discussed the concept of the dynamic unconscious at length in Chapter 3, exploring its conceptual origins and its role in the mind and in the formation of symptoms and dreams. However, aside from some general ideas about "unacceptable sexual wishes, often from childhood," we have not discussed much about unconscious wishes, thoughts, and feelings.

2. The oedipus complex represents a change in Freud's theory from one that emphasized external causes of mental events to one that emphasized internal psychological motivation. For example, as mentioned in Chapter 4 ("Core Dimensions of Mental Functioning"), Freud's initial theory of hysteria was based on his *seduction hypothesis*, which posited that experiences of sexual seduction (or abuse) perpetrated on children by caretakers led to overstimulation and later illness (Freud 1894/1962, 1896/1962). One of the seminal events in the birth of psychoanalysis was Freud's abandonment of the seduction hypothesis in favor of a new theory emphasizing the inner psychological life of the normal child as a source of stimulation (in normal development) or overstimulation (in cases of hysteria) (Freud 1897/1962). The oedipus complex took the place of the seduction hypothesis in the developing psychoanalytic model of the mind.

3. The oedipus complex represents Freud's first effort to describe in detail how the psychological life of the child lives on in the adult. Aside from his having asserted that it does, we know little about it. The oedipus complex is the first of several universal problems that we

face as children and that affect our psychological life forever (see section "The Universality of the Oedipus Complex" later in this chapter).

4. The oedipus complex includes some of Freud's first ideas about the importance of the body and of sexuality, leading to his later descriptions of the oral and anal phases of psychosexual development, drives, and libido (see Chapter 9, "The Id and the Superego").

5. The oedipus complex includes some of Freud's first ideas about the importance of early caretakers in the development of psychological life.

6. The oedipus complex represents Freud's first complete account of the mind's storytelling capacity. The importance of this aspect of the psychoanalytic model of the mind will be discussed later in this chapter (see section "The Oedipus Complex and the Importance of Narrative and Fantasy").

Freud's Theory: Terms and Concepts

Let us begin our discussion of the oedipus complex with a more detailed description of some terms and concepts developed by Freud. Because so many of Freud's ideas are closely connected with his ideas about the oedipus complex, it will be easiest if we address these terms and concepts as a group. We can then move on to discuss which ideas continue to be important and which have been updated.

Freud named the oedipus complex after the myth of Oedipus, as told in the play *Oedipus Rex*, by Sophocles. He explained the dramatic impact of this play as resulting from the empathy that we all feel with Oedipus' tragic fate, in which, despite his best efforts, he accidentally marries his mother and kills his father. In Freud's view, this fate is inescapable because Oedipus is acting out what we all wish for, by virtue of having once been children. Despite the term's having been named after a mythical male hero, Freud used *oedipus complex* to refer to both men and women.

Freud borrowed the word *complex* from his friend and colleague Carl Gustav Jung (1875–1961), who used the term to mean any set of unconscious associated feelings and ideas that form a network or template in the mind (Jung 1934/1960). Jung made use of the word *complex* in word-association experiments in which subjects were asked to say what words came to mind in response to a stimulus word, thereby revealing the organization of complexes (Jung 1906/1919). When Freud broke with Jung around 1910, he also ceased to use the word *complex.* However, the term *oedipus complex* has persisted as the name by which the concept became famous. Because the oedipus complex contains many thoughts and feelings that contradict one another, such as wishes and fears, we often refer to oedipal *conflict* when talking about its influence on mental life.

Although Freud asserted that the oedipus complex is universal, appearing in both male and female children, he had many ideas about the difference between the genders, some of which have to do with how each gender negotiates the oedipal period. In Freud's view, preoedipal children of both genders are most always involved with and attached to the mother. For the little boy, this attachment becomes more romantic and sexual as he enters the oedipal stage, and he develops a full-blown oedipal complex. Then the oedipal boy, in the grip of what Freud called *castration anxiety* (see below) regarding actual or imagined threats to his penis, relinquishes his sexual/romantic longings for his mother. In the process, he develops a conscience that thereafter tells him how to behave (Freud 1924/1962).

For the little girl, who also enters the oedipal phase attached to her mother, things are quite different. Her recognition of the genital difference between males and females leads to her feeling disappointed, as she develops what Freud famously called *penis envy*. In his view, the little girl blames her mother for her lack of a penis and turns to her father, who has the desired and admired organ. In this way, the little girl changes her love object from her mother to her father, and in turn, goes on to develop a full-blown oedipus complex. However, in Freud's view, the impetus for the girl's renunciation of oedipal strivings is not so complete as is the boy's, as she feels that she has already been castrated and therefore has less to fear. Her oedipal wishes are never fully repressed, and her conscience is never fully formed (Freud 1925/1962). We find here a first presentation of Freud's notorious views of women, which immediately got him (and, through association, much of psychoanalysis) into trouble with those who felt that his views of women were seriously wrong.

Freud's ideas about the oedipus complex also overlap with his ideas about the development of sexual orientation, particularly about the development of homosexuality. He used the term *positive oedipus complex* when he wanted to talk about sexual wishes for the opposite-sex parent, accompanied by hatred and fear of the same-sex parent. He used the term *negative oedipus complex* when talking about sexual longings for the parent of the same sex, accompanied by hatred and fear of the opposite-sex parent. In Freud's view, the child's sexual and romantic longings develop under the influence of what he called *innate bisexuality*. Because of this innate bisexuality, the positive oedipal complex and the negative oedipal complex invariably coexist, and the child experiences ambivalence toward each parent. However, most of the time, either the positive or the negative oedipus complex prevails, with the child preferring one parent or the other. The prevailing complex corresponds to sexual orientation in the adult. In Freud view, sexual orientation was immutable. It resulted from a *fixation* (see Chapter 9, "The Id and the Superego") at an early phase of development, but it is not pathological.

Although we know that the oedipus complex is universal, leaving a lasting imprint on the psyche of all of us, we find few adults who are consciously aware of having romantic and sexual feelings toward a parent, however beloved that parent may be. This is because the oedipus complex becomes increasingly unconscious as repression sets in. Oedipal feelings are driven from awareness by several factors: fears of retaliation by the rival parent, experienced as a threat of bodily harm, which (for both sexes) Freud termed *castration anxiety;* fear of the loss of love of the parent(s) and/or of abandonment by them; and fear of the feeling of guilt. The fear of guilt becomes increasingly important as the child grows older.

In the course of repression, the oedipus complex leaves behind both unconscious wishes and unconscious fears. It also leaves behind a new psychic structure, which Freud eventually named the *superego,* formed as the child internalizes parental prohibitions against oedipal strivings (see Chapter 9, "The Id and the Superego"). It is this newly formed superego, or conscience, that generates the feeling of guilt. Finally, the oedipus complex also leaves behind important modifications in self-image, or *identifications,* formed as the child begins to copy his or her parents instead of pursuing his or her wishes for romantic attachment to them (see Parts III and IV).

Contribution of the Oedipus Complex to Theory of Psychopathology and Therapeutic Action in the Topographic Model

In classical psychoanalytic thinking, the oedipus complex was seen as the major cause of all neurosis. Nowadays this view is no longer common, because contemporary psychodynamic clinicians understand that many conflicts stemming from various stages of early life leave a lasting imprint on the mind of the adult. However, the oedipus complex is still very important in the genesis of much of the psychological suffering seen in adulthood. In other words, many neurotic struggles and inhibitions of adult patients can be traced to lingering conflicts over oedipal fears and wishes.

For example, a middle-aged man presents to treatment with troubles in many areas of initiative, repeatedly failing at work and in other activities. In his marriage, he is excessively submissive to his wife, with whom he has sexual intimacy only rarely. In treatment it emerges that as a little boy, the patient feared retaliation from an aggressive and bullying father. The boy imagined (probably somewhat correctly) that this bullying was punishment for his romantic strivings directed toward his mother. Because this boy needed to appease his father, he came to fear and avoid any kind of pleasurable activity, resigning himself to a dreary, dull life. In this way he not only placated his father (and all persons in authority) but also made himself less attractive to his mother (and all desirable women).

In another example, a woman in her late 30s presents to treatment, anxious about whether she will ever find a husband. She has a history of repeated love affairs with married men but has had trouble finding a man of her own. In treatment it emerges that as a little girl, she felt (probably accurately) that her distant and cold father could not return her love. As a result, she learned to squander her romantic attentions on unavailable men, in a vain effort to get what she never was able to get from her father. A final example is the young woman with panic attacks described in Chapter 5 ("The Mind's Topography"), who avoided all efforts to make herself more attractive because these efforts reminded her of oedipal strivings to outdo her mother (and all other women).

In contemporary psychodynamic psychotherapy, exploration and management of oedipal conflict is almost always important, and therapists continue to look for its lasting effects. They search for these lasting effects in the patient's choice of whom to love; in his or her attitudes toward sexuality and pleasure of all kinds; in all aspects of the patient's self-image, especially those related to gender; in the patient's attitudes toward morality (whether overly strict or too lenient); in the patient's capacities for initiative, curiosity, and strivings for success; in his or her attitudes toward competition; and in fears of all kinds, especially those related to bodily injury.

Throughout the life cycle, many events trigger oedipal feelings and conflicts, which must be worked out again and again. As an example, let us look at the young woman whose dream of the doll on the shelf was described in Chapter 6 ("The World of Dreams"). Early in her adult life, this young woman was content to focus on her career, seemingly uninterested in men. However, when her married older sister gave birth to a child, this event stirred up envy and a wish to have a husband and a baby of her own. She began treatment, worried that these wishes would never come true. As her psychodynamic psychotherapy deepened, it became clear that an early version of her wish for romantic love had been driven from awareness in response to the sudden death of her mother when the patient was 4 years old, at the height of the oedipal period. She responded to her mother's death with a profound sense of loss and grief, which she tried to control with efforts to "rise above it all." To make matters worse, however, she imagined that her mother's death from a rapidly growing cancer was caused by her own competitive oedipal feelings. In other words, at the time of her mother's death, this little girl experienced herself as having triumphed over her mother (or, as it is often called, as an *oedipal victor*). She felt that she deserved punishment for her competitive transgression, and she doled out this punishment to herself in the form of a loss of pleasure in all "female pursuits." She focused on becoming a good, studious girl who would cause no further trouble to anyone, and who paid attention only to her career. Her feelings about the plastic doll turned out to have many sources, including her repressed wishes to have a baby of her own, her thoughts about her mother's dying body, her own grief characterized by feelings of lifelessness and being unreal, and her distant, lifeless relationship with her father, heightened by their shared need to retreat from each other after her mother's death. In other words, exploration of her grief at the time of her mother's death was complicated by oedipal feelings. We will return to this patient later in this book, when we discuss how conflicts other than oedipal ones also affect the psyche in lasting ways.

The Oedipus Complex Updated

The Mind of the Developing Child

Let us now have a look at the many ways in which the oedipus complex and related ideas have changed in contemporary psychodynamic theory. Many of these changes point to important developments in theory and practice. To begin with, contemporary developmental psychologists have a vastly broader view of the oedipal period in children, taking into account many aspects of development in addition to the development of new desires and fears. These aspects include many related to the cognitive maturation of the child, emphasizing the child's increased capacity for self-regulation, problem solving, reality testing, theory of mind, language, episodic memory, symbolization, private speech, and narrative and fantasy (Gilmore and Meersand 2013). When we explore the concept of the ego introduced in the Structural Model of the mind (see Chapter 8,

"A New Configuration and a New Concept: The Ego"), we will see that many of these functions are called *ego functions.*

All of these developing capacities can be drawn into and affected by oedipal conflict, so that psychodynamic psychotherapists will often understand inhibitions and/or difficulties in any of these capacities as being related to lingering oedipal conflict. For example, a young woman suffering from oedipal conflicts may act very flustered, confused, and downright ignorant about many things that appear obvious to everyone around her, and that are not consistent with her high level of intelligence. Upon exploration, her confusion may turn out to be related to a fear of knowing too much about the "facts of life" for fear of the oedipal feelings that this knowledge would arouse.

Nevertheless, as developmental psychologists have shown us, the oedipal child will confront the challenge of new wishes and fears about the body and relationships, morality, gender, love, and hate with new capacities for dealing with these challenges. For example, we see that oedipal boys and girls love to tell stories, which are often related to their struggles to come to terms with a new situation. Their conversation becomes more complex, they become more curious, they engage with others in imaginative play, and they are beginning to love fairy tales. As we shall see at the end of this chapter, perhaps this is why Freud named the oedipus complex after one of the most famous stories of all time.

Finally, it is important to remember that although the mind of the oedipal child is becoming more mature, it is still very undeveloped and naïve. The thinking of oedipal children is characterized by cognition that is concrete, with a poorly developed capacity for differentiating fantasy from reality. Freud himself was aware that oedipal thoughts and feelings were influenced by the mind of the child. He wrote about the many daydreams that children have about sex between the parents (or *the primal scene,* as he called it). Primal-scene daydreams are universal scenarios, both real and imagined, about what takes place in the parents' bedroom. An example of a primal-scene daydream is the idea, common among children, that the parents are involved in some kind of violent activity. He also described children's ideas about "where babies come from" (Freud 1908b/1962). Common examples of such ideas are that pregnancy results from having eaten something, and that birth takes place through the anus. Finally, Freud emphasized that castration anxiety need not be the result of real threats to the child's genitals, but is most often the result of the child's primitive psychological life, in which he or she imagines that frightening things could happen, often in response to "bad deeds." In addition, penis envy results from the little girl's childish reaction to the awareness of gender difference, in which she might imagine that she lacks something important, or that she has been "castrated" for some misdeed.

As noted earlier, the oedipus complex in adults bears the mark of this cognitive immaturity of the child. In other words, oedipal wishes not only maintain the intensity of wishes left over from childhood but also are arranged in a way that reflects the mind of a child. For example, the young man described earlier with persistent oedipal conflict has intense fears of retaliation for any sign of initiative. These fears vastly exceed the real dangers of his current situation. One explanation for the intensity of his fears is that they reflect the terrors that torment even the average child. In the same vein, the young woman who dreamt of the doll on the shelf imagined, even as an adult, that her mother would disapprove of her or punish her, even though her mother had been dead for many years. Another young woman came to treatment because she was unusually interested in dangerous and/or violent sex with men. In her treatment, she discovered that as a child, she confused her parents' frequent fights with their lovemaking, which she had already imagined might include violence. Feeling intensely left out, she wanted to "get into the act," which she imagined as brutal and dangerous.

Other Events That Affect the Oedipal Situation

In addition to placing a greater emphasis on the cognitive development of children, contemporary theorists are also more aware of many other issues that are likely to be on the mind of adult patients, contributing to suffering and complicating the experience of the oedipal complex. First of all, contemporary theorists are acutely aware of the impact of prior stages of life on how each patient has negotiated oedipal challenges. Every child enters the oedipal period having already had important experiences that affect feelings of attachment to his or her parents, feelings about him- or herself, and attitudes toward bodily experience. He or she will have already had considerable experience with pleasure, pain, fear, and anxiety. The period of development from birth to the onset of the oedipal period is called the *preoedipal stage* of development. (We will discuss the preoedipal period in greater depth in Chapter 11, "Object Relations Theory.") Second, contemporary psychodynamic psychotherapists are more likely to be aware of the impact of the parents' reactions to the child's oedipal wishes (Anthony 1970). For example, an adult whose parents accepted and were amused by his or her competitive strivings during the oedipal period will look very different from an adult whose parents became angry and vindictive when challenged (Britton 1989). Finally, contemporary practitioners are aware of the importance of other factors such as adoption, same-sex parenting, single parenting, the death of a parent, divorce, and any other atypical situation. For example, a young man who was adopted may grow into an adult with intense fears of abandonment in response to any transgression, including any stemming from the oedipal period. Contemporary psychodynamic therapists are also aware of the impact of cultural attitudes toward romance and sexuality, morality, gender roles, and a host of other important issues.

Gender Development and Homosexuality Reconsidered

Contemporary theorists and practitioners have very different ideas than did Freud about gender development and homosexuality. Although a full discussion of these important issues would take us far afield, we will discuss them briefly here, because, as noted above, we cannot easily separate Freud's well-known views on these topics from his views on the oedipus complex. Also, theories about gender development and about homosexuality are among the most important errors made by psychoanalytic theory makers. During the several decades when these theories were widely believed and applied, they caused great pain to many women and gay people in psychodynamic psychotherapy.

In Freud's views of the oedipus complex, we find the seeds of his view that the average woman 1) is plagued with residual penis envy (i.e., is narcissistic), 2) constitutes her femininity in response to a feeling of inferiority (i.e., is masochistic), and 3) never really relinquishes her oedipal strivings and has a poorly formed conscience (i.e., is immature and easily led astray). Indeed, as is well known, Freud understood little girls to be an inferior, or "castrated," version of little boys. The application of these ideas had disastrous consequences for many women in treatment. Indeed, many women in treatment were made to feel as if their ambitious strivings were "unfeminine." Pathological masochism and narcissism were seen as "normal" and were not treated as vigorously as they should have been. The guilty feelings from which many women suffer were poorly understood.

Although Freud's ideas were challenged immediately by some of his followers (Horney 1924, 1926), it was not until the 1960s and 1970s that the field of psychoanalysis fully reviewed and revised his theories of female gender development (Blum 1976; Mitchell 1974; Schuker and Levinson 1991). Since then, contemporary theorists have offered important new versions of female development that emphasize *primary femininity,* in contrast to Freud's view that femininity develops in reaction to a feeling of being castrated (Stoller 1976). They also posit normal, albeit somewhat different, moral development (Gilligan 1982). The experience of penis envy is no longer seen as universally important for the development of little girls, and its importance can be influenced by a host of factors, such as the experience of power distribution among the genders in a given family, or prior experiences of loss and bodily damage that affect self-esteem (Grossman and Stewart 1976). At the same time, awareness that little boys feel envy in reaction to the attributes of their mother and sisters offers contemporary practitioners a more balanced view (Jaffe 1977). In contemporary theory, both genders must face the experience of envy in response to the feeling of loss that accompanies awareness that one cannot have everything (Klein 1957/1975). These and many other advances in the psychoanalytic theory of gender development are now widely accepted.

Views about homosexuality have also been challenged, especially in the 1970s and 1980s, as the entire field of mental health revised its views on homosexuality. As almost everyone knows, in response to new data from many neighboring fields, and to political activism, the American Psychiatric Association removed all references to homosexuality as a disorder from the Third Edition of the *Diagnostic and Statistical Manual of Mental Disorders* in 1973, and the fields of psychiatry, psychology, and social work revised their theory and practice. In what was one of the most unfortunate episodes in its history, psychoanalysis was among the last holdouts in the field of mental health, with many theorists asserting ideas such as the following: 1) homosexuality represents a defense against oedipal (or other) fears; 2) homosexuality is always accompanied by narcissistic personality; and 3) homosexuality can be changed in treatment that addresses the motivations and defenses that underlie the psychological choice of same-sex attraction, to mention just a few. Many of these views were vastly more extreme in their antihomosexual bias then were those of Freud himself. Indeed, Freud's own views on the subject were varied and included the following: 1) everyone has innate bisexuality, 2) homosexuality cannot be changed, 3) homosexuality does not represent psychopathology, 4) the negative oedipus complex is a defense against the positive oedipus complex, and 5) homosexuality represents a *fixation* at an early stage of development, among others. When applied to homosexual men and women in treatment, these views had many disastrous consequences as homosexual people in treatment tried to change their orientation, deepened their self-hatred, and were denied the many opportunities that come with greater self-understanding (Bayer 1981; Lewes 1988).

Today, psychodynamic psychotherapists understand that same-sex romance and sexual attraction is not pathology and is mostly immutable. They also understand that clinical data alone cannot lead to a complete theory of the development of sexual orientation (Auchincloss and Vaughan 2001; Downey and Friedman 1998; Friedman 1988; Isay 1989). Contemporary psychodynamic psychotherapists are interested in how all patients, whatever their primary orientation may be, face the challenges presented by intimacy and sexuality. Aware that some problems are specific to those with same-sex orientation, psychodynamic psychotherapists are alert to how patients with same-sex orientation consolidate identity (or not); manage the problem of being different from (most) parents; deal with homophobia, either from the surrounding culture or in the form of *internalized homophobia* (Friedman 1998); and/or raise children under atypical circumstances, to mention a few issues. As with the psychoanalytic theory of gender development, human sexuality of all kinds is now understood in vastly more inclusive terms, with developmental theorists considering findings from behavioral genetics, psychoneuroendocrinology, and many other neighboring disciplines in addition to data from the clinical situation (Britton et al. 1989; Friedman and Downey 1995).

The Universality of the Oedipus Complex

Contemporary psychodynamic practitioners have a complex view of oedipal-phase issues that includes an appreciation of innate factors and the influence of the environment. However, despite the fact that many concepts related to the oedipus complex have changed in the face of new information, psychodynamic psychiatrists continue to feel that the oedipus complex describes an important and universal set of thoughts and feelings that have lasting effects on everyone. To begin with, psychodynamic psychotherapists retain much of the terminology associated with the oedipus complex, adhering to a long tradition beginning with Freud. For example, although the complex was named for a male hero, the term is used when talking about both genders. Although attempts to correct this male-centered bias in terminology have been made (for example, the suggestion of analogous concepts such as the Electra complex), these efforts did not catch on. Some theorists have proposed that the myth of Persephone offers a better story to describe the conflicts of a little girl (Kulish and Holtzman 1998).

In the face of the many changes and developments in oedipal theory, the best way to explain the universality of the complex is to understand that in every culture, and in every mind, there are always at least three problems that must be addressed by every individual. First, everyone in every culture must deal with the problem that other people with whom we are emotionally involved may have a relationship with each other that excludes us. Second, everyone in every culture must deal with the problem that certain strivings are forbidden. Finally, everyone in every culture must deal with the fact of having once been a child and with the many lasting feelings that accompany that fact. Understood in this way, although the oedipal configuration may differ among cultures and individuals, no human being escapes the psychic effects of these universal problems. Everyone must find a way to manage the challenges presented by these problems, and as a result, everyone must contend with feelings of competition and exclusion; desire, fear, and guilt; and helplessness and powerlessness. In Western culture, the oedipus complex (as described by psychoanalytic theory) is the most common way that this scenario presents itself in childhood. Although variations in this configuration are common, the oedipal scenario and its accompanying emotional challenges are universal.

Evidence for the universality and continued relevance of the oedipus complex continues to come from the growing field of developmental psychology (Gilmore and Meersand 2013). In addition, cognitive psychologists have devised ingenious experiments to explore the influence of oedipal fantasies on performance of a variety of tasks (Britton 1989; Eagle 1959; Palumbo and Gillman 1984). However, the most compelling evidence for the ongoing significance of this concept comes from clinical experience with individuals in psychodynamic psychotherapy who struggle with the persistent effects of oedipal conflict as evinced by neurotic suffering.

The Oedipus Complex and the Importance of Narrative and Fantasy

Freud's interest expanded from the study of hysteria and psychopathology to the study of dreams and of normal psychology. His attention also moved from a focus on external events (seduction hypothesis) to a focus on the internal workings of the mind. In the process, Freud developed the Topographic Model. He began to write about art and literature, in which he found many examples of stories illustrating how this model of the mind works. Freud came to see that neurotic suffering and dreams are linked to art and literature through the shared structure of the story. His explication of the oedipus complex was the first (and perhaps most famous) example of how to understand that a dramatic story appears in both the work of poets and playwrights and in the ordinary human mind. Moving back and forth from the exploration of neurotic and normal human psychology to the study of literature, art, and artists, Freud used his new theory of mind to reveal the ordinary psychology hidden in artistic creation and the dramatic scenarios expressed in everyday life. In his writings about literature, Freud suggested that creative writers are individuals who have special access to an innate storytelling capacity of the mind (Freud 1908a/1962).

This innate storytelling aspect of mental life is reflected in the growing importance of the concept of *fantasy* as children approach the oedipal period. In the human mind, all experience is organized in the form of fantasies—scenarios in narrative form that usually feature the fantasizer in a major role. With regard to the narrative framework of experience, the psychoanalytic model of the mind posits the following process: experience begins as a feeling; a feeling develops into a wish and/or fear; wishes and fears are grouped into complexes; and complexes are organized into networks of fantasy. Again, the oedipus complex is the first of these networks of fantasy to be described. Throughout this book, we will describe many more. This aspect of the mind's shaping of experience is called the *narrative structure of the mind*. The emphasis placed by the psychoanalytic model of the mind on the mind's storytelling capacity brings it into closer contact with neighboring mind science, which has become increasingly interested in the narrative structure of mind and brain.

The most obvious examples of fantasy in mental life include the phenomenon of daydreaming and the fantasies that accompany masturbation and sexual activity. Also, earlier in this chapter we saw that oedipal-stage children become increasingly interested in storytelling. However, the creation of fantasy is a more or less continuous process, most of which goes on outside of awareness, so that we often refer to *unconscious fantasy*. The most elaborate of our fantasies is the life story (or stories) by which each of us lives. Much of psychoanalytic psychotherapy is devoted to the tasks of exposing and exploring the unconscious fantasy life of the mind and organizing this fantasy life into a life story. Indeed, in the autobiographical subplot of *The Interpretation of Dreams*, we find the first full-length exposition of how the workings of the unconscious mind are connected not just to the creation of symptoms, or even of dreams, but also to the narration of personal details of the entire life story of a single striving individual—in this case the life story of Sigmund Freud himself.

Revision of the Topographic Model: Freud's Structural Model of the Mind

Part of Freud's genius was to see the similarities between apparently disparate human activities such as symptoms, jokes, bungled actions, dreams, and daydreams, finding in these seemingly unimportant bits of human mental activity the key to understanding some of the deepest of human concerns. It is part of the lasting appeal of Freud's work that he was able to link the ordinary to the extraordinary, discovering the common humanity between the suffering neurotic and the creative artist, alike in their struggle to reconcile the demands of the unconscious with the constraints imposed by everyday reality. The Topographic Model of the mind, initially presented in *The Interpretation of Dreams* and developed over the subsequent 20-odd years, represents Freud's first attempt to build a theoretical model that would organize and account for his extraordinary observations. This model opened the door to ways of thinking about what human mental life is like—and about how it expresses itself in many diverse ways—that had never been considered before.

However, in this description of the Topographic Model of the mind we find many contradictions. The alert reader may have already noticed these many contradictions. Although Freud struggled for more than two decades to fit his many observations about human mental life into the Topographic Model, he was finally forced to offer a radical revision of this model, known as the Structural Model. In Part III, we will begin with an exploration of the many contradictions in the Topographic Model that led to its being revised. As we will see, one of these contradictions is the structure of fantasy itself, which according to the Topographic Model of the mind should not exist in the unconsciousness. Nevertheless, let us end Part II with a reminder that much of the Topographic Model remains useful, especially the understanding of the power of the dynamic unconscious to affect everything that we do. Clinicians must remember that unacceptable thoughts and feelings pushed from awareness are often the cause of neurosis, and that bringing these thoughts and feelings to light can assist their patients in combating mental suffering.

Chapter Summary and Chart of Core Dimensions

Table 7–1 shows our Topographic Model chart of core dimensions with the addition of key concepts for Motivation, Structure/Process, and Development.

- **Topographic point of view:** The oedipus complex is almost entirely unconscious.
- **Motivational point of view:** *Oedipal strivings* (the wish to be the primary recipient of the desired parent's love, along with the wish to be rid of the other, competing parent) are part of what motivates each of us all the time. *Oedipal fears* (including fear of abandonment or loss of love, fear of retaliation [i.e., castration anxiety], and fear of guilt feelings) are also important to each of us.
- **Structural point of view:** The oedipus complex creates a structure in the mind that influences all later experience. (The term *complex* refers to any set of unconscious associated feelings and ideas that form a network, or template, in the mind.) The oedipus complex illustrates the innate storytelling capacity of the human mind. In his writings, Freud vividly described how the mind organizes its experience by means of *fantasy* scenarios in *narrative* form. Finally, the oedipal complex leads to some important changes in the mind. As the child gradually internalizes parental prohibitions against oedipal strivings, a new structure—the superego (or *conscience*)—emerges that generates the feeling of guilt. Important modifications in self-image, or *identifications*, also form as the child begins to emulate the parents instead of pursuing wishes for romantic attachment to them.
- **Developmental point of view:** The oedipal phase—between the ages of 3 and 6 years old—is the time when *oedipal strivings and fears* predominate. However, these strivings and fears last forever, persisting into adolescence and adulthood. In other words, the life of the child lives on the adult mind.
- **Theory of psychopathology:** Oedipal conflicts stemming from early life leave a lasting imprint and contribute to psychological suffering (neurosis) in adulthood.
- **Theory of therapeutic action:** Exploration of the oedipus complex is part of almost all psychodynamic psychotherapies.

TABLE 7–1.   Topographic Model Part 3: The Oedipus Complex

Topography	Motivation	Structure/Process	Development	Psychopathology	Treatment
The mind is divided into three regions: Conscious Preconscious Unconscious	The unconscious mind consists of wishes always striving for expression Unacceptable wishes are kept in check by forces of repression from the preconscious/conscious mind **Oedipal strivings Oedipal fears**	The unconscious operates according to primary process; the preconscious/conscious operates according to secondary process A censor separates the unconscious and the conscious/preconscious mind Dreams **Complex Fantasy Narrative** **Conscience Identifications**	Primary process is the earliest mode of mental functioning; secondary process develops later Wishes come from childhood and form the basis of infantile sexuality **Oedipal strivings and fears persist into adolescence and adulthood** Wishes become increasingly unacceptable Censoring capacity grows	Neurosis arises from conflict between the conscious/preconscious domains and the unconscious domain Return of the repressed Repetition compulsion	Free association ("fundamental rule") Examination of transference and resistance Therapeutic interpretation and reconstruction Insight ("Make the unconscious conscious") Dream exploration

References

Anthony EJ: The reactions of parents to the oedipal child, in Parenthood: Its Psychology and Psychopathology. Edited by Anthony EJ, Benedek T. Boston, MA, Little, Brown, 1970, pp 275–288

Auchincloss EL, Vaughan SC: Psychoanalysis and homosexuality: do we need a new theory? J Am Psychoanal Assoc 49:1157–1186, 2001

Bayer R: Homosexuality and American Psychiatry: The Politics of Diagnosis. Princeton, NJ, Princeton University Press, 1981/1987

Blum HP (ed): Female Psychology: Contemporary Psychoanalytic Views. New York, International Universities Press, 1976

Britton R: The missing link: parental sexuality in the Oedipus complex, in The Oedipus Complex Today: Clinical Implications. Edited by Britton R, Feldman M, O'Shaughnessy E. London, Karnac, 1989, pp 83–101

Britton R, Feldman M, O'Shaughnessy E (eds): The Oedipus Complex Today: Clinical Implications. London, Karnac, 1989

Downey J, Friedman R: Female homosexuality reconsidered. J Am Psychoanal Assoc 46:471–506, 1998

Eagle M: The effects of subliminal stimulation with aggressive content on conscious cognition. J Pers 27:678–688, 1959

Freud S: The neuro-psychoses of defense (1894), in The Standard Edition of the Complete Psychological Works of Sigmund Freud, Vol 3. Translated and edited by Strachey J. London, Hogarth Press, 1962, pp 41–61

Freud S: Further remarks on the neuro-psychoses of defense (1896), in The Standard Edition of the Complete Psychological Works of Sigmund Freud, Vol 3. Translated and edited by Strachey J. London, Hogarth Press, 1962, pp 157–185

Freud S: Letter 70 (Extracts from the Fliess Papers) (1897), in The Standard Edition of the Complete Psychological Works of Sigmund Freud, Vol 1. Translated and edited by Strachey J. London, Hogarth Press, 1962, pp 261–263

Freud S: The interpretation of dreams (1900), in The Standard Edition of the Complete Psychological Works of Sigmund Freud, Vol 4/5. Translated and edited by Strachey J. London, Hogarth Press, 1962, pp 1–626

Freud S: Creative writers and day-dreaming (1908a), in The Standard Edition of the Complete Psychological Works of Sigmund Freud, Vol 9. Translated and edited by Strachey J. London, Hogarth Press, 1962, pp 141–154

Freud S: On the sexual theories of children (1908b), in The Standard Edition of the Complete Psychological Works of Sigmund Freud, Vol 9. Translated and edited by Strachey J. London, Hogarth Press, 1962, pp 205–226

Freud S: The dissolution of the Oedipus complex (1924), in The Standard Edition of the Complete Psychological Works of Sigmund Freud, Vol 19. Translated and edited by Strachey J. London, Hogarth Press, 1962, pp 171–180

Freud S: Some psychical consequences of the anatomical distinction between the sexes (1925), in The Standard Edition of the Complete Psychological Works of Sigmund Freud, Vol 19. Translated and edited by Strachey J. London, Hogarth Press, 1962, pp 241–258

Friedman RC: Male Homosexuality: A Contemporary Psychoanalytic Perspective. New Haven, CT, Yale University Press, 1988

Friedman RC: Internalized homophobia, pathological grief, and high-risk sexual behavior in a gay man with multiple psychiatric disorders. Journal of Sex Education and Therapy 23:115–120, 1998

Friedman RC, Downey JI: Biology and the Oedipus complex. Psychoanal Q 64:234–264, 1995

Gilligan C: In a Different Voice: Psychological Theory and Women's Development. Cambridge, MA, Harvard University Press, 1982

Gilmore KJ, Meersand P: Normal Child and Adolescent Development: A Psychodynamic Primer. Arlington, VA, American Psychiatric Publishing, 2013

Grossman W, Stewart W: Penis envy: from childhood wish to developmental metaphor. J Am Psychoanal Assoc 24 (5 suppl):193–212, 1976

Horney K: On the genesis on the castration complex in women. Int J Psychoanal 5:50–65, 1924

Horney K: The flight from womanhood: the masculinity complex in women, as viewed by men and by women. Int J Psychoanal 7:324–339, 1926

Isay R: Being Homosexual: Gay Men and Their Development. New York, Farrar, Strauss & Giroux, 1989

Jaffe DS: The masculine envy of a woman's procreative function, in Female Psychology: Contemporary Psychoanalytic Views. Edited by Blum HP. New York, International Universities Press, 1977, pp 361–392

Jung CG: Studies in Word-Association (1906). New York, Moffat, Yard, 1919

Jung CG: A review of the complex theory (1934), in The Collected Works of C.G. Jung, Vol 8. New York, Pantheon Books, 1960

Klein M: Envy and gratitude (1957), in Envy and Gratitude, and Other Works, 1946–1963. London, Hogarth Press, 1975

Kulish N, Holtzman D: Persephone, the loss of virginity and the female oedipal complex. Int J Psychoanal 79 (Pt 1):57–71, 1998

Lewes K: The Psychoanalytic Theory of Male Homosexuality. New York, Simon & Schuster, 1988

Mitchell J: Psychoanalysis and Feminism: Freud, Reich, Laing, and Women. New York, Random House, 1974

Palumbo R, Gillman I: Effects of subliminal activation of oedipal fantasies on competitive performance: a replication and extension. J Nerv Ment Dis 172:733–741, 1984

Schuker E, Levinson NA (eds): Female Psychology: An Annotated Psychoanalytic Bibliography. Hillsdale, NJ, Analytic Press, 1991

Stoller R: Primary femininity. J Am Psychoanal Assoc 24 (suppl):59–78, 1976

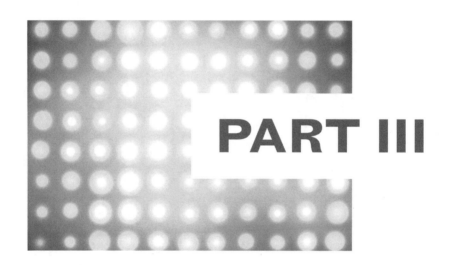

PART III

The Structural Model

CHAPTER 8

A New Configuration and a New Concept: The Ego

This chapter introduces readers to the Structural Model of the mind, briefly defining the concepts id, ego, and superego. It reviews the reasons why the psychoanalytic model of the mind needed to be changed. It explores the concept of ego in greater depth. Vocabulary introduced in this chapter includes the following: *adaptation, autonomous ego functions, average expectable environment, ego, ego functions, ego identity/identity, ego psychology, ego strength, ego weakness, homeostasis, id, identification, internalization, reality testing, superego,* and *tripartite model.*

The Structural Model of the mind was the second version of the psychoanalytic model of the mind. Freud introduced the Structural Model in 1923, in his book *The Ego and the Id* (Freud 1923/1962). As we will see, Freud offered his revised model of the mind in response to his growing awareness that the Topographic Model of the mind had many theoretical inconsistencies, and most important, that it failed to help him explain the ever-wider range of clinical problems with which he was confronted. As a result of this awareness, Freud began to question whether the best way to understand the psychological struggles of his patients was to explore them along topographic lines. He proposed that mental life might be best understood not as the result of a struggle between unconscious and preconscious/conscious domains of the mind but instead as the result of the interaction between three structures of the mind, which he called *ego, id,* and *superego.* These structures are distinguished from one another by their different motivations, structural properties, modes of operation, and development. To summarize briefly, *ego* is the name for the executive function of the mind responsible for maintenance of homeostasis and adaptation; *id* is the name for the motivational forces in human psychic life, called the *drives;* and *superego* is the name for the moral imperatives and ideals that we commonly call the *conscience.*

In the 1950s, especially in the United States, the Structural Model of the mind became the dominant model of mental functioning used by psychodynamic clinicians. Over time, it became synonymous with the term *ego psychology,* the branch of psychoanalysis that emphasizes the ego and its role in psychological functioning. In addition, the Structural Model of the mind is considered to be synonymous with the term *tripartite model of the mind* and also often with the term *conflict theory,* which emphasizes how the ego manages the competing aims of the id and the superego in accord with external reality by forging compromises that affect all of mental life. Finally, the Structural Model of the mind (and/or Ego Psychology/Conflict Theory) has often been considered to be synonymous with what has been called *classical psychoanalysis* or even simply *Freudian psychoanalysis.* Beginning in the 1970s and continuing into the present, the Structural Model of the mind (and Ego Psychology) has often been in competition with Object Relations Theory and/or Self Psychology (and, more recently, with Relational Psychoanalysis) for dominance in the world of psychodynamic psychiatry (see Part IV). Among the aims of this book is to show that these models can be combined (along with the Topographic Model) into an integrated point of view.

Problems Leading to Revision of the Topographic Model

What problems led Freud to revise his theory in the form of the Structural Model of the mind? Although we have seen that the Topographic Model is useful in many ways, Freud soon discovered that his division of the mind into unconscious and preconscious/conscious s was not adequate to describe all of the complexities of mental life. To review briefly, in the Topographic Model, conflict occurs between unconscious wishes seeking expression and preconscious/conscious forces of repression, which respond to the demands of reality, society, and morality. The unconscious is entirely wishful and uninhibited, and the preconscious/conscious includes all capacities for organization, appraisal, planning, and delay. This model presents several problems.

First of all, the model was challenged by Freud's observation, perhaps already obvious to the astute reader, that both the defenses against the emergence of unconscious wishes and the censor at whose behest these defenses operate are themselves unconscious. They cannot be brought to consciousness simply by attending to them, as we can with the preconscious. For the most part (with some exceptions), we are not aware of deliberately excluding thoughts from consciousness or of censoring them. Indeed, if we were, the whole purpose of a defense intended to produce "not knowing" would be defeated. In the clinical situation, the patient shows evidence of resistance, but this resistance is not mounted consciously. In other words, *the psychoanalytic model of the mind must include an unconscious that is capable of appraisal and defense.*

Second, Freud began to observe that in more than a few instances, the thoughts and feelings defended against are not wishes at all; rather, they are moral concerns. Freud's work with patients suffering from *melancholia* (the term that he used for depression), obsessional symptoms, and masochism led to his understanding that moral imperatives and self-punitive tendencies can also operate unconsciously. These moral imperatives may include ideals, taboos, punishments, and rewards. In other words, *the psychoanalytic model of the mind must include an unconscious that contains moral imperatives in addition to wishes.*

Finally, as we have seen in Chapter 7 in our exploration of the oedipus complex, the unconscious is replete with stories organized in narrative form. When Freud first began clinical work, he did not worry much about the structure or organization of psychological experience. However, as his theory developed, he began to recognize that certain mental contents are organized in ways that, in themselves, influence the nature of experience. As we have seen, Freud recognized early on that thoughts in the form of wishes had a special place in mental life. Soon, with the help of ideas borrowed from colleagues (including Carl Jung and others), Freud began to understand that these wishes are organized into *complexes*—groups of associated ideas, feelings, and wishes—that are stored together in the mind. He went on to develop the idea that mental experience, especially emotionally charged experience, is organized in the form of fantasies, or imaginative story-like narratives featuring the imagining subject in a major role. The concept of unconscious fantasy began to take on major importance in the psychoanalytic approach to understanding subjective experience (see Chapter 7, "The Oedipus Complex"). However, the idea that unconscious mental life is organized as a story contradicts the Topographic Model of the mind, which asserts that unconscious mental life can only be wishful, organized by primary process. In other words, *the psychoanalytic model of the mind must include an unconscious that can be organized in narrative form.* Ultimately, for these three reasons, the Topographic Model had to be revised (Arlow and Brenner 1964).

As the Topographic Model Collapses, the Unconscious Expands

Another way to look at the transition from the Topographic Model to the Structural Model of the mind is to recognize that the important concept of the unconscious has itself changed dramatically. Contemporary psychodynamic psychiatrists no longer refer to the original idea, central to the Topographic Model, of a unified unconscious domain of the mind characterized by a single type of childish, wishful content or a single kind of mental processing. We can see from our earlier look at the Topographic Model how the Freudian unconscious got its widespread and false reputation as a "cauldron full of seething excitations" (Freud 1933/1962, p. 73; Park and Auchincloss 2006). However, when Freud formulated the Structural Model of the mind, he dismantled the Topographic Model, with its "seething cauldron" view of the unconscious. This dismantling was largely in response to his own growing awareness that unconscious mental life includes not only peremptory wishes but also moral, strategic, and reality-oriented strivings, many organized in ways that are logical and goal directed. In other words, with the introduction of the Structural Model, the idea of the unconscious as an underworld full of primitive, irrational, and wishful strivings, hell-bent on seeking expression at all costs, was no longer viable. In the new model, the dynamic unconscious was envisioned as including strivings for self-preservation, capacities for appraisal and choice, and moral imperatives, as well as childish, pleasure-seeking wishes (see Chapter 3, "Evolution of the Dynamic Unconscious").

The Ego

This brings us to the new and important concept of the ego, or the executive agency of the mind. Among the most important novel features of the Structural Model of the mind is its greater emphasis on our psychological capacities for *self-regulation* (sometimes called *homeostasis*) and for *adaptation*. Although these capacities are implied in the Topographic Model, with a censor capable of judgment and delay, they are given vastly greater attention in the new Structural Model—all posited to be capacities of this new structure called the ego. The word *ego* was coined by

James Strachey in his translation of Freud's *das Ich* or "the I." Strachey was the editor in chief of the English language edition of Freud's writings, *The Standard Edition of the Complete Psychological Works of Sigmund Freud*, published between 1956 and 1974. Strachey and his team of editors are responsible for coining familiar words such as *ego, id, parapraxis, cathexis,* and others. Prior to 1923, Freud had used the term *ego* in variety of ways, but mostly to designate the whole mind or the whole person. He did not formally assert that the ego is the executive function of the mind—or, as he put it, "a coherent organization of mental processes"—until his introduction of the Structural Model (Freud 1923/1962, p. 9).

When Freud developed this formal concept of the ego, he launched the beginning of an enormous interest in the processes of homeostasis and adaptation and in the *ego functions* that comprise these important processes. These ego functions include capacities previously attributed to the conscious/preconscious mind in the Topographic Model, such as censorship and defense, as well as characteristics assigned to secondary process in the Topographic Model, such as reason, logic, and judgment. The ego functions also include cognition, perception, memory, motility, affect, thinking, language, symbolization, reality testing, evaluation, impulse control, and affect tolerance, to mention an important few. Ego functions include the vital tasks of mediating conflict and forging compromise (see Chapter 10). They also include the key tasks of forming and maintaining mental representations, including representations of self and object (see Chapters 11 and 12). The ego has conscious, preconscious, and unconscious aspects; however, for the most part, ego functions operate outside of awareness. Only a few ego functions operate preconsciously and consciously (Auchincloss and Samberg 2012, p. 69).

Let us explore the processes of self-regulation/homeostasis and adaptation in greater detail. To begin with, *homeostasis* is a concept borrowed by psychoanalysis from general biology, which explores this important function in every organism. Recently, the field of cognitive science has contributed a great deal to our understanding of how this function works (see section "The Rise of Cognitive Psychology" in Chapter 3). We also mentioned some aspects of this function in Chapter 7 when we discussed contemporary views of the oedipus complex. As we saw then, the psychoanalytic model of the mind helps us understand the capacity to regulate conflicting motives by appraising them, deciding on priorities, and forging compromises among them.

The Structural Model of the mind marks a vast improvement over the Topographic Model in terms of delineating conflicting motivations, explaining how we at arrive at compromises, and explicating the ego functions necessary for forging these compromises. For example, in the

Structural Model, *defense* is defined as both a capacity of the ego and one of the most important elements of compromise. In the new model, the range of possible defenses expands beyond repression to include an almost infinite array of strategies by which the mind can manage conflict. Managing the subjective experience of psychic conflict requires additional ego functions, such as impulse control and affect tolerance. As noted previously, we will discuss conflict, defense, and compromise in greater detail in Chapter 10.

In addition to having the function of self-regulation, the ego is defined as the mental structure with the capacity for adaptation to external reality. *Adaptation* is another concept borrowed by psychoanalysis from general biology and refers to the survival needs of every organism and how these survival needs are met in interaction with the environment. Adaptation includes the fit between an individual and the environment and the psychological processes that enhance this fit by changing, controlling, and/or accommodating to the environment (Auchincloss and Samberg 2012, p. 6). When applied to psychoanalytic psychology, the concept of adaptation emphasizes the fact that human psychology is shaped not only by conflicting internal motivations but also by interactions with the relevant environment. For the most part, psychoanalysis stresses the caregiving environment, the family, and sometimes the surrounding culture. As we will see in Chapter 10, adaptation to external reality plays an important role in mediation of conflict and forging of compromise. As we will see in Part IV, in both Object Relations Theory and Self Psychology, exploration of how the growing child develops psychological structures in interaction with the care taking environment becomes ever more important as the psychoanalytic model of the mind develops.

The earlier Topographic Model of the mind does include some awareness of the importance of adaptation to external reality in psychological life. For example, the Topographic Model posited that unconscious wishes are in conflict with the demands of external reality or society as perceived by the preconscious/conscious. Furthermore, Freud argued that the secondary processes of the preconscious/conscious regions of the mind develop in response to the infant's growing awareness that the primary processes are not enough to achieve satisfaction in the real world. Finally, arguing within the Topographic Model of the mind, Freud also argued that motives for *self-preservation* (an early version of what would soon become the ego) were in conflict with unconscious wishes. However, the Topographic Model of the mind places strongest emphasis on the unconscious wishes themselves. Indeed, most of the writing of Freud consisted of his attempts to characterize the nature of the unconscious. In other words, although the Topographic Model of the mind did acknowledge the impact of the external world, as delineated above, this impact was poorly conceptualized.

The new Structural Model of the mind marked a vast improvement over the Topographic Model in terms of understanding the mind's capacity to adapt to external reality. For example, the capacity for *reality testing*, defined as an ego function, can now be studied in greater depth. In addition, we find a growing interest in processes of *internalization*, also an ego function, which can also be studied in greater depth. Internalization is another concept borrowed from general biology, defined (often in opposition to *externalization*) as an organism's tendency to take in aspects of the external world. Indeed, Freud first described the ego itself as developing under the impact of perceptual stimuli, or awareness of external reality. Later he described how the ego gains strength and *character* from the internalization of interpersonal relationships (see Chapters 9 and 10 for an introduction to the concept of *character*). For example, *identification* is defined as a modification of the self-image that results from internalizing the traits of others. We have seen how oedipal strivings are managed through the development of identifications with parents who have previously been experienced as rivals. Understanding the many aspects of internalization (including identification) will become increasingly important as the psychoanalytic model of the mind develops, and as we explore Object Relations Theory and Self Psychology in Part IV (Vaillant 1977, 1983).

Contribution of the Ego to Theory of Psychopathology and Therapeutic Action in the Structural Model

The Structural Model of the mind, and the concept of the ego in particular, has had a profound effect on how psychodynamic psychiatrists think about mental health, psychopathology, and treatment. Delineation of the various ego functions allowed clinicians to evaluate them individually and to thereby give a richer description of mental health expressed as *ego strengths,* and psychopathology expressed as *ego weaknesses.* Although these concepts have been refined over time, they are in widespread use in the contemporary mental health professions to describe the level at which our patients function.

In the Topographic Model of the mind, neurotic psychopathology was understood as resulting from the inflexible, stereotyped influence of unconscious wishes in situations where repression was too rigid or wishes too strong. The goal of treatment was the search for hidden but pathogenic unconscious striving with the aim of "mak[ing] conscious everything that is pathogenically unconscious" (Freud 1901/1962, p. 238; Freud 1916–1917/1962, p. 282). What Freud meant by this statement was that by subjecting unconscious wishes to conscious judgment rather than to repression, the patient would have greater control over his or her mind (Freud 1905/1962). With the introduction of the Structural Model, neurotic psychopathology came to be understood as the result of inflexible or maladaptive efforts on the part of the ego to forge compromise among competing aims. Under the new model, the goal of treatment was to understand how the ego manages (or fails to manage) conflict, with the aim of strengthening the ego's adaptive capacity. With this in mind, we can better understand Freud's famous statement, "Where id was, there ego shall be" (Freud 1923/1962, p. 56; Freud 1933/1962, p. 80). These new ways of thinking about psychopathology and treatment will be explored in greater depth in Chapter 10 ("Conflict and Compromise").

The Work of Well-Known Ego Psychologists

Anna Freud

The Topographic Model of the mind was largely the creation of one man, Sigmund Freud. However, although introduced by Freud, the Structural Model of the mind was elaborated by many others. For example, Freud's youngest daughter, Anna Freud (1895–1982), explored the defensive capacities of the ego in her book *The Ego and the Mechanisms of Defense* (A. Freud 1936/1974). Anna Freud is probably best known as a major proponent of the field of psychodynamic child psychiatry and psychotherapy, but in this role, she also made many contributions to the study of normal and pathological ego development (A. Freud 1965/1975). We will not explore the field of psychodynamic child psychiatry in depth, or even the vast field of ego development, as such an exploration would take us far afield. However, it is useful to notice that Ego Psychology developed alongside the growth of psychoanalytic developmental theory and child observation and that the two are closely related (Gilmore and Meersand 2013).

Heinz Hartmann

Another important contributor to the field of Ego Psychology was Heinz Hartmann (1894–1970), whose book *Ego Psychology and the Prob-*

lem of Adaptation (1939/1958) made explicit the importance of the mind's capacity for adaptation to external reality. In Hartmann's view, the ego develops in the course of interactions between the mind's inborn potential and what he called the *average expectable environment*. The average expectable environment includes aspects of the usual caregiving environment, such as love, nurturing, and safety. Hartmann was also important for having described *autonomous ego functions*—inborn capacities of the mind that develop independently, or autonomously, from conflict and that include thought, memory, perception, cognition, and motility. As we have seen in some of the examples in Chapter 7 on the oedipus complex, autonomous ego functions can be drawn into conflict and become distorted. As we will see below, the delineation of autonomous ego functions, and the concept of the ego in general, allows psychoanalytic psychology to develop in close contact with the rest of psychology, including cognitive neuroscience.

Erik Erikson

A final ego psychologist familiar to most of our readers is Erik Erikson (1902–1994), who after Sigmund Freud is possibly the best known psychoanalyst in the United States (Park and Auchincloss 2006). Erikson is famous for his eight-stage theory of human development throughout the life cycle, which includes the stages *trust/mistrust, autonomy/shame and doubt, initiative/guilt, industry/inferiority, identity/role confusion* (or *diffusion*), *intimacy/isolation, generativity/stagnation,* and *ego integrity/despair.* In the successful negotiation of each of these stages, the developing individual acquires the psychological capacity for which each stage is named (e.g., trust); if this capacity is not attained, a pathological state of mind ensues (e.g., mistrust). Capacities result from interactions among inborn capacities, external reality, interpersonal relationships, and the surrounding culture. One of Erikson's most important contributions was the concept of *ego identity,* later shortened to *identity,* which is defined as the consolidation of a stable sense of oneself as a unique individual in society (Erikson 1950, 1956, 1959; see also Auchincloss and Samberg 2012, p. 70). Erikson's argument that ego development can only be understood in the context of the surrounding culture has allowed psychoanalytic psychology to develop in close contact with the rest of the social sciences, including sociology, anthropology, and others. In addition, Erikson's interest in the importance of the object in each stage and the importance of developing a healthy sense of identity presages the development of Object Relations Theory and Self Psychology (see Chapters 11 and 12).

Points of Convergence Between the Structural Model and General Psychology

As we have seen, the Structural Model of the mind and Ego Psychology brought with them an interest in a wide array of mental processes and capacities. Some of these capacities—such as many related to the management of conflict (see Chapter 10)—operate outside of awareness because they are repressed. However, the ego also includes many processes and capacities that operate outside of awareness not because they are repressed but because they are designed to operate this way. These capacities are part of what Freud called the descriptive unconscious (see Chapters 3 and 5). Indeed, with the emphasis of the Structural Model on the mind's capacities for homeostasis and adaptation, Ego Psychology brings the psychoanalytic model of the mind into closer contact with the rest of general psychology (Kagan 1983; Mischel et al. 1989; Piaget and Inhelder 1969; White 1959). The Structural Model of the mind also brings the psychoanalytic model of the mind into contact with aspects of neuroscience (Casey et al. 2011; Ochsner and Gross 2005; Ochsner et al. 2002). The National Institute of Mental Health, which aims to arrive at a new way of classifying psychopathology based on dimensions of observable behavior and neurobiological measures, has introduced Research Domain Criteria that include the domain "Cognitive Systems," which in the psychoanalytic model of the mind are defined as ego functions (Cuthbert and Insel 2013).[1]

During a period in the development of the psychoanalytic model of the mind in the 1950s and 1960s, proponents of Ego Psychology, including Hartmann and others, went so far as to argue that psychoanalysis was on its way to becoming a "general psychology" (Hartmann 1964). These ego psychologists understood that a complete psychology should include many things, including findings from the clinical situation, experimental psychology, developmental psychology, cognitive neuroscience, and the social sciences. They argued that the Structural Model of the mind, especially the concept of the ego with its autonomous functions, brought psychoanalysis closer to developing such a general psychology, or a complete understanding of the mind. For those readers interested in history, this view of psychoanalysis coincides with a period of relative hegemony of psychoanalysis in American psychiatry. How-

---

[1]See nimh.nih.gov/research-priorities/rdoc/index.shtml (accessed January 12, 2014).

ever, this broad, expansive view of the possibilities of the psychoanalytic model of the mind has fallen out of favor. Most contemporary psychoanalysts (the author included) feel that psychology is a composite field that includes many kinds of knowledge, from experimental psychology, developmental psychology, cognitive psychology, linguistics, artificial intelligence, philosophy of mind, neuroscience, and others. This book seeks not to delineate a complete theory of mind, but rather to delineate the special contributions of the psychoanalytic model of the mind to a theory of mind. It also seeks to outline a psychoanalytic model of the mind that is consistent with information from neighboring disciplines, especially from the cognitive neurosciences. At the same time, as we saw in Part I, the rest of general psychology is slowly but surely inching its way toward the psychoanalytic model of the mind, in a quiet process that continues to this day. In the next chapter we will discuss the other components of the Structural Model of the mind: the id and the superego, emphasizing how in these structures, also, we can find links to neighboring disciplines.

Chapter Summary and Chart of Core Dimensions

Table 8–1 introduces our Structural Model chart of core dimensions, in which we have placed the following key concepts:

- **Topographic point of view:** The ego and superego have both conscious/preconscious and unconscious aspects. The id is defined as entirely unconscious.
- **Motivational point of view:** The ego seeks both *homeostasis* (self-regulation) and *adaptation*. The id is the seat of our basic pleasure-seeking motives, called *drives*. The superego is concerned with *moral imperatives*. These motivations are always in conflict; as a result, compromise among them must be forged.
- **Structural point of view:** The mind is divided into three structures: ego, id, and superego. The ego has capacities—termed *ego functions*—that include faculties previously attributed to primary process in the Topographic Model, such as censorship and defense, as well as characteristics associated with secondary process, such as cognition,

perception, memory, evaluation (encompassing reality testing), affect and impulse tolerance, and the ability to form mental representations. The ego also has capacities for *internalization* (an organism's tendency to take in aspects of the external world), *identification* (modification of the self-image that results from internalizing the traits of others), and the formation of *ego identity* (the consolidation of a stable sense of oneself as a unique individual in society).

- **Developmental point of view:** The ego develops throughout the life cycle, especially during childhood. In Erikson's eight-stage theory of human development, each stage represents a specific psychological capacity that must be acquired for the ego to develop successfully: *trust/mistrust, autonomy/shame and doubt, initiative/guilt, industry/inferiority, identity/role confusion* (or *diffusion*), *intimacy/isolation, generativity/stagnation,* and *ego integrity/despair.*

- **Theory of psychopathology:** In the Structural Model, mental health is assessed in terms of ego strength, and psychopathology in terms of ego weakness.

- **Theory of therapeutic action:** Exploration of the strategies by which the ego maintains homeostasis and adaptation in the face of conflict is part of every psychodynamic psychotherapy—hence the phrase "Where id was, there ego shall be."

TABLE 8–1. Structural Model Part 1: A New Configuration and a New Concept: The Ego

Topography	Motivation	Structure/Process	Development	Psychopathology	Treatment
The ego and the superego have both conscious/preconscious and unconscious aspects	The ego, superego, and id each have separate aims: The ego—homeostasis and adaptation	The mind is divided into three structures: ego, superego, and id	Ego development Erikson's stages	Ego strength/ego weakness serves as an index of mental health/illness	Strengthening the ego "Where id was, there ego shall be"
	The superego—moral imperatives	The ego Ego functions Defense Internalization Identification Ego identity			
The id is entirely unconscious	The id—drives				
	Conflict is always present because of competing aims				

References

Arlow J, Brenner C: Psychoanalytic Concepts and the Structural Theory. New York, International Universities Press, 1964

Auchincloss EL, Samberg E: Psychoanalytic Terms and Concepts. New Haven, CT, Yale University Press, 2012

Casey BJ, Somerville LH, Gotlib IH, et al: Behavioral and neural correlates of delay of gratification 40 years later. Proc Natl Acad Sci U S A 108:14998–15003, 2011

Cuthbert BN, Insel TR: Toward precision medicine in psychiatry: the NIMH research domain criteria project, in The Neurobiology of Mental Illness, 4th Edition. Edited by Charney DS, Sklar P, Buxbaum JD, et al. New York, Oxford University Press, 2013, pp 1076–1088

Erikson E: Childhood and Society. New York, WW Norton, 1950

Erikson E: The problem of ego identity. J Am Psychoanal Assoc 4:56–121, 1956

Erikson E: Identity and the Life Cycle: Selected Papers. New York, International Universities Press, 1959

Freud A: The ego and the mechanisms of defense (1936), in The Writings of Anna Freud. Vol 2. New York, International Universities Press, 1974, pp 3–176

Freud A: Normality and pathology in childhood: assessments of development (1965), in The Writings of Anna Freud, Vol 6. New York, International Universities Press, 1975, pp 3–230

Freud S: The psychopathology of everyday life (1901), in The Standard Edition of the Complete Psychological Works of Sigmund Freud, Vol 6. Translated and edited by Strachey J. London, Hogarth Press, 1962, pp vii–296

Freud S: Fragment of an analysis of a case of hysteria (1905), in The Standard Edition of the Complete Psychological Works of Sigmund Freud, Vol 7. Translated and edited by Strachey J. London, Hogarth Press, 1962, pp 1–122

Freud S: Introductory lectures on psycho-analysis (1916–1917), in The Standard Edition of the Complete Psychological Works of Sigmund Freud, Vol 16. Translated and edited by Strachey J. London, Hogarth Press, 1962, pp 241–463

Freud S: The ego and the id (1923), in The Standard Edition of the Complete Psychological Works of Sigmund Freud, Vol 19. Translated and edited by Strachey J. London, Hogarth Press, 1962, pp 1–66

Freud S: New introductory lectures on psycho-analysis (1933), in The Standard Edition of the Complete Psychological Works of Sigmund Freud, Vol 22. Translated and edited by Strachey J. London, Hogarth Press, 1962, pp 1–182

Gilmore KJ, Meersand P: Normal Child and Adolescent Development: A Psychodynamic Primer. Arlington, VA, American Psychiatric Publishing, 2013

Hartmann H: Ego Psychology and the Problem of Adaptation (1939). New York, International Universities Press, 1958

Hartmann H: Essays on Ego Psychology. New York, International Universities Press, 1964

Kagan J: Stress and coping in early development, in Stress, Coping, and Development in Children. Edited by Garmezy N, Rutter M. New York, McGraw-Hill, 1983, pp 191–216

Mischel W, Shoda Y, Rodriguez ML: Delay of gratification in children. Science 244:933–938, 1989

Ochsner KN, Gross JJ: The cognitive control of emotion. Trends Cogn Sci 9:242–249, 2005

Ochsner KN, Bunge SA, Gross JJ, et al: Rethinking feelings: an fMRI study of the cognitive regulation of emotion. J Cogn Neurosci 14:1215–1229, 2002

Park S, Auchincloss EL: Psychoanalysis in introductory textbooks of psychology: a review. J Am Psychoanal Assoc 54:1361–1380, 2006

Piaget J, Inhelder B: The Psychology of the Child. New York, Basic Books, 1969

Vaillant GE: Adaptation to Life. Boston, MA, Little, Brown, 1977

Vaillant GE: The Wisdom of the Ego. Cambridge, MA, Harvard University Press, 1983

White RW: Motivation reconsidered: the concept of competence. Psychol Rev 66:297–333, 1959

CHAPTER 9

The Id and the Superego

This chapter describes the concepts of id and superego in greater detail. It also explains drive theory, libido theory, and psychosexuality. The advantages and disadvantages of a drive view of motivation are explored. Vocabulary introduced in this chapter includes the following: *aggression, aggressive drive, anal stage, autoerotic, drive, drive theory, ego ideal, erotogenic zone, fixation, genital stage, guilt, infantile sexuality, instinct, latency, libido, libido theory, object seeking, oedipal period, oral stage, phallic stage, preoedipal period, psychic energy, psychosexual stages, psychosexuality, reaction formation, regression, separation anxiety, sexuality, shame, stranger anxiety,* and *sublimation.*

To understand how the Structural Model of the mind helps us to understand normal and pathological mental functioning, we must move on to explore the id and the superego. As noted in Chapter 8 ("A New Configuration and a New Concept: The Ego"), the ego has the job not only of self-regulation/homeostasis and adaptation but also of mediating conflict and forging compromise between the demands of id and superego, in accord with external reality. What are the id and the superego? How do they function, and what do they help us to understand about the mind?

The Id

In the Structural Model of the mind, the id is the part of the mind that contains our basic pleasure-seeking motives. In the Structural Model, the forces of the id are called *drives.* These drives consist of the drive for psychosexual satisfaction and the drive for aggression. Drive theory was the first fully developed theory of motivation in the psychoanalytic model of the mind. In this chapter, we explain what *drive theory* is, along with its well-known corollary *libido theory.* We also explain what the *aggressive drive* is. We explain which aspects of drive theory are important and how this theory has been updated in contemporary psychoanalysis.

The word *id* (like the word *ego*) was coined by James Strachey in his translation of Freud's term *das Es* (literally "the It"[1]). The *id* is the structure of the mind most closely associated with biological needs of the human organism, including sexual and aggressive urges. The id is defined as entirely unconscious. It is made up of inborn needs and acquired passions, both of which can be repressed.

In the Structural Model of the mind, the concept of the id inherits almost all of the properties of the unconscious as described in the Topographic Model of the mind. For example, the id includes the quality of wishfulness, it is often unacceptable to consciousness, and it is kept from awareness by the force of repression. It operates according to the primary process mode of functioning, seeking satisfaction and pleasure without concern for the consequences. Finally, it seeks always to escape repression and to influence thought and behavior. In the service of this escape from repression, the id assumes many disguises. We will explore all of these features in greater detail here and also in Chapter 10, where we discuss how the id contributes to conflict and compromise.

The id is always in close contact with the ego, with which it functions in a tight symbiosis. Each structure is dependent on the other. The id lacks the organizational and rational capacities of the ego, and unlike the ego, it cannot recognize the world outside the mind. Therefore, the id can express itself only through the activities of the ego. The ego lacks the motivational power of the id. Therefore, in order to accomplish anything, the ego must borrow this power from the id. Freud represented the tight relationship between ego and id in his famous metaphor of the rider (ego) and the horse (id). In the functioning of this team, most of the power is provided by the horse, and most of the planning is pro-

---

[1]Here Freud acknowledged his adaptation of the term from the German psychiatrist Georg Groddeck (1923/1949), who employed *das Es* to describe the way that man is "lived by" unknown and uncontrollable forces. Freud also linked this use with Friedrich Nietzsche, who used *das Es* to refer to the component of human nature that is under the control of natural law (Auchincloss and Samberg 2012).

vided by the rider. However, the uneasiness of their relationship is also represented in the metaphor. Imagine what happens when the rider is unable to direct the horse to go where he wants it to go. If the rider fails, the team runs into trouble. In other words, if the ego fails, the person develops psychopathology (Freud 1923/1962). Again, we will explore the contributions of the id (and of the ego and the superego) to psychopathology in both this chapter and Chapter 10.

For several reasons, most contemporary psychoanalytic practitioners do not use the word *id* very much anymore. First of all, the id is defined as consisting of wishful desires alone, without any organization beyond that of the primary process. Therefore, we cannot experience the contents of the id directly; we can only infer its existence from its contribution to compromises forged by the ego. In addition, the id and the drives are associated with the language of *psychic energy* in which these concepts were first described by Freud. This language has been much criticized both within and outside of psychoanalysis (Brenner 1982; Holt 1976; Klein 1976; Rosenblatt and Thickstun 1970; Schafer 1976). In other words, in the Structural Model of the mind, the id is conceived of as a place in the mind made up of purely wishful drive energy. For these reasons, even theorists who use the word *drive* rarely invoke the term *id*. However, work in the neurosciences has provided some support for the concept of a deep level of motivation and reward that seems to correspond to aspects of the concept of id (LeDoux 1996; Olds and Forbes 1981; Panksepp 1998). There are also links between the concept of id and the domain "Positive Valence Systems" of the National Institute of Mental Health Research Domain Criteria.[2] The concept of id (and drive) is also still useful as a way of conceptualizing important aspects of motivation. We will say more about these below.

Freud's Drive Theory

Let us turn now to the concept of *drive,* without which we cannot understand the id. As we have said above, the id consists of the sexual and aggressive drives. A *drive* is defined as a psychological representation of a motivational force that emerges from the body as a result of an individual's biological needs. Indeed, we cannot improve on Freud's own definition of *drive* as "a concept on the frontier between the mental and the somatic, as the psychical representative of the stimuli originat-

---

[2]See nimh.nih.gov/research-priorities/rdoc/index.shtml (accessed January 12, 2014).

ing from within the organism and reaching the mind, as a measure of the demand made upon the mind for work in consequence of its connection with the body" (Freud 1915/1962, p. 122). A drive exerts a constant pressure on the psychological system, continuously stimulating mental activity. It serves as the motivating force behind all human psychological experience and activity (Auchincloss and Samberg 2012, pp. 65–67). The term *instinct,* with which *drive* is often confused, is defined in general biology as a species-specific, inherited pattern of behavior that does not have to be learned, rather than as an inborn motivational force (Lorenz 1937, 1949/1979; Tinbergen 1951).

Where does the concept of *drive* come from? At first, in the Topographic Model of the mind, the psyche is forced into action by wishes, many of which are unacceptable to the censor. In the Structural Model, these same wishes are unacceptable to the ego. In 1905, in his book *Three Essays on the Theory of Sexuality,* Freud (1905/1962) organized his observations about wishes into his new and more elaborate *drive theory.* Drive theory includes discussion of the role of drive in development, in normal functioning, and in psychopathology. Because Freud formulated drive theory in 1905, when the Topographic Model of the mind was still new and the Structural Model of the mind had not yet been developed, the concept of drive spans both models and is important to both. Originally, in the Topographic Model of the mind, Freud conceptualized only one drive, which he called *libido.* Later, with the introduction of the Structural Model, he added a second drive, *aggression* (Freud 1920/1962). As we will see, the concept of drive was modified in later versions of the psychoanalytic model of the mind. For example, we will see some of these modifications when we study Object Relations Theory in Chapter 11. The concept of drive is not used at all in Self Psychology (discussed in Chapter 12). Certainly the concept of *motivation* has moved beyond sexuality and aggression as the only two forces active in the human mind. Nevertheless, an aim of this book is to show how the concept of drive continues to be useful, even if our view of motivation has expanded.

The Sexual Drive

Libido and Psychosexuality. *Libido* is the name that Freud gave to the drive for sexual pleasure. The word *libido* is derived from the Latin for "wish" or "desire." Sometimes Freud used the word *libido* in much the same way we do today, to mean sexual desire or sexual appetite. However, the term also has a more specific use in the psychoanalytic model of the mind, where it is synonymous with the drive for sexual satisfaction. Ideas about the origins, transformations, and effects of libido have been collectively referred to as *libido theory*. When we discuss libido theory, it might be helpful to refer to Appendix A. Almost everyone associates Freud with the idea that "Everything we do is because of sex." In other words, by explaining what libido is, we can explain why Freud has the reputation for thinking so much about sex, and, more important, what his ideas actually were.

In order to understand what is meant by libido, we need to understand what Freud meant by *sexuality* (or what he often called *psychosexuality*). In Freud's view, sexuality meant much more than the sexual coupling of adults during intercourse. Freud equated psychosexuality with the human search for sensual bodily pleasure in all its forms. In his view, this search begins immediately at birth and reflects an inborn tendency to seek bodily pleasure. Bodily pleasure is attached to the survival needs of the organism, which vary with each stage of development. For example, in the infant's earliest days, the search for bodily pleasure is centered in the mouth or oral cavity, thus ensuring that the infant will find nourishment; next, the search becomes centered in the anus (and urethra), ensuring that the child will defecate and urinate; and finally the search becomes centered in the genitals, ensuring that the child (or adolescent) will become interested in his or her genitals, ultimately using them to have sexual intercourse and thereby procreate. In other words, throughout development, the search for bodily pleasure takes different forms, depending on what is most important at each stage of life.

We will discuss the oral, anal, and genital stages in greater detail later in this chapter. However, according to libido theory, the quest for pleasure at every stage is always fueled by the same drive, called *libido*. In other words, when Freud talked about sexuality, he meant a great deal more than just adults engaging in sexual liaisons. We are correct when we say that Freud asserted that everything we do is caused by our interest in sex. However, we are not correct when we say that Freud asserted that everything we do is the result of our interest in sexual intercourse. In Freud's view, sexual intercourse is merely one manifestation of the workings of libido and is far too narrow a term to capture all that is meant by the concept of psychosexuality. As we will see, in this early period Freud did use the concept of libido to explain just about everything, from adult sexual behavior, to neurosis and character, to culture. Indeed, libido theory is Freud's early "theory of everything," which has led to most people's associating Freud with sex (Freud 1915/1962) (see Appendix A, "Libido Theory").

Psychosexual Phases of Development.   Let us go on to explain more about how libido develops. According to libido theory, libido has its source in any one of a number of *erotogenic zones,* which develop according to a predetermined maturational sequence. These erotogenic zones are the *oral zone,* the *anal zone,* the *phallic zone,* and the *genital zone.* In response to the continuous demand for pleasure created in each of these zones, the mind creates wishes, fantasizes about how these wishes will be satisfied, and ultimately plans for how satisfactions will be achieved. These plans are called *libidinal aims.* Libidinal aims reflect the influence of each zone on a series of psychosexual phases—also named oral, anal, phallic, and oedipal/genital—that each child must transverse. By the way, when Freud delineated a stage/zone that he called *phallic,* he named it that way because he believed that both sexes conceived of only one type of (male) genitalia; in response to revisions in theory, this phase was renamed the *early genital phase.* (For further discussion of the problems in Freud's views of female development, see Chapter 7, "The Oedipus Complex".) Libidinal aims may be directed toward the child's own body (*autoerotic*) or toward another person (*object seeking*). Because stimulation of the erotogenic zones by parents or other caretakers occurs in the course of normal childhood, caretakers always become the first *libidinal objects* of the child's libidinal aims.

The first evidence of the libido at work is the infant's obvious pleasure and satisfaction while sucking either his mother's breast or his own thumb (in what is known as the oral phase). Pleasurable pursuit of anal and genital satisfactions is also easily observed in the activities of young children, who often play games with their own feces (during the anal phase) and who love to show off their genitals (during the early genital [phallic] phase). The early genital/phallic phase is followed by the genital/oedipal phase, which (as we have seen in Chapter 7) reflects the child's erotic/romantic interest in his or her caretakers. Indeed, as we can see, the oedipus complex has the distinction of being the first scenario about infantile sexuality to be invented by Freud, but it is not the first in terms of the development of the child. The oral, anal, and early genital (phallic) phases are often referred to collectively as the *preoedipal* stage of development. The preoedipal and oedipal stages of development are often referred to collectively as *infantile sexuality.* The oedipal period is followed by the stage of *latency,* a period of relative quiescence during which the force of repression holds the sexual drive in check until the hormonal changes of adolescence bring it to the fore again. The many aspects or components of libido finally come together in the service of reproduction at a relatively late stage of development, adolescence and/or adulthood.

Although originally attached to the survival needs of the species, libidinal aims quickly become independent of these needs. Through complex transformations, they become a powerful source of motivation in their own right, serving as a constant source of stimulation to which the mind must respond. In other words, as with the oedipus complex (see Chapter 7), libidinal aims from all stages of development do not go away, but continue to act in the mind of the adult, influencing later psychological experience and activity. First of all, we detect clear evidence of the influence of libidinal aims from the oral, anal, and early genital (phallic) zones during adult sexual activity and foreplay. If infantile sexuality is totally repressed, we see sexual inhibition (see Appendix A). However, most often we see the influence of early psychosexual stages in more disguised forms. Indeed, among the most intriguing aspect of libido theory is that it alerts us to the existence of sexual pleasure hidden in behavior that is apparently nonsexual. Many neurotic symptoms represent forbidden sexual fantasies in a disguised form. For example, hysterical difficulties swallowing or eating may reflect fellatio fantasies; obsessional rituals involving touching may reflect conflicts over masturbation (see Appendix A, "Libido Theory").

Infantile sexuality is transformed not just into neurotic symptoms but also into character traits through the processes of sublimation and reaction formation, new defenses that Freud described for the first time in relation to the development of character (Freud 1908/1962). In *sublimation*, a forbidden wish is deflected from its original aim to one with a higher social value. For example, a "voracious reader" may satisfy an oral wish to devour food through a love of reading. In *reaction formation*, a forbidden wish is transformed into its opposite. For example, the anal pleasure that accompanies playing with feces may be transformed into character traits such as fastidious cleanliness and compulsive orderliness. If a person evinces symptoms or character traits that reflect the overwhelming influence of a particular stage, he or she is often said to have a *fixation* on that stage. Fixation may be caused by either overstimulation or deprivation during a particular stage. If a person substitutes pleasures from an earlier stage for those at a later stage that are either frightening or forbidden, he or she is said to be showing evidence of *regression*. For example, a woman who always picks a fight with her husband on Friday night because "he isn't helping her clean the bathroom" may be *regressing* to a preoccupation with anal concerns in order to avoid the possibility of a sexual encounter at the genital/oedipal level. We find here the basis for Karl Abraham's (1877–1925) oral, anal, early genital/phallic, and genital character types to which we still refer today (Abraham 1921/1948, 1924/1948, 1925/1948). We often describe people with *oral character* as those who appear fixated on finding satisfaction or pleasure in being cared for or fed, or in eating and/or drinking too much. We describe people with *anal character* in much the same way as Freud did, as characterized by "parsimony, orderliness, and obstinacy" (Freud 1908/1962). Finally, we often encounter people who seem to have an excessive interest in exaggerated displays of genital prowess without being much interested in relationships; we are likely to refer to these people with the later term *phallic narcissistic character* (Reich 1933/1945). In Chapter 10 ("Conflict and Compromise"), we will explore the concept of character in greater depth, discussing how Ego Psychology improved upon this early theory. Later, in Chapters 11 and 12, we will see how the concept of character is improved upon even more by the advances of Object Relations Theory and Self Psychology. Later in this chapter we will see how Freud goes on with libido theory to explain aspects of culture itself (again, see Appendix A, "Libido Theory").

The Aggressive Drive

Whereas Freud originally attempted to describe aggressive thoughts and actions as expressions of the libidinal drive, eventually he modified this theory of motivation by adding a separate aggressive drive (Freud 1920/1962). Freud was moved to make this change by his clinical observations of patients in whom aggressive motives appeared to predominate, as well as by his observations of the fighting that engulfed Europe during World War I. By the time that Freud introduced the Structural Model, he argued that the aggressive drive is of equal importance to libido as a motivational force in human psychology. Although theorists disagree about the extent to which the aggressive drive is innate (as opposed to being a response to frustration), all agree that aggression is a ubiquitous force in mental life.

Aggression can be expressed in many forms, both normal and pathological. These expressions vary in intensity, ranging from self-assertion and mastery through irritation, anger, and resentment and on to extreme fury, overt sadism, combat, and murderous rage. As with libido, aggressive "aims" can be expressed in oral, anal, or genital/phallic form. As with libido, aggressive objects are most often caretakers from the child's early life. For example, during the oral phase, aggression may be expressed as biting and/or spitting; during the anal phase, aggression may be expressed in power struggles over control; during the early genital/phallic phase, aggression may be expressed as wishes to dominate others with displays of genital prowess. We find remnants of preoedipal aggression in our language: aggression is often described in such phrases as "biting sarcasm," treating someone "like shit," "pissing" on someone, or "fucking [someone] over." Many developmental psychologists have explored how aggression is expressed during childhood (Parens 1979). Many have also explored the factors contributing to the intensity of aggression, including early experiences of intense pain, deprivation, loss, abuse, enforced passivity, overstimulation, and/or sexual abuse (Furst 1998).

Like libido, aggression is subject to repression and is often expressed in disguised form. Examples of common disguises are jokes or seemingly harmless pranks. Another example is *passive aggressive behavior,* which often includes procrastination that interferes with the aims of other people. Aggression can be *turned against the self,* as in self-hatred (see Appendix B, "Defenses"). Extreme forms of self-hatred may appear as self-mutilation or suicide. Like libido, aggression also makes a contribution to character style. For example, aggression can be sublimated in the form of initiative and ambition and/or intense demands for morality and justice. It can be observed in activities such as some kinds of organized sports, military service, police work, and of course medical practice. In an example from psychopathology, the paranoid personality is organized around the projection onto others of one's own aggression. Finally, aggression plays a prominent role in many kinds of severe psychopathology, such as borderline personality disorder, perversions, and violence (Auchincloss and Samberg 2012, pp. 11–13).

Contribution of the Drives (the Id) to Theory of Psychopathology and Therapeutic Action in the Structural Model

Understanding every individual's relationship to the search for bodily pleasure and/or the expression of aggression plays an important role in psychodynamic psychotherapy. As id demands make a contribution to every kind of psychopathology, all psychodynamic psychotherapy must include an exploration of how each patient experiences and manages his or her most primitive urges. The fantasies through which urges are expressed should be explored, as should any points of fixation and/ or regression. Fantasies about sexual and aggressive urges are often a source of resistance, or not knowing about oneself. In addition, the patient often turns to the therapist in his or her quest to express these urges. In other words, exploration of transference wishes for the gratification of libidinal wishes or for the expression of aggressive impulses constitutes an important part of every psychodynamic psychotherapy. In Chapter 10, when we explore the concepts of conflict and compromise, we will learn more about the contributions of libido and aggression to both normal mental life and psychopathology, as well as how these forces are expressed in the clinical situation.

Role of the Drives in Human Motivation

There are many problems with the drive theory of motivation as expressed in the Structural Model. The most obvious problem is that we no longer think of human beings as struggling with only two motivational forces—sexuality and aggression. Indeed, explaining all of human activity as representing the vicissitudes of these two urges is difficult. In Part IV, we will consider additional motives, such as needs for attachment, separation, and all varieties of self-enhancement. We will see how these motives are described in Object Relations Theory and Self Psychology in Chapters 11 and 12. In addition, contemporary psychodynamic theorists know that even with this greater complexity in our understanding of motivation, a compete theory of motivation requires a broad interdisciplinary dialogue among all kinds of psychologists, neuroscientists, evolutionary biologists, as well as social and political scientists.

Nevertheless, despite the limitations of this conceptualization, there is much to be gained from the idea of motivation conceptualized as a drive. This conceptualization allows us to talk about three important observations that clinicians have made about human motivation: 1) human beings appear to be under continuous pressure from certain kinds of desire; 2) human beings express desire in many forms, which can often be substituted for each other; and 3) human beings have desires that seem to derive from the body. Let us talk about these three observations one by one.

First, the concept of drive captures what appears to be a continuous and demanding force in the human mind to achieve its aims. In other words, human motivation does not appear to be a sporadic or intermittent force; instead, it seems to be ongoing. In addition, human motivation often seems imperative, demanding satisfaction at every turn. The drive concept captures this aspect of human desire, stressing the ongoing peremptory nature of the pressure for mental activity created by some motivational forces. Efforts to meet this demand can be seen in character traits and life patterns that are enduring, repetitive, and stable. Indeed, the ongoing quest for pleasure underlies some of the most basic aspects of personality, such as a sense of "aliveness," vivacity, or enjoyment and appreciation of the "spice of life." Too much dampening of this quest can lead to inertia, inhibition, or feelings of "deadness." The ongoing wish to express aggression underlies such basic aspects of personality as initiative, assertiveness, and activity. Again, too much dampening of this wish can lead to excessive meekness or passivity. (In Chapter 10, we will see an example of how this passivity might be expressed in a man who suffers from a marked inhibition of aggression.)

Second, the concept of drive captures the fact that human strivings appear in many forms and can be substituted for one another. Indeed, Freud's expansion of the concept of sexuality beyond sexual intercourse in adults was one of his most revolutionary contributions to the understanding of human psychology. By postulating that a single drive—libido—lies behind such disparate phenomena as sucking, defecating, and genital interest, Freud asserted that pleasure-seeking behaviors in children are on a continuum. Pleasure-seeking behaviors in children are also on a continuum with pleasure-seeking behaviors in adults, including sexual activity such as foreplay, sexual intercourse, and atypical sexual activities (which are often called "perversions"). When we assert that these diverse behaviors result from a single motivational force, it follows that they can be substituted for one another. Such substitutions take place when one form of pleasure seeking (or aggression) is deemed to be unacceptable. Pleasure seeking and aggression may also disguise themselves in the form of apparently nonsexual or nonaggressive behavior, including symptoms (in neurotic people) and character traits (in all people). Finally, pleasure seeking and aggression can disguise themselves in the form of culturally acceptable activities such as art, science, or religion. In other words, widely diverse phenomena such as sexuality and aggression in children, sexuality and aggression in adults, perverse sexuality, neurotic symptoms, character traits, and cultural activities, which appear to be dissimilar, are all related to each other, in that each represents a disguised form of libido or aggression, or more usually, a combination of the two. The fact that Freud pointed to the similarities among these widely disparate phenomena is responsible for the fact that his ideas are considered so revolutionary. This fact is also responsible for much of why Freud's ideas have been so controversial. People still have trouble accepting that children have sexual wishes, that the division between "normal" and "perverse" sexuality is arbitrary, and that character traits and cultural activities might have sexual and/or aggressive origins (see Appendix A, "Libido Theory").

Finally, the concept of drive allows us to talk about aspects of the important connection between the mind and the body. Indeed, as noted in Chapter 1 ("Overview: Modeling the Life of the Mind"), a feature of the psychoanalytic model of the mind important to the rest of mind science is its emphasis on *embodiment*. The concept of embodiment includes the idea that the mind is intrinsically shaped by its connection to the body, or that the body is an essential determinant of the nature of mind. The drive theory of motivation asserts that all motivational forces in the mind derive from bodily needs. In other words, the id emerges from and is shaped by the experience of the body, as in the experience of the erotogenic zones. Indeed, the Structural Model asserts that the ego also is shaped by its contact with the body. For example, as we have already seen in our description of bodily expressions of aggression, metaphor is a powerful way that we organize thought and language; in metaphor, the body literally provides us with "food for thought" (Lakoff and Johnson 1980, 1999; Melnick 1997). Finally, as we will see in our next discussion, even the superego is shaped by its relationship to the body.

The Superego

In the Structural Model of the mind, the superego is the part of the mind that is commonly known as the conscience. In stark contrast to the id, which represents the pleasure-seeking aspect of mental life, the superego represents those aspects of mental life that are concerned with morality. The superego consists of a set of values and ideals by which we measure ourselves, called the *ego ideal*. It also includes a set of prohibitions and commands that guide our behavior. For the most part, the superego operates unconsciously, although many of its derivatives can be observed easily with simple introspection. Indeed, almost all of us are aware of a large part of our experience that deals with our ideas and feelings about right and wrong.

When we measure up to the ideals held by our superego, we have a sense of well-being and self-esteem. In other words, we feel good about ourselves. When we fail to meet our ideals or violate a superego prohibition, we feel a painful sense of inferiority, *shame* (the feeling that "I am judged to be bad by other people"), or *guilt* (the feeling that "I judge myself to be bad") (Lansky 1994). The superego also prescribes punishment for bad thoughts or behaviors. Some of these punishments are overt, as in acts of appeasement or reparation. Many are disguised, participating in the formation of symptoms, character traits, and other activities. Feelings of shame, guilt, and self-punishing behavior are a unique aspect of self-regulation. Indeed, Freud argued often that the superego is the aspect of psychic functioning that most clearly differentiates human beings from other animals (Auchincloss and Samberg 2012, pp. 252–255; Freud 1900/1962).

The concept of morality played an important role in the Topographic Model, long before the Structural Model (and the concept of the superego) was invented. In this earlier model of the mind, we see morality at work in the fact that unconscious wishes are often judged to be "unacceptable" by the censor. However, in the Topographic Model, morality was only vaguely defined, as roughly equivalent to the injunctions imposed by society, transmitted from generation to generation by parental authority. In the Structural Model, this vague description gives way to a more sophisticated view of morality. Superego development is understood to be a complex process involving several aspects of experience, including the internalization of parental ideals, demands, and threats; the structuring of the child's primitive fantasies about these parental ideals, demands, and threats; and the harnessing of the child's own aggressive wishes, all in the service of policing the self.

Originally, the superego was thought to emerge at the end of the oedipal stage and to represent an admixture of the child's internalization of parental prohibitions and the child's own aggression toward the rival parent. As Freud said, the superego is "the heir to the Oedipus complex" (Freud 1923/1962, p. 48) (see Chapter 7). However, it is more common for contemporary psychodynamic practitioners to see the oedipal stage not as marking the first appearance of the superego, but rather as marking an important consolidation of many earlier experiences and feelings, both positive and negative, that play a role in the development of thinking about morality. Contemporary psychodynamic theory draws from the observations of developmental psychologists, who trace superego development back to infant–caregiver affective communications beginning immediately at birth. Children between 18 and 36 months of age have already internalized some superego functions, as demonstrated by empathy for others, affective reactions to wrongdoing, prosocial behaviors and attitudes, and the capacity to struggle with moral dilemmas (Blum and Blum 1990; Decety and Ickes 2009; Emde and Buchsbaum 1990; Gilmore and Meersand 2013). Other theorists stress the development and change of the superego throughout the rest of the life cycle (Blos 1979; Bornstein 1951, 1953; A. Freud 1936/1974; Gilmore and Meersand 2013; Sarnoff 1976). In any case, because the superego so obviously results, in part, from the internalization of the relationship with caregivers, it points the way to the next model of the mind, Object Relations Theory (described in Chapter 11), in which the process of internalization of relationships plays a central role in the establishment of all psychological structures.

The Superego and the Mind of the Child

Because the superego develops during childhood, it bears the imprint of the child's immature mind. For example, because it develops in the course of our interactions with our parents, the superego never completely loses its personal quality. We tend to experience our conscience as an inner "voice" or "eye" that monitors and judges our behavior. We also tend to experience our conscience as omnipresent and omniscient, like we do our parents. Indeed, we often treat our conscience as we would a parent whom we can make deals with, hide from, or seduce. The superego also includes archaic irrational elements that correspond to the fantasy life of the child. For example, our ideals often lie far beyond what is realistic for us to achieve. This fact reflects both our nostalgia for feelings of omnipotence from infancy and our wish to hang onto an idealized view of our parents from childhood.

Fears of judgment and punishment are also archaic and irrational. They include fears of castration, mutilation, or abandonment, which correspond to the greatest fears of children. Usually these threats are considerably more savage than the behavior of the average parent, a fact that reflects the input into the superego of the child's own untamed aggressive fantasies (Freud 1923/1962). The superego judges thoughts and actions as though they are the same, reflecting the fact that young children cannot easily distinguish between thoughts and deeds. Indeed, this is a major reason why Freud felt that human beings are usually "discontent" (Freud 1930/1962). Superego imperatives are often contradictory, and are therefore impossible to meet. For example, as a lingering effect of the oedipus complex, many men struggle with conflicting demands, both emanating from the superego: the demand to live up to the image of the father as a successful male, and, at the same time, the threatening injunction that being too much like the father will lead to punishment. In other words, the superego has qualities that make it difficult to feel 100% good about oneself, no matter what one does!

Because we recognize these archaic and primitive aspects of the superego, we often speak about the conscience as if it were an animal, or in metaphors that refer to animals. Think of the book *Pinocchio*, with the puppet's conscience incarnated as "Jiminy Cricket!" Thus, a person might complain that his conscience is "buzzing like a mosquito" in the back of his mind, or she may experience her conscience as "gnawing" or "nipping" at her. We remember that Freud depicted the id as a horse in the famous metaphor of the horse and rider by which he represented the relationship between id and ego, and we are not surprised to find him representing the id as our "animal nature." We may be more surprised to realize that we also represent the superego as an animal. The fact that we often compare both the id and the superego to an animal makes us understand more clearly what Freud meant when he argued that id and superego are closely related to each other (Freud 1923/1962). He meant that they share primitive origins in childhood and that the superego is fueled by aggression from the id. Indeed, Freud's argument that we use our own aggression, turned against the self, to police and control ourselves in the form of morality was another one of his most useful contributions to the study of psychology.

Contribution of the Superego to Theory of Psychopathology in the Structural Model

Under normal circumstances, over the course of development, the superego becomes more impersonal, more temperate, and more realistic, resulting in a coherent and manageable set of ideals. These ideals can be met well enough with a reasonable degree of self-monitoring and self-control. Under pathological circumstances, the superego may be poorly structured and weak, resulting in psychopathic and criminal behavior. The superego may also be overly harsh and sadistic, resulting in excessive self-punishment or moralistic rigidity. Self-punishment is easily observed in the form of self-mutilation or suicidal behaviors, inhibition of pleasure, depression, and masochism of all kinds (Brenner 1959). Superego pathology is seen in almost every character style, including several famous "types" described by Freud, such as "Those Wrecked by Success" (people with intense unconscious guilt who punish themselves by stumbling on the threshold of accomplishment), "The Exceptions" (people who feel that because they have had an unfair life and have suffered so much already, they need not adhere to the usual moral standards), and "Criminals Out of a Sense of Guilt" (people with intense unconscious guilt who commit crimes so that they will be caught and punished) (Freud 1916/1962). In Chapter 10, we will explore the concepts of conflict and compromise, learning more about how the superego (and the id) contributes to normal mental life and to psychopathology.

However, again, it is important to notice that most of the examples cited here emphasize the effects of the harsh, punitive aspects of the superego. Indeed, Freud himself was most aware of this negative, punishing side of the conscience, writing rarely about the positive side (Freud 1927/1962). He has often been criticized for failure to theorize much about other, more loving aspects of the superego, which are equally important. Other, more recent theorists, including many from Object Relations Theory, have emphasized the importance of the loving superego (Schafer 1960) or (as we will see in Chapter 11) an internalized good object that makes us feel good about ourselves when we do the right thing, which, arguably, is most of the time. Indeed, when we discuss the impact of Object Relations Theory on our theories of psychopathology and psychodynamic technique, we will learn more about the importance of the ability to maintain a good internal object in the face of negative feelings. When we discuss Self Psychology (in Chapter 12), we will see how the concept of the ego ideal is amplified, as we learn how positive feelings between mother and child lead to the development of goals and ideals that are central to a healthy self.

Contribution of the Superego to Theory of Therapeutic Action in the Structural Model

Psychodynamic psychotherapists spend a lot of time trying to understand the workings of the patient's superego. The superego makes a contribution to almost every thought, feeling, and behavior, big or small, in everyone. Irrational superego demands as well as irrational and contradictory ideals make a contribution to almost every kind of psychopathology. Sometimes, as we have seen, superego pathology dominates the presentation of psychopathology, as in masochism, depression, and many kinds of inhibitions.

Therefore, all psychodynamic psychotherapy must include an exploration of the patient's attitudes toward morality, the patient's ideals, and the circumstances that lead to feeling guilt or shame, or to feeling good about the self. The circumstances leading to self-punishment must also be understood. The complex consequences of shame, guilt, and self-punishment must be explored. Because the superego so obviously develops in the context of relationships with caregivers, it is prone to being externalized onto authority figures, including the therapist. This fact is of particular clinical significance in understanding the transference because the therapist is frequently experienced as the arbiter of right and wrong, or as someone who is likely to disapprove, forgive, and/or otherwise judge the patient. Indeed, one of the most influential early views of the therapeutic action in psychodynamic psychotherapy argues that over time, the patient's superego is modified through internalization of interactions with the therapist, whose attitudes toward the patient's wishes are often less harsh and moralistic (Strachey 1934). When we move on to Chapter 10, we will learn more about how the superego (and the id) is expressed in the clinical situation and how psychodynamic psychotherapy works by helping the patient find better ways to regulate morality in the forging of compromise.

Understanding Moral Development: Contributions From General Psychology and Cognitive Neuroscience

Contemporary psychodynamic practitioners recognize that a complete theory of morality (or of any important aspect of mental life) requires input from many disciplines, including social psychology (Appiah 2008; Blasi 1980; Haidt 2008), anthropology (Gilmore 1991), and developmental psychology (Eisenberg 2000; Emde et al. 1991; Gilligan and Wiggins 1988; Kohlberg 1963, 1976; Turiel 1998; Zahn-Waxler et al. 1992). Indeed, the famous thought experiment called the "trolley problem," introduced by philosopher Philippa Foot, which asked subjects whether, under a variety of circumstances, they would act to save people endangered by a runaway trolley, has spawned a whole generation of "trolleyologists" who are interested in using empirical methods to study how we handle issues of right and wrong (Grimes 2010). For example, in studies related to the concept of the superego, social psychologists have found that individuals who are encouraged to imagine that authority figures are "watching you from the back of your mind" have lower self-esteem (Baldwin et al. 1989); in studies related to the concept of the ego ideal, social psychologists have found that individuals' self-worth is highly contingent and varied (Crocker and Wolfe 2001) and that whether or not people behave according to their ego ideal affects their self-esteem (Higgins 1987). Neuroscientists, too, are interested in the study of morality, offering strong evidence for the biological basis of the sense of right and wrong, or the lack of it, in studies of brain function and genetics (Delgado et al. 2005; Greene et al. 2001; Grigsby and Stevens 2000; Koenigs et al. 2007; Weston and Gabbard 2002). (For an interesting review of evidence from both general psychology and neuroscience on the development and functioning of morality, see Paul Bloom's book *Just Babies: The Origins of Good and Evil* [2013].)

Chapter Summary and Chart of Core Dimensions

Table 9–1 shows our Structural Model chart of core dimensions with the addition of key concepts for Motivation, Structure/Process, and Development.

- **Topographic point of view:** The id is defined as entirely unconscious. The superego has both conscious/preconscious and unconscious aspects.
- **Motivational point of view:** The id is the seat of the *drives—libido* and *aggression*. A *drive* is the mental representation of a bodily need or urge; it exerts a continuous demand on the mind for satisfaction. Drive aims can appear in disguised forms and can be substituted for one another. Superego aims include all motivations concerned with morality.

- **Structural point of view:** The id is the structure of the mind most closely associated with biological needs of the human organism. It operates according to the primary process mode of functioning, seeking satisfaction and pleasure without concern for the consequences. The superego—the part of the mind commonly known as the conscience—consists of prohibitions and commands that guide our behavior; it also contains a set of values and ideals by which we measure ourselves, called the *ego ideal.*
- **Developmental point of view:** Libido develops according to a hard-wired set of psychosexual phases: the oral, anal, and early genital (phallic) phases (comprising the preoedipal period); the genital/oedipal phase (i.e., the oedipal period); the latency phase; and adolescence. The preoedipal and oedipal stages of development are often referred to collectively as *infantile sexuality.* Infantile sexuality can sometimes manifest as symptoms or character traits, especially when transformed by defenses such as sublimation or reaction formation. Both symptoms and character traits can show evidence of *fixation* (the overwhelming influence of a particular stage) or of *regression* (the substitution of pleasures from an earlier stage for those of a later stage). Aggression also undergoes stages of development.

  Whereas the superego was originally considered to emerge at the end of the oedipal stage, contemporary theorists commonly view superego development as beginning considerably earlier, with the oedipal stage marking not the first appearance of the superego, but rather a period of important consolidation of earlier experiences and feelings that play a role in the development of thinking about morality. Other theorists believe that the superego undergoes development and change throughout the life cycle.
- **Theory of psychopathology:** The primitive urges of the id—both the search for bodily pleasure and the expression of aggression—make a contribution to every kind of psychopathology. Under pathological circumstances, the superego may be poorly structured and weak, resulting in psychopathic and criminal behavior, or may be overly harsh and sadistic, resulting in excessive self-punishment or moralistic rigidity.
- **Theory of therapeutic action:** All psychodynamic psychotherapies include exploration of the id (e.g., transference wishes for gratification of libidinal wishes or for expression of aggressive impulses) and the superego (e.g., attitudes toward morality, ideals, and circumstances leading to feeling guilt or shame).

TABLE 9–1. Structural Model Part 2: The Id and the Superego

Topography	Motivation	Structure/Process	Development	Psychopathology	Treatment
The ego and the superego have both conscious/preconscious and unconscious aspects	The ego, superego, and id each have separate aims: The ego—homeostasis and adaptation The superego—moral imperatives	The mind is divided into three structures: ego, superego, and id The ego Ego functions Defense Internalization Identification Ego identity	Ego development Erikson's stages Superego development Development of the drives (Id)	Ego strength/ego weakness serves as an index of mental health/illness	Strengthening the ego "Where id was, there ego shall be"
The id is entirely unconscious	The id—drives Libido Aggression Conflict is always present because of competing aims	The superego Ego ideal The id	Psychosexual phases (oral, anal, early genital [phallic], genital/oedipal, latency, adolescence) Fixation Regression		

References

Abraham K: Contributions to the theory of the anal character (1921), in Selected Papers of Karl Abraham, MD. Edited by Jones E. London, Hogarth Press, 1948, pp 370–392

Abraham K: The influence of oral eroticism on character-formation (1924), in Selected Papers of Karl Abraham, MD. Edited by Jones E. London, Hogarth Press, 1948, pp 393–406

Abraham K: Character-formation on the genital level of the libido (1925), in Selected Papers of Karl Abraham, MD. Edited by Jones E. London, Hogarth Press, 1948, pp 401–417

Appiah KA: Experiments in Ethics: The Flexner Lectures. Cambridge, MA, Harvard University Press, 2008

Auchincloss EL, Samberg E: Psychoanalytic Terms and Concepts. New Haven, CT, Yale University Press, 2012

Baldwin MW, Carrell SE, Lopez DF: Priming relationship schemas: my advisor and the pope are watching me from the back of my mind. J Exp Soc Psychol 26:435–454, 1989

Blasi A: Bridging moral cognition and moral action: a critical review of the literature. Psychological Bulletin 88:1–45, 1980

Bloom P: Just Babies: The Origins of Good and Evil. New York, Crown, 2013

Blos P: The Adolescent Passage. New York, International Universities Press, 1979

Blum E, Blum H: The development of autonomy and superego precursors. Int J Psychoanal 71:585–595, 1990

Bornstein B: On latency. Psychoanal Study Child 6:279–285, 1951

Bornstein B: Masturbation in the latency period. Psychoanal Study Child 8:65–78, 1953

Brenner C: The masochistic character: genesis and treatment. J Am Psychoanal Assoc 7:197–226, 1959

Brenner C: The Mind in Conflict. Madison CT, International Universities Press, 1982

Crocker J, Wolfe CT: Contingencies of self-worth. Psychol Rev 108:593–623, 2001

Decety J, Ickes W (eds): The Social Neuroscience of Empathy. Cambridge, MA, MIT Press, 2009

Delgado MR, Frank RH, Phelps EA: Perceptions of moral character modulate the neural systems of reward during the trust game. Nature Neuroscience 8:1611–1618, 2005

Eisenberg N: Emotion, regulation, and moral development. Annual Review of Psychology 51:665–697, 2000

Emde R, Buchsbaum H: "Didn't you hear my mommy?" Autonomy with connectedness in moral self-emergence, in The Self in Transition: Infancy to Childhood. Edited by Cicchetti D, Beeghly M. Chicago, IL, University of Chicago Press, 1990, pp 35–60

Emde R, Biringen Z, Clyman R, et al: The moral self of infancy: affective core and procedural knowledge. Dev Rev 11:251–270, 1991

Freud A: The ego and the mechanisms of defense (1936), in The Writings of Anna Freud. Vol 2. New York, International Universities Press, 1974, pp 3–176

Freud S: The interpretation of dreams (1900), in The Standard Edition of the Complete Psychological Works of Sigmund Freud, Vol 4/5. Translated and edited by Strachey J. London, Hogarth Press, 1962, pp 1–626

Freud S: Three essays on the theory of sexuality (1905), in The Standard Edition of the Complete Psychological Works of Sigmund Freud, Vol 7. Translated and edited by Strachey J. London, Hogarth Press, 1962, pp 123–246

Freud S: Character and anal erotism (1908), in The Standard Edition of the Complete Psychological Works of Sigmund Freud, Vol 9. Translated and edited by Strachey J. London, Hogarth Press, 1962, pp 167–176

Freud S: Instincts and their vicissitudes (1915), in The Standard Edition of the Complete Psychological Works of Sigmund Freud, Vol 14. Translated and edited by Strachey J. London, Hogarth Press, 1962, pp 109–140

Freud S: Some character-types met with in psycho-analytic work (1916), in The Standard Edition of the Complete Psychological Works of Sigmund Freud, Vol 14. Translated and edited by Strachey J. London, Hogarth Press, 1962, pp 309–333

Freud S: Beyond the pleasure principle (1920), in The Standard Edition of the Complete Psychological Works of Sigmund Freud, Vol 18. Translated and edited by Strachey J. London, Hogarth Press, 1962, pp 1–64

Freud S: The ego and the id (1923), in The Standard Edition of the Complete Psychological Works of Sigmund Freud, Vol 19. Translated and edited by Strachey J. London, Hogarth Press, 1962, pp 1–66

Freud S: Humour (1927), in The Standard Edition of the Complete Psychological Works of Sigmund Freud, Vol 21. Translated and edited by Strachey J. London, Hogarth Press, 1962, pp 159–166

Freud S: Civilization and its discontents (1930), in The Standard Edition of the Complete Psychological Works of Sigmund Freud, Vol 21. Translated and edited by Strachey J. London, Hogarth Press, 1962, pp 57–146

Furst S: A psychoanalytic study of aggression. Psychoanal Study Child 53:159–178, 1998

Gilligan C, Wiggins G: The origins of morality in early childhood relationships, in Mapping the Moral Domain: A Contribution of Women's Thinking to Psychological Theory and Education. Edited by Gilligan C, Ward JV, McLean Taylor J. Cambridge, MA, Harvard University Press, 1988, pp 111–137

Gilmore DD: Manhood in the Making: Cultural Concepts of Masculinity. New Haven, CT, Yale University Press, 1991

Gilmore KJ, Meersand P: Normal Child and Adolescent Development: A Psychodynamic Primer. Arlington, VA, American Psychiatric Publishing, 2013

Greene JD, Sommerville RB, Nystrom LE, et al: An fMRI investigation of emotional engagement in moral judgment. Science 293:2105–2108, 2001

Grigsby J, Stevens D: The Neurodynamics of Personality. New York, Guilford, 2000

Grimes W: Philippa Foot, renowned philosopher, dies at 90. New York Times, October 9, 2010

Groddeck G: The Book of the It (1923). New York, Knopf, 1949

Haidt J: Morality. Perspectives in Psychological Science 3:65–72, 2008

Higgins ET: Self-discrepancy theory: a theory relating self and affect. Psychol Rev 94:319–340, 1987

Holt R: Drive or wish? A reconsideration of the psychoanalytic theory of motivation, in Psychology vs. Metapsychology: Psychoanalytic Essays in Memory of George S. Klein. Edited by Gill M, Holzman P. New York, International Universities Press, 1976, pp 158–197

Klein GS: Psychoanalytic Theory: An Exploration of Essentials. New York: International Universities Press, 1976

Koenigs M, Young L, Adophs R, et al: Damage to the prefrontal cortex increases utilitarian moral judgments. Nature 446:908–917, 2007

Kohlberg L: Moral development and identification. National Society for the Study of Education Yearbook 62(I):277–332, 1963

Kohlberg L: Moral stages and moralization: the cognitive-developmental perspective, in Moral Development and Behavior: Theory, Research, and Social Issues. Edited by Lickona T. New York, Holt, Rinehart, & Winston, 1976, pp 31–55

Lakoff G, Johnson M: Metaphors We Live By. Chicago, IL, University of Chicago Press, 1980

Lakoff G, Johnson M: Philosophy of the Flesh: The Embodied Mind and Its Challenge to Western Thought. New York, Basic Books, 1999

Lansky M: Shame: contemporary psychoanalytic perspectives. J Am Acad Psychoanal 22:433–441, 1994

LeDoux J: The Emotional Brain: The Mysterious Underpinnings of Emotional Life. New York, Simon & Schuster, 1996

Lorenz K: The concept of instinctive action. Folia Biotheoretica 2:17–50, 1937

Lorenz K: King Solomon's Ring (1949). New York, Harper-Collins, 1979

Melnick B: Metaphor and the theory of libidinal development. Int J Psychoanal 78:997–1015, 1997

Olds ME, Forbes JL: The central basis of motivation: intracranial self-stimulation studies. Annu Rev Psychol 32:523–574, 1981

Panksepp J: Affective Neuroscience: The Foundations of Human and Animal Emotions. Oxford, UK, Oxford University Press, 1998

Parens H: The Development of Aggression in Early Childhood. New York, Jason Aronson, 1979

Reich W: Character Analysis (1933). New York, Simon & Schuster, 1945

Rosenblatt A, Thickstun J: A study of the concept of psychic energy. Int J Psychoanal 51:265–278, 1970

Sarnoff C: On Latency. New York, Jason Aronson, 1976

Schafer R: The loving and beloved superego in Freud's structural theory. Psychoanal Study Child 15:163–188, 1960

Schafer R: A New Language for Psychoanalysis. New Haven, CT, Yale University Press, 1976

Strachey J: The nature of the therapeutic action of psycho-analysis. Int J Psychoanal 15:127–159, 1934

Tinbergen N: The Study of Instinct. Oxford, UK, Clarendon Press, 1951

Turiel E: The development of morality, in Handbook of Child Psychology, Vol 3: Social, Emotional, and Personality Development. New York, Wiley, 1998, pp 863–932

Westen D, Gabbard G: Developments in cognitive neuroscience, I: conflict, compromise, and connectionism. J Am Psychoanal Assoc 50:53–98, 2002

Zahn-Waxler C, Radke-Yarrow M, Wagner E, et al: Development of concern for others. Dev Psychol 28:126–136, 1992

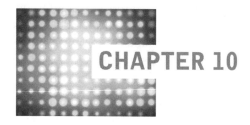

CHAPTER 10

Conflict and Compromise

This chapter introduces readers to the concepts of conflict and compromise. It explores the concept of defense. It also surveys important concepts related to appraisal and defense from neighboring mind sciences. Vocabulary introduced in this chapter includes the following: *affect, character, character disorder, compromise/compromise formation, conflict, danger situations, defense, defense mechanism, defensive style, deficit, ego dystonic, ego syntonic, intersystemic conflict, intrasystemic conflict, mentalization, metacognition, observing ego, reflective function, signal affect/signal anxiety,* and *somatic marker hypothesis.*

In Chapters 8 ("A New Configuration and a New Concept: The Ego") and 9 ("The Id and the Superego"), readers were introduced to the three components of the Structural Model of the mind: the *ego,* the *id,* and the *superego.* We looked at each component from the topographic point of view, learning that each has an unconscious aspect. We saw how these three components differ from each other in terms of motivation and structure. Finally, we also learned a bit about their development. Because the Structural Model was derived from the Topographic Model of the mind, all three components have inherited aspects of the previous model. The id is conceptually close to the unconscious of the Topographic Model. The ego and the superego both include aspects of the conscious/preconscious, especially if we include the censor and the concept of defense.

In this chapter, we explore how id, superego, and ego work together. Although these structures have competing aims, their competition is worked out through compromise forged by the ego. Compromise takes many forms, including symptoms, inhibitions, and a wide variety of character traits, both pathological and adaptive. This chapter examines the concepts of conflict and compromise and what the Structural Model has to say about how psychodynamic psychotherapy works.

The Mind in Conflict

From the beginning, as we have seen, the psychoanalytic model of the mind posits that everyone is struggling with *conflict* over competing thoughts and feelings. In the Topographic Model of the mind, conflict can be detected in the formation of symptoms. Even when there is no apparent psychopathology, conflict can be detected in parapraxes, slips of the tongue, dreams, and/or character traits. However, whereas the Topographic Model describes conflict between the unconscious and the conscious/preconscious mind, the Structural Model of the mind describes conflict between the id and the superego, both operating within the constraints imposed by external reality. In the Structural Model, the ego has responsibility for mediating conflict. In Chapter 8 ("A New Configuration and a New Concept: The Ego"), we defined the ego as the part of the mind responsible for homeostasis and adaptation. Both of these responsibilities are carried out during the process of conflict mediation, which includes both the ability to modulate inner tension (homeostasis) and the ability to assess and deal with external reality (adaptation).

The ego must mediate many different conflicts. There is conflict between the id and the superego (*intersystemic conflict*)—for example, a man may wish to be sexually powerful like his father (id), but this wish may compete with feelings of guilt (superego). There is conflict within the id or within the superego (*intrasystemic conflict*)—for example, a man's wish to replace his father (id) may compete with his wish to love and be loved by his father (id). Or a man's feeling that he should be highly successful at work (superego/ego ideal) may compete with his feeling that he should be perfectly available to his children (superego/ego ideal). Finally, either the id, the superego, or both may be in conflict with the demands of external reality—for example, a man's wish to replace his father (id) may compete with the awareness that his father is the source of knowledge important for success (external reality). Although the Structural Model divides the mind into only three parts, we can see that motivational forces are many, maybe even infinite, and that the convolutions of conflict are complex. To make matters even more difficult, motivational forces are at work in the mind all of the time, and external reality never goes away. Therefore, the mind is in conflict all of the time.

Conflict Mediation and Compromise Formation

In Chapter 8 ("A New Configuration and a New Concept: The Ego"), we delineated many functions available to the ego. In this chapter, we examine how these functions are used in the mediation of conflict. The Structural Model posits the following sequence of events: 1) wishes and moral prohibitions are aroused; 2) the ego appraises the situation, sending information to itself; 3) defenses are mobilized; and 4) compromises are formed. This process goes on continuously and unconsciously.

In the process of conflict mediation described above, we find at least two important ego capacities: appraisal and defense.

Appraisal: Signal Affect/Signal Anxiety

If the ego is to mediate between competing demands, it must be able to appraise the situation, or to understand what is going on. In other words, the ego must be able to figure out what is likely to happen in various scenarios, or the consequences of acting on various motivations. For example, what will happen to the boy/man mentioned above if he expresses his wish to replace his father? On the other hand, what will happen to him if expresses his need to be loved by his father?

The appraisal system of the mind is complicated, and much of general psychology is devoted to understanding how we know what is going on inside ourselves and in the outside world. In the psychodynamic approach, we use terms such as *reality testing* to describe an individual's ability to understand external reality. We use terms such as *psychological mindedness, observing ego, mentalization* (Fonagy et al. 2002), and *reflective function* (Levy et al. 2006) to talk about an individual's ability to understand internal psychological processes. When we use these terms, we are talking about ego functions, or appraisal processes, important in the mediation of conflict. In Chapter 3 ("Evolution of the Dynamic Unconscious"), we mentioned how cognitive psychologists in general psychology are investigating what they call *unconscious scanning operations,* or *metacognition,* appraisal processes by which we can monitor our own minds and thereby choose among priorities (Metcalfe and Shimamura 1994; Roseman and Smith 2001; Scherer 2001; Uleman 2005).

However, the ego uses not just cognitive capacities but also emotional capacities to evaluate and manage situations both inside the mind and between the mind and the outside world. This process makes use of *affects,* or feelings—our basic, inborn ability to experience varieties of pleasure and pain (Auchincloss and Samberg 2012, pp. 8–10). Here's how the affective, or emotional, aspect of the appraisal system works.

During the course of development, the child learns that sometimes the expression of wishes leads to satisfaction and pleasure. For example, much of the time, a hungry child with the wish to suck or eat has the experience of being fed, accompanied by an experience of satisfaction and pleasure. At other times, this same child learns that the expression of wishes leads to pain, in the form of disappointment and suffering. For example, a hungry child with the wish to suck or eat may, for various reasons, be met with frustration and/or pain. Throughout the life cycle, affective experiences of pleasure or pain accompany every wish or aim, in increasingly complex and nuanced forms.

Over time, the child learns to remember the experiences of pleasure or pain that accompany his or her wishes and to use these memories in decisions about how to manage wishes. Beginning in childhood, the ego subjects all wishes to a process of evaluation in which the amount of pleasure that will likely result from pursuit of a wish is compared with the amount of pain that will likely result. In this process of evaluation, the ego uses a *signal affect*—an attenuated version of the experience of an affect (either pleasure or pain) remembered from the past (Auchincloss and Samberg 2012, p. 9). The ego makes use of all kinds of pleasurable affects (e.g., happiness, satisfaction, pride) to signal that pleasure will ensue if a wish is pursued. It makes use of all kinds of negative affects (e.g., anxiety, shame, guilt) to signal that pain will ensue if a wish is pursued. If the ego receives a signal that pleasure will result from the expression of a wish, it gives the wish a green light. If it receives a signal that pain will result, it gives a red light. Because there is almost invariably conflict among competing wishes, the ego will need to find a compromise. This compromise must be made quickly, as from moment to moment, the ego makes split-second decisions about the situation. Furthermore, if we remember that motivations are many and emanate from many parts of the mind, we realize that the process of appraisal is complex. Affects work well as components of the appraisal system because they transmit a lot of information quickly and forcefully. Affects also work well because they are able to mobilize defense.

When he first described this system of appraisal, Freud focused on painful experience in the form of anxiety, suggesting that the ego uses *signal anxiety* to evaluate various outcomes and make decisions. Freud described a universal developmental sequence of *danger situations* that trigger anxiety in all human beings. These danger situations include loss of an important object, loss of an object's love, castration anxiety (the name given to the fear of physical punishment), and ultimately superego disapproval, or the feeling of guilt (Freud 1926/1962). As the psychoanalytic model of the mind developed, others contributed to the list of typical anxieties, adding separation anxiety (Bowlby 1960), stranger anxiety (Spitz 1950), and persecutory and depressive anxiety (Klein 1940; see Chapter 11, "Object Relations Theory"). Freud was arguably somewhat pessimistic, and this may have played a role in his emphasis on anxiety and unpleasure. Indeed, we have seen in our discussion of the superego that Freud rarely emphasized the positive. However, there is research suggesting that we remember negative experience more intensely than we do pleasurable experience, so perhaps Freud's negative emphasis was appropriate (Christianson and Loftus 1987; Kahneman and Tversky 1979; Ochsner 2000). However, whereas Freud emphasized painful affects in the system of appraisal, other theorists have emphasized the positive feelings used by the ego to signal that we are on the right track. For example, the ego uses the good feelings that come from knowing that we are "doing the right thing" or a feeling that we will be "safe" if we pursue our wishes (Sandler 1960; Schafer 1960; Stern 2003). Developmental psychoanalysts have also emphasized the important role of positive feelings such as interest, curiosity, pleasure, and pride in the formation of the appraisal system used by adults (Emde 1983, 1991).

Many have pointed to similarities between the concept of *signal anxiety* from the psychoanalytic model and the concept of *learned expectations* from learning theory in general psychology (Bandura 1977). In addition, there is much evidence from cognitive neuroscience about the importance of different parts of the brain in the formation of the reward systems that determine much of our behavior (Olds and Forbes 1981).[1] There is also much evidence from cognitive neuroscience about the role of brain structures such as the amygdala in creating fear, and the importance of fear signals in determining behavior (Aggleton 1992; Armony

---

[1]See also National Institute of Mental Health Research Domain Criteria, domains "Positive Valence Systems," "Negative Valence Systems," and "Cognitive Systems" (nimh.nih.gov/research-priorities/rdoc/index.shtml; accessed January 12, 2014).

and LeDoux 2000; LeDoux 1996; Phelps 2006; Phelps and LeDoux 2005). For a system of appraisal that uses both positive and negative signal affects, see Damasio's *somatic marker hypothesis,* in which attenuated affective experiences generated by the body play a central role in the regulation of mental life. The somatic marker hypothesis is very similar to the signal affect hypothesis from the Structural Model of the mind. In the somatic marker hypothesis, we also see an important example of how cognitive neuroscience (and psychoanalysis) argues that the mind is embodied in important ways (see Chapter 1, "Overview: Modeling the Life of the Mind") (Damasio 1984).

Defense

In almost every situation, the ego must deal with conflict among competing motivations, with each motivation leading to different imagined consequences, often involving fear of an unpleasant feeling. Here is where defense, one of the most important ideas in the psychoanalytic model of the mind, comes in. The concept of *defense* is not new to us. From the beginning, Freud differed from his predecessors in his approach to patients suffering from hysteria, when he asserted that hysterical symptoms result not from a diseased brain (or a neurodegenerative disorder) but rather from "the motive of defense" (Breuer and Freud 1893/1895/1962, p. 285). As he moved from the study of hysteria to the study of all people, Freud based his new Topographic Model on conflict between regions of the mind separated from each other by repression. The Topographic Model emphasized the defense of repression; indeed, in this model, defense and repression are often interchangeable. In the Structural Model of the mind, we see the concept of *defense* becoming increasingly complex and increasingly central to how the mind works. Let us back up and explain what we mean by defense.

Defense is defined as any unconscious psychological maneuver used to avoid the experience of a painful feeling (Auchincloss and Samberg 2012, pp. 51–52). The mind is capable of an infinite variety of such maneuvers, and any thought, feeling, or behavior can be used in the service of defense. Furthermore, defense can be directed not only against wishes but also against any mental activity that might give rise to unpleasurable feelings, including thoughts, memories, actions, and feelings themselves. Defensive operations are always mixed together. They begin early in childhood and continue to operate throughout the life cycle. Developmental psychologists have tried to describe the chronological development of defenses (Gilmore and Meersand 2013). Everyone uses defenses, and defenses play an important role in both normal functioning and psychopathology (see Appendix B, "Defenses").

Some defenses are fleeting, called into action when a short-lived situation threatens to stir up pain. For example, a defense called *denial* is commonly used by otherwise realistic people who have recently been diagnosed with a fatal illness. Other defenses form long-standing patterns that may be enacted over extended periods of time. For example, in a defense called *identification with the aggressor*, a person adopts the behavior of a former tormenter so as to *turn passive into active* and thereby avoid the pain evoked by feelings of weakness, pain, and helplessness. Another defense that can be enacted over a long period of time is *altruistic surrender*, exemplified by the behavior of a shy teenager who devotes all her energies to furthering the love interest of her best friend, with the aim of avoiding awareness of her own dangerous competitive feelings. Every individual develops patterns of defense that are relatively stable over time.

Although any psychological experience may serve a defensive function, there are many specific and commonly used *defense mechanisms*. Defense mechanisms with which readers may be familiar include *repression, reaction formation, sublimation, conversion, displacement, projection, isolation, undoing, denial/disavowal, splitting, negation,* and *turning against the self,* all described first by Sigmund Freud. Anna Freud added the defenses *introjection, idealization, asceticism, intellectualization, altruistic surrender,* and *identification with the aggressor,* to mention a few (A. Freud 1936/1974). Melanie Klein added *primitive idealization, projective identification,* and *reparation* (Klein 1932, 1945, 1975a, 1975b). Another well-known defense mechanism is called *regression in the service of the ego* (Kris 1950). Definitions and examples of these and other defense mechanisms are provided in Appendix B.

General psychology is converging on psychoanalytic concepts of defense when it posits analogous concepts such as *motivated forgetting, coping mechanisms, biased attribution, defensive nonattending, compensatory mechanisms/processes,* and *safeguarding tendencies* (Bornstein 1996; Park and Auchincloss 2006). Many investigators have applied empirical methods to the study of defense, both within psychoanalysis and in cognitive and social psychology. For example, some investigators have developed research instruments that can objectively and reliably measure the use of specific defenses (Cooper 1992; Perry and Lanni 2008). Other investigators have studied how defenses operate in a variety of contexts (Westen 1999). For example, studies demonstrate that the concept of defense can be applied across cultures (Tori and Bilmes 2002), can differ according to gender (Bullitt and Farber 2002), and can change in treatment (Roy et al. 2009). Cramer (2006) has reviewed what we know about how defenses develop, function, and change, as well as research methods for their assessment. Finally, cognitive psychologists have used empirical methods to study defense (Adams et al. 1996; Anderson et al. 2004; Newman and Stone 1996; Newman et al. 1995; Rotton 1992; Simons and Chabris 1999; Singer 1990; Stein and Young 1997; Weinberger et al. 1979), and neuroscientists have turned their attention to understanding the biological underpinnings of defense (Anderson et al. 2004; Aybek et al. 2014; Moscarello and LeDoux 2013; Northoff et al. 2007).

Conflict and Compromise in Operation: An Example

According to the Structural Model of the mind, every experience, however big or small, represents a compromise between competing demands of id, superego, and external reality. The ego has the task of forging compromise after appraising the situation and mobilizing defenses to make the situation manageable. Having said this, and explained a bit about how the system of conflict mediation and compromise formation works, it is time for an example:

> Dr. A, a 28-year-old unmarried physician, is seeing Dr. B two times a week in psychodynamic psychotherapy. He came to treatment with a chief complaint of intense anxiety that threatens to overwhelm him whenever he becomes romantically interested in a woman. In addition, Dr. A's personality is marked by diffidence bordering on obsequiousness, which is especially pronounced with "authority figures." Although he is highly intelligent and skilled, he is not advancing professionally.
>
> One day, several years into treatment, as Dr. A is walking to his psychotherapy session, he spies Dr. B on the other side of the street approaching her office. Dr. A arrives at the office door just before his therapist. While he is waiting, he suddenly imagines himself hurling insults at Dr. B for being late. In his mind, these insults are accompanied by angry and derisive thoughts. As they meet at the door, Dr. A quickly "forgets" his earlier thoughts of anger and derision. In a markedly subservient manner, he bows slightly to Dr. B and offers to carry her bags. In the process, he drops and breaks his mobile phone.

How does the Structural Model help us to understand this scenario? The ego has the task of mediating the competing demands of the id, the superego, and external reality, forging compromise among them. In other words, Dr. A's behavior must serve to satisfy his wishes, gratify the imperatives of his superego, and meet the demands of external reality. Having instantaneously and unconsciously evaluated his angry thoughts as potentially damaging to his relationship with Dr. B, Dr. A defends against this danger through repression and reaction formation. In addition, he turns his aggression against himself in a submissive gesture of appeasement. In his behavior at the door, we can see Dr. A's fear of his own aggressive thoughts, his defense against them, and his need for self-punishment. The satisfaction of aggressive wishes is also provided by his obsequious behavior. In addition, we can see a glimpse of Dr. A's forbidden wishes for romantic intimacy with Dr. B—wishes that are partially satisfied by the closeness he feels with her in the act of carrying her bags. In fact, when Dr. A later "confesses" to Dr. B, with great anxiety, that he had imagined saying "Fuck you" to her, we see that aggression may itself defend against sexual wishes, as both are expressed in this highly ambiguous phrase. As it turned out, Dr. A was afraid that he would suffer punishment more severe than a broken mobile phone if he were to openly express his sexual and romantic thoughts about Dr. B.

Drs. A and B still had much work to do in exploring Dr. A's feelings and thoughts. They needed to understand them, Dr. A's fears about them, his defenses against them, their interactions, and their origins. However, this brief vignette provides a first glimpse of how conflict leads to compromise. Later in this chapter, when we examine the Structural Model's contribution to our understanding of how psychodynamic psychotherapy works, we will return to the case of Dr. A.

Contribution of Conflict and Compromise to Theory of Psychopathology in the Structural Model

The Structural Model teaches us that all behavior and experience represents compromise, which may take many forms, including some kinds of psychopathology. The Structural Model makes a major contribution to the study of psychopathology, representing an advance over the Topographic Model. In Chapter 8, when we discussed the ego, we learned that, using the Structural Model, we can examine neurotic symptoms for the ego weaknesses that are in evidence. In this chapter, we discover that we can also examine such symptoms for what they reveal about the adaptiveness or maladaptiveness of the compromises forged by the individual. Furthermore, we also see how the Structural Model expands the concept of neurosis to encompass psychopathology without overt symptoms—in other words, psychopathology in the form of *character.*

The Concept of Character

Character is defined as an individual's stable and enduring behaviors, attitudes, cognitive styles, and moods. It also includes the individual's typical modes of self-regulation, adaptation, and relating to others. In contrast to the popular usage of the term, *character* in the psychoanalytic model places no special emphasis on moral values (although traits involving thoughts about right and wrong are an aspect of every individual's character). In short, everyone has a character or a character style (Auchincloss and Samberg 2012, p. 32). Indeed, because Dr. A is submissive not just occasionally but much of the time, we describe him as having a character marked by extreme diffidence even to the point of passivity.

The concept of character is roughly analogous to what psychologists and psychiatrists (especially when using the DSM system) usually call *personality,* the major difference being that character, as a psychoanalytic concept, links external manifestations of an individual's functioning to the psychoanalytic model of the mind (Baudry 1984). When we define the concept of character, we quickly find ourselves using terms that are closely associated with the Structural Model, such as self-regulation, adaptation, and ego. Indeed, most of the best definitions of character define it as representing the ego's stable and preferred solution to conflict among the id, the superego, and external reality (Fenichel 1954; Reich 1933/1945).

In Chapter 9 ("The Id and the Superego") we had a brief look at the first concept of character (developed by Sigmund Freud and Karl Abraham) as reflecting the predominance of one or another of the erotogenic zones—oral, anal, or early genital (phallic). However, when we define character in terms of ego, we are using a much more successful strategy. Indeed, the study of character became something of a growth industry in the Ego Psychology of the 1950s, as psychoanalysts generated many theories about character functioning, classification, and development. Contemporary theories emphasize the many factors leading to character formation, including interactions with caregivers, parental character traits and ideals, family style, culture or society, biological endowment, temperament, cognitive style, mood, and early loss or trauma. However, the concept itself continues to focus on the functioning of the ego.

An individual's stable *defensive style* is an important feature of his or her character. A rigid defensive style contributes to character pathology, with specific defensive maneuvers associated with specific character types. For example, we typically think of hysterical/histrionic character as marked by use of the defenses of *repression* and *somatization*. We think of obsessional character as marked by the use of *reaction formation, isolation, intellectualization,* and *undoing.* We think of paranoid character as marked by the use of *projection* (Shapiro 1965, 1984). In Chapter 11 when we talk about Object Relations Theory, we will see how theorists have linked use of certain defenses with psychopathology, including neurotic, borderline, and psychotic psychopathology (Kernberg 1970; see also Appendix B, "Defenses"). When we reach Chapter 12 on Self Psychology, we will see how the concept of self influences the formation of character (Kohut and Wolf 1978).

Character Disorders

Whereas the term *character* itself implies neither health nor pathology, to the extent that someone's character is inflexible and maladaptive, he or she may be diagnosed with a *character disorder.* Traditionally, pathological character traits are distinguished from symptoms by the fact that they are experienced as part of the self (*ego-syntonic*), whereas symptoms are experienced as alien to the self (*ego-dystonic*).

Character is considered pathological if it involves weaknesses in the areas of reality testing and social judgment, abstract thinking, affect tolerance (Kernberg 1970; Krystal 1975; Zetzel 1949), or impulse control (Kernberg 1970). It is also considered pathological if it involves too much disturbance in the capacity for pleasure. Certain defensive strategies are seen as healthier or more adaptive than others because they come with less "cost" in terms of ego functioning. For example, altruism and humor are considered higher-level defenses because they do not include narrowed reality testing, whereas projection and denial are considered lower-level defenses because they do include distortions in the experience of reality (see Appendix B, "Defenses").

Theories of Ego Weakness: Defense Versus Deficit

There are two major theories that explain ego weakness. The first of these theories describes ego weakness as the result of a maladaptive use of *defense.* For example, an individual who is afraid that the expression of oedipal strivings will lead to retaliation and/or punishment may defend against them by limiting all forms of initiative, developing severe inhibitions in many areas of ego functioning. The second of these theories describes ego weakness as the result of a *deficit* caused either by innate biological factors or by environmental factors such as deprivation. For example, a patient may be low on initiative because he or she has a passive temperament. Another patient may have trouble experiencing pleasure because he or she experienced so many deprivations as a child that he or she simply does not recognize positive feelings. Indeed, clinicians will often argue among themselves about whether a specific ego weakness is caused by defense or by deficit. For example, does a patient feel confused because she creates confusion in her mind as a defense against painful awareness? Or is she confused because her lack of experience means that she simply does not understand what is going on? Is another patient inattentive as a way to defend against painful awareness, or is he inattentive because of some form of attention-deficit disorder?

In Chapter 11, we will see a famous example of the defense/deficit argument in debates over the etiology of borderline psychopathology. We will see another famous example in Chapter 12 when we explore differences in how Kernberg and Kohut conceptualized narcissistic problems. For the most part, however, contemporary psychodynamic practitioners do not take an either/or point of view in the debate over defense versus deficit as the cause of ego weakness, but instead recognize that psychopathology must be understood from multiple perspectives and that combined treatment approaches are often required.

Contribution of Conflict and Compromise to Theory of Therapeutic Action in the Structural Model

Having explored how the Structural Model helps us to understand psychopathology, we can see that this new model also makes an important contribution to the theory of psychoanalytic psychotherapy. The Structural Model adds complexity to our therapeutic goals. In the Topographic Model, successful psychotherapy aimed at increasing self-awareness by making the unconscious conscious, with the goal of increasing our ability to use rational judgment in regard to our wishes. In the Structural Model, successful psychotherapy aims not only at bringing unconscious mental life into awareness but also at increasing ego strength. If we understand this aim better, we can better understand Freud's famous statement, "Where id was, there ego shall be" (Freud 1923/1962, p. 56; Freud 1933/1962, p. 80).

In the course of psychodynamic psychotherapy, the therapist and the patient use the therapeutic setting to explore compromises forged by the ego in the process of mediating conflict. Exploration of the ego's ways of forging compromise is called *defense analysis*. Compromises are expressed not only in the form of symptoms and character traits but also in the patient's way of behaving in the psychotherapeutic situation.

Exploration of the patient's habitual modes of resistance as he or she defends against the emergence of wishes, impulses, feelings, fears, and fantasies within the treatment setting provides important clues as to the ego's habitual modes of defense and conflict resolution in everyday life. Indeed, one of the hallmarks of treatment using the Structural Model is the therapist's greater emphasis on the methods of and reasons for resistance, rather than on simply what is being warded off. Many of the patient's habitual modes of conflict resolution are also expressed in the transference, or in the patient's way of experiencing the therapist. For example, a woman who becomes childlike, helpless, and forgetful in her psychotherapy sessions whenever she is threatened with the emergence of sexual fantasies directed toward her therapist is demonstrating the use of repression and regression typical of the hysterical histrionic character style. As we have seen with Dr. A, a man who becomes overly polite and deferential to his therapist when threatened with the emergence of aggressive or sexual fantasies is showing the reaction formation and isolation of affect typical of the obsessive character style.

Many of these habitual modes of defense represent the persistence into adult life of strategies for conflict resolution that were used by the ego during childhood that are no longer adaptive in the adult. In psychodynamic psychotherapy, patient and therapist explore these outdated strategies. In the course of such exploration, the growth of new ego capacities for affect tolerance and reality testing allows the patient to make new attempts at conflict resolution, using defenses that are more adaptive. For example, a chronically self-defeating woman may learn in therapy that she has destroyed her successes out of unconscious guilt for hidden aggressive fantasies toward an overbearing mother and out of fear of retaliation from parental "authority figures." A greater tolerance for feelings of fear, guilt, and anger, as well as a more realistic view of the actual nature of both her imagined "crimes" and the danger she faces, will enable this woman to tolerate greater success in life. Although conflict and defense can never be eliminated, psychotherapy helps the patient find new compromises among competing wishes, fears, and environmental constraints that are less self-punishing, have a higher yield of pleasure, and are better adapted to the realities of present-day life. To illustrate:

> After treatment in psychotherapy, Dr. A learned to accept his hostile feelings toward women and his fears of assertive sexuality. As a result of this greater acceptance, he was able enjoy a mutually satisfying relationship with his new wife. He was also able to find greater success at work. Residual aggression and unconscious sadism were expressed in a successful career as a plastic surgeon whose patients were largely women.

Chapter Summary and Chart of Core Dimensions

Table 10–1 shows our Structural Model chart of core dimensions with the addition of key concepts for Motivation, Structure/Process, Psychopathology, and Treatment.

- **Topographic point of view:** Conflict and compromise are, for the most part, unconscious.
- **Motivational point of view:** All motivations are in conflict. The sources of conflict are many, including the differing aims of the ego, id, and superego. Conflict also includes attempts to avoid *danger situations*—specific scenarios that trigger anxiety in all human beings.
- **Structural point of view:** *Compromise formation* is the result of the ego's mediation of conflict among the id, the superego, and external reality. To forge compromise, the ego uses its many capacities for appraisal and defense. (*Defense* is defined as any unconscious psychological maneuver used to avoid the experience of a painful feeling.) *Appraisal* through use of a *signal affect* (also called *signal anxiety*)—an attenuated version of the experience of an affect (either pleasure or pain) remembered from the past—as an information system is an important part of compromise formation. *Character* has been defined as an individual's stable and enduring behaviors, attitudes, cognitive styles, and moods. Importantly, the concept of character also includes the individual's typical mode of mediating conflict.
- **Developmental point of view:** Like many aspects of the mind, compromise has a developmental history. What may have been adaptive for one phase of life may no longer be adaptive for a later phase. Danger situations also have a developmental history, as does character.
- **Theory of psychopathology:** Certain defensive strategies are seen as healthier or more adaptive than others because they come with less "cost" in terms of ego functioning. *Maladaptive compromise* can lead to symptoms and/or character disorders. There is disagreement regarding whether ego weakness is best conceptualized as resulting from a maladaptive use of *defense* or from a *deficit* due to innate biological or environmental factors. For the most part, however, contemporary psychodynamic practitioners do not take an either/or stance in the debate over *defense versus deficit*, but instead recognize that psychopathology must be understood from multiple perspectives.
- **Theory of therapeutic action:** The exploration of compromise (including the nature of conflict and defense) is an important part of all psychodynamic psychotherapies.

TABLE 10–1.   Structural Model Part 3: Conflict and Compromise

Topography	Motivation	Structure/Process	Development	Psychopathology	Treatment
The ego and the superego have both conscious/preconscious and unconscious aspects	The ego, superego, and id each have separate aims: The ego—homeostasis and adaptation The superego—moral imperatives The id—drives Libido Aggression **Avoidance of danger situations**	The mind is divided into three structures: ego, superego, and id The ego Ego functions Defense Internalization Identification **Signal affect** **Compromise formation** Ego identity **Character**	Ego development Erikson's stages Superego development Development of the drives (Id) Psychosexual phases (oral, anal, early genital [phallic], genital/oedipal, latency, adolescence) Fixation Regression	Ego strength/ego weakness serves as an index of mental health/illness **Maladaptive compromise may lead to character disorders** **Defense versus deficit theories of psychopathology**	Strengthening the ego **Exploring conflict, defense, and compromise** "Where id was, there ego shall be"
The id is entirely unconscious	Conflict is always present because of competing aims	The superego Ego ideal The id			

References

Adams HE, Wright LW, Lohr BA: Is homophobia associated with homosexual arousal? J Abnorm Psychol 105:440–445, 1996

Aggleton E (ed): The Amygdala: Neurobiological Aspects of Emotion, Memory, and Mental Dysfunction. New York, Wiley-Liss, 1992

Anderson MC, Ochsner KN, Kuhl B, et al: Neural systems underlying the suppression of unwanted memories. Science 303:232–235, 2004

Armony JL, LeDoux JE: How danger is encoded: toward a systems, cellular, and computational understanding of cognitive emotive interactions in fear, in The New Cognitive Neurosciences, 2nd Edition. Edited by Gazzaniga MS. Cambridge, MA, MIT Press, 2000, pp 1067–1080

Auchincloss EL, Samberg E: Psychoanalytic Terms and Concepts. New Haven, CT, Yale University Press, 2012

Aybek A, Nicholson TR, Zelaya F, et al: Neural correlates of recall of life events in conversion disorder. JAMA Psychiatry 71:52–60, 2014

Bandura A: Social Learning Theory. Englewood Cliffs, NJ, Prentice Hall, 1977

Baudry F: Character: a concept in search of an identity. J Am Psychoanal Assoc 32:455–477, 1984

Bornstein RF: Psychoanalytic research in the 1990s: reclaiming what is ours. Bulletin of the Psychoanalytic Research Society 5:1–3, 1996

Bowlby J: Separation anxiety. Int J Psychoanal 41:89–113, 1960

Breuer J, Freud S: Studies on hysteria (1893/1895), in The Standard Edition of the Complete Psychological Works of Sigmund Freud, Vol 2. Translated and edited by Strachey J. London, Hogarth Press, 1962, pp 1–335

Bullitt C, Farber B: Gender differences in defensive style. J Am Psychoanal Assoc 30:35–51, 2002

Christianson SA, Loftus EE: Memory for traumatic events. Applied Cognitive Psychology 1:225–239, 1987

Cooper SH: The empirical study of defensive processes: a review, in The Interface of Psychoanalysis and Psychology. Edited by Barron W, Eagle MN, Wolitzky DL. Washington, DC, American Psychological Association, 1992, pp 327–346

Cramer P: Protecting the Self: Defense Mechanisms in Action. New York, Guilford, 2006

Damasio A: Descartes' Error: Emotion, Reason, and the Human Brain. New York, Putnam, 1984

Emde R: The prerepresentational self and its affective core. Psychoanal Study Child 38:165–192, 1983

Emde R: Positive emotions for psychoanalytic theory: surprises from infancy research and new directions. J Am Psychoanal Assoc 39 (suppl):5–44, 1991

Fenichel O: Psychoanalysis of character, in The Collected Papers of Otto Fenichel (2nd series). Edited by Fenichel H, Rapaport D. New York, WW Norton, 1954, pp 198–214

Fonagy P, Gergely G, Jurist E, et al: Affect Regulation, Mentalization, and the Development of the Self. New York, Other Press, 2002

Freud A: The ego and the mechanisms of defense (1936), in The Writings of Anna Freud. Vol 2. New York, International Universities Press, 1974, pp 3–176

Freud S: The ego and the id (1923), in The Standard Edition of the Complete Psychological Works of Sigmund Freud, Vol 19. Translated and edited by Strachey J. London, Hogarth Press, 1962, pp 1–66

Freud S: Inhibitions, symptoms and anxiety (1926), in The Standard Edition of the Complete Psychological Works of Sigmund Freud, Vol 20. Translated and edited by Strachey J. London, Hogarth Press, 1962, pp 75–176

Freud S: New introductory lectures on psycho-analysis (1933), in The Standard Edition of the Complete Psychological Works of Sigmund Freud, Vol 22. Translated and edited by Strachey J. London, Hogarth Press, 1962, pp 1–182

Gilmore KJ, Meersand P: Normal Child and Adolescent Development: A Psychodynamic Primer. Arlington, VA, American Psychiatric Publishing, 2013

Kahneman D, Tversky A: Prospect theory: an analysis of decision under risk. Econometrica 47:263–291, 1979

Kernberg O: A psychoanalytic classification of character pathology. J Am Psychoanal Assoc 18:800–822, 1970

Klein M: The Psycho-Analysis of Children. London, Hogarth Press, 1932

Klein M: Mourning and its relation to manic-depressive states. Int J Psychoanal 21:125–153, 1940

Klein M: The Oedipus complex in the light of early anxieties. Int J Psychoanal 26:11–33, 1945

Klein M: Love, Guilt and Reparation, and Other Works, 1921–1945. London, Hogarth Press, 1975a

Klein M: Envy and Gratitude, and Other Works, 1946–1963. London, Hogarth Press, 1975b

Kohut H, Wolf ES: The disorders of the self and their treatment: an outline. Int J Psychoanal 59:413–426, 1978

Kris E: On preconscious mental processes. Psychoanalytic Quarterly 19:540–560, 1950

Krystal H: Affect tolerance. Annual of Psychoanalysis 3:179–219, 1975

LeDoux J: The Emotional Brain: The Mysterious Underpinnings of Emotional Life. New York, Simon & Schuster, 1996

Levy KN, Meehan KB, Kelly KM, et al: Change in attachment patterns and reflective function in a randomized control trial of transference-focused psychotherapy for borderline personality disorder. J Consult Clin Psychol 74:1027–1040, 2006

Metcalfe J, Shimamura AP (eds): Metacognition: Knowing About Knowing. Cambridge, MA, MIT Press, 1994

Moscarello JM, LeDoux JE: Active avoidance learning requires prefrontal suppression of amygdala-mediated defensive reactions. J Neurosci 33:3815–3823, 2013

Newman LS, Baumeister RF, Duff KJ: A new look at defensive projection: thought suppression, accessibility and biased person perception. J Pers Soc Psychol 72:980–1001, 1995

Newman MG, Stone AA: Does humor moderate the effects of experimentally induced stress? Ann Behav Med 18:101–109, 1996

Northoff G, Bermpohl F, Schoeneich F, et al: How does our brain constitute defense mechanisms? First-person neuroscience and psychoanalysis. Psychother Psychosom 76:141–153, 2007

Ochsner KN: Are affective events richly collected or simply familiar? The experience and process of recognizing feelings past. J Exp Psychol Gen 129:242–261, 2000

Olds ME, Forbes JL: The central basis of motivation: intracranial self-stimulation studies. Annu Rev Psychol 32:523–574, 1981

Park S, Auchincloss EL: Psychoanalysis in introductory textbooks of psychology: a review. J Am Psychoanal Assoc 54:1361–1380, 2006

Perry J, Lanni F: Observer-rated measures of defense mechanisms. J Pers 66:993–1024, 2008

Phelps EA: Emotion and cognition: insights from studies of the human amygdala. Annu Rev Psychol 24:27–53, 2006

Phelps EA, LeDoux: Contributions of the amygdala to emotional processing: from animal models to human behavior. Neuron 48:175–187, 2005

Reich W: Character Analysis (1933). New York, Simon & Schuster, 1945

Roseman IJ, Smith CA: Appraisal theory: overview, assumptions, varieties, and controversies, in Appraisal Process in Emotion: Theory, Methods, Research. Edited by Scherer KR, Schorr A, Johnstone T. New York, Oxford University Press, 2001, pp 3–19

Rotton L: Trait humor and longevity: do comics have the last laugh? Health Psychol 11:262–266, 1992

Roy C, Perry J, Luborsky L, et al: Changes in defensive functioning in completed psychoanalyses: the Penn psychoanalytic treatment collection. J Am Psychoanal Assoc 57:399–415, 2009

Sandler J: The background of safety. Int J Psychoanal 41:352–356, 1960

Schafer R: The loving and beloved superego in Freud's structural theory. Psychoanal Study Child 15:163–188, 1960

Scherer KR: The nature and study of appraisal: a review of the issues, in Appraisal Process in Emotion: Theory, Methods, Research. Edited by Scherer KR, Schorr A, Johnstone T. New York, Oxford University Press, 2001, pp 369–391

Shapiro D: Neurotic Styles. New York, Basic Books, 1965

Shapiro D: Autonomy and Rigid Character. New York, Basic Books, 1984

Simons DJ, Chabris CF: Gorillas in our midst: sustained inattentional blindness for dynamic events. Perception 28:1059–1074, 1999

Singer JL (ed): Repression and Dissociation: Implications for Personality, Psychopathology, and Health. Chicago, IL, University of Chicago Press, 1990

Spitz R: Anxiety in infancy: a study of its manifestations in the first year of life. Int J Psychoanal 3:138–143, 1950

Stein DJ, Young JE: Rethinking repression, in Cognitive Science and the Unconscious. Edited by Stein DJ. Washington, DC, American Psychiatric Press, 1997, pp 147–176

Stern DN: The Present Moment in Psychotherapy and Everyday Life. New York, WW Norton, 2003

Tori C, Bilmes M: Multiculturalism and psychoanalytic psychology: the validation of a defense mechanisms measure in an Asian population. Psychoanal Psychol 19:701–721, 2002

Uleman JS: Introduction: becoming aware of the new unconscious, in The New Unconscious. Edited by Hassin RR, Uleman JS, Bargh JA. New York, Oxford University Press, 2005, pp 3–18

Weinberger D, Schwartz G, Davidson R: Low-anxious, high-anxious, and repressive coping styles: psychometric patterns and behavioral and physiological responses to stress. J Am Psychoanal Assoc 88:369–380, 1979

Westen D: The scientific status of unconscious processes: is Freud really dead? J Am Psychoanal Assoc 47:1061–1106, 1999

Zetzel E: Anxiety and the capacity to bear it. Int J Psychoanal 30:1–12, 1949

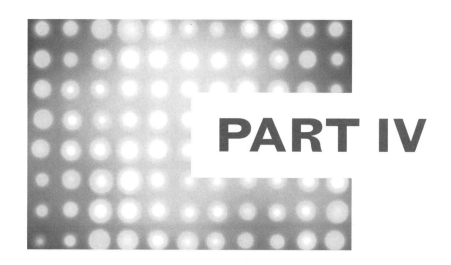

PART IV

Object Relations
Theory and
Self Psychology

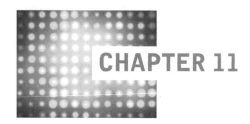

CHAPTER 11

Object Relations Theory

This chapter introduces readers to Object Relations Theory. It outlines the basic assertions of this model of the mind, comparing it with previous models. It discusses some famous object relations theories, pointing to similarities and areas of overlap with neighboring disciplines and fields of research. Finally, it explores the contributions of Object Relations Theory to our understanding of psychopathology and treatment. Vocabulary introduced in this chapter includes the following: *Adult Attachment Interview, attachment, attachment behavioral system, attachment theory, borderline personality organization, co-created experience, container/contained, corrective emotional experience, countertransference, depressive anxiety, depressive position, differentiation, envy, good-enough mother, holding environment, identity diffusion, individuation, internal working models of attachment, interpersonal, Mentalization-Based Treatment, midlife crisis, need-satisfying object, object, object permanence, object relations, on the way to object constancy, paranoid position, part object, persecutory anxiety, position, practicing, rapprochement, rapprochement crisis, representation, schema, schizophrenogenic mothering, self constancy, separation, separation-individuation, Strange Situation, therapeutic alliance, Transference-Focused Psychotherapy,* and *whole object.*

After its introduction in the early 1920s, the Structural Model, along with Ego Psychology, dominated thinking about the psychodynamic approach to mental heath in America for almost half a century. However, in the 1960s and 1970s, it gradually became clear to many theorists that some behavior and many states of mind are best described not in terms of conflict among the structures of ego, id, and superego but rather in terms of internal representations of self and other. It also became increasingly clear to developmental psychologists that many mental capacities previously attributed to the ego could be better understood as developing in the infant–caregiver matrix. In the midst of these two developments, Object Relations Theory was invented.

Object Relations Theory: Terms and Concepts

Object Relations Theory models the mind in terms of internal representations of self and other. *Object* is the word that psychoanalytic theorists use mainly to describe another person. An *object relation* is defined as a psychological configuration consisting of three parts: a self representation, an object representation, and a representation of an affectively charged interaction between the two. The word *representation* as used in psychoanalysis is roughly analogous to the word *schema* as used in cognitive psychology; both mean "an organized and persistent pattern of thought" (Weinberger and Weiss 1997). When we use the term *object relations,* we are referring to psychological representations. In other words, object relations must be distinguished from interpersonal relationships, a term that refers to the interactions between an individual and another person in the outside world. The term *object relations* is often erroneously assumed to be synonymous with interpersonal relationships.

Object Relations Theory attempts to understand how self and object representations develop in childhood, how they are maintained throughout life, how they influence and are influenced by other structures and motivations, and how they affect psychic functioning and behavior. The basic tenets of Object Relations Theory may be summarized as follows:

- Object relations are largely unconscious.
- Human beings are object seeking from birth; object seeking is not reducible to any other motivation.
- All psychological phenomena, from the most fleeting experience to the most stable structure, are organized by object relations.
- Object relations evolve through internalization of the infant's interactions with the object world, developing from an admixture of innate factors (including affect dispositions and cognitive capacities) and interactions with caregivers.
- Interpersonal relationships reflect internalized object relations; psychopathology, especially serious psychopathology, is best conceptualized in terms of disturbances in object relations.

In placing object relations at the center of psychological life, Object Relations Theory emphasizes the fact that psychic life develops in the context of the social or interpersonal environment and is adapted to that environment.

Comparison of Object Relations Theory With the Topographic and Structural Models

Sigmund Freud used the term *object* throughout his writing life. In fact, there is no aspect of either the Topographic Model or the Structural Model—including those related to motivation, structure, development, and psychopathology/treatment—that does not include understanding of the role of the object. For example, in our discussion of oedipal conflict (see Chapter 7, "The Oedipus Complex"), we saw how early objects, including father and mother, are important in the developing mind of the child. When drive theory was introduced (see Chapter 9, "The Id and the Superego"), we explored how almost all forms of libido and aggression (except those that are autoerotic) require an object for the attainment of satisfaction. Throughout our discussion of the Structural Model, we saw how both the ego and the superego develop in interaction with caregivers. In addition, in the developmental sequence of danger situations important in the mediation of conflict, loss of the object—or of the love of the object—is an important fear (see Chapter 10, "Conflict and Compromise"). Finally, in all models of the mind, theories of therapeutic action emphasize the role of the transference as revealing important aspects of the mind. It should not be surprising to us then that there is considerable overlap between the earlier models of the mind and Object Relations Theory. Indeed, it is important to remember that maintenance of stable and realistic self and object representations is defined as an ego function. In other words, one way of conceptualizing Object Relations Theory is to think of it as a model of the mind that specifically focuses on the ego functions responsible for developing and maintaining object relations.

A brief comparison of several of the basic tenets of Object Relations Theory with those of the Structural Model of the mind may be useful in clarifying how the Object Relations model of the mind differs from the earlier model:

- **Topographic point of view**—In Object Relations Theory, object relations are conceptualized as being largely unconscious. By contrast, in the Structural Model, the id was defined as unconscious, and the ego and superego were conceptualized as having both unconscious and conscious/preconscious aspects.

- **Motivational point of view**—According to Object Relations Theory, the pursuit of objects is not reducible to the pursuit of bodily and/or aggressive pleasure (as is asserted in the Structural Model). In other words, we do not seek attachment to our mother because she is a source of pleasure; rather, we seek the attachment for its own sake. Wish and drive may be important motivators in psychic life, but they must always be as embedded in self and object representations.

- **Structural point of view**—In Object Relations Theory, the basic unit of experience is a package consisting of a self representation, an object representation, and the interaction between the two—an *object relation*—rather than a package consisting of a conflict between a wish and a prohibition (as in the Structural Model). All psychic structures—not just the superego—are made up of object relations.

- **Developmental point of view**—In Object Relations Theory, infant–caregiver interactions are central to all aspects of the developing mind, not just the superego (as is posited in the Structural Model); preoedipal interactions involving the infant–mother relationship are just as important to the development of the mind as are oedipal interactions; and the establishment of stable object relations during the preoedipal period of development is a necessary forerunner to development of the oedipal phase. In other words, Object Relations Theory places more emphasis on the preoedipal period than does the Structural Model.

- **Theory of psychopathology and theory of therapeutic action**—In Object Relations Theory, psychopathology is conceptualized primarily in terms of disturbances in object relations, rather than in terms of oedipal conflict (neurosis) (as in the Structural Model). In regard to the mechanism of therapeutic action, Object Relations Theory posits that it is the patient–therapist relationship itself that brings about change, as opposed to insight derived from interpretation (per the Structural Model). Contributions of the Object Relations model to psychoanalytic theories of psychopathology and therapeutic action are discussed in greater detail later in this chapter (see sections "Object Relations Theory and Adult Psychopathology" and "Object Relations Theory and Psychodynamic Treatment").

The Birth of Object Relations Theory

The most important object relations theorists are Klein, Mahler, Bowlby, and Kernberg. Bion and Winnicott are discussed briefly in this chapter and will be mentioned again in Chapter 12 when we talk about Self Psychology. Each of these theorists emphasized a different aspect of Object Relations Theory.

Anna Freud: The Need-Satisfying Object

After Sigmund Freud's death in 1939, the psychoanalytic model of the mind developed in several directions, in large measure differentiated from the Freudian model by the place given to the role of the object and object relations in psychological life. Anna Freud (1895–1982), Freud's youngest child, remained loyal to her father's Structural Model of the mind, broadening this model (later called Ego Psychology) through her work with children and the study of defense. However, her interest in development led her to study object relations in childhood, although she did not use that term. In her work, Anna Freud described a natural progression from object dependency to self-reliance. She posited a series of predictable stages through which normal children pass: an early stage of undifferentiated self and object representations; a stage in which the object is experienced as *need-satisfying*; a stage marked by the attainment of *object constancy*, in which stable object representations are maintained even in the face of feelings of anger; an oedipal stage marked by conflicts over rivalry and possessiveness; and a stage marked by the adolescent struggle to find new, nonincestuous objects (A. Freud 1963). We will discuss the important concepts of *need-satisfying object* and *object constancy* in greater depth in a moment.

Melanie Klein: The Paranoid and Depressive Positions

At roughly the same time that Anna Freud was doing her work, Melanie Klein (1882–1960) proposed a very different theory, which has had a lasting effect on the psychoanalytic model of the mind. Klein's theory is considered the first real Object Relations Theory.[1] Building on ideas about the development of the superego, understood as resulting from internalization of interactions between child and caregiver, Klein proposed that the entire mind is built out of similar internalizations, which

---

[1]Although the term itself—*object relations theory*—was invented by Ronald Fairbairn (1954), who was a student of Klein's.

lead to the formation of representations of both self and object. Let us explain a bit more about how Klein's theory works.

In her theory, Klein described the feelings and thoughts of young children that influence the development of object relations. For example, if the young child experiences the object as "bad," this experience of "badness" is as much the result of projection of the child's angry thoughts and feelings onto the representation of the object as it is the result of any actual bad qualities of the object. By the same token, if the young child experiences the object as "good," this "goodness" is the result of an admixture of the projection of the child's experience of happy satisfaction onto the object and the object's own good qualities. According to Klein's Object Relations Theory, the child's efforts to manage the good and bad aspects of experience lead to the development of his or her inner world. As we can see, Klein adhered to Sigmund Freud's concept of drive (libido and aggression); however, in Klein's theory, drive is always experienced in the context of relationships with others.

In the process of managing these good and bad experiences, every child must progress through what Klein called *positions,* analogous to Sigmund Freud's and Anna Freud's developmental stages. These positions—the *paranoid position* (also known as the *paranoid-schizoid position*) and the *depressive position*—are defined as stable configurations of self and object representations built from the combined influence of wishes, thoughts, and feelings; and interactions with caregivers. In Klein's view, successful development is defined as the capacity to tolerate conflicting feelings of love and hate toward the same object, as expressed in movement from the paranoid to the depressive position.

The paranoid position is the earliest organization of the psyche. It is characterized by the splitting apart of good (satisfying and loving) from bad (frustrating and aggressive) aspects of experience, accompanied by the use of projection and projective identification of bad aspects of experience onto the object. *Splitting* and *projection/projective identification* serve to protect the good self and good object from angry, hostile feelings. (We will say more about splitting and projective identification in a moment when we talk about patients with borderline psychopathology.) In the paranoid position, the child fears that he or she is in danger of being destroyed by the bad object, who has become the repository for all of the child's own projected aggression. The child is also threatened by his or her own experience of envy, which is also projected onto the object. In other words, the paranoid position is marked by *persecutory anxiety.*

During the course of normal development, in the context of supportive maternal care and the absence of too much frustration, the child begins to move into the depressive position. This movement progresses as the child develops the capacity to tolerate conflicting feelings of love and hate toward the same object, so that he or she does not have to resort to splitting and projective identification to manage bad experience. In the depressive position, a child fears that his or her own angry feelings may threaten the object, now experienced as loved and needed. In other words, the depressive position is marked by *depressive anxiety.* However, the child's new capacity for gratitude toward the object, along with growing confidence that envy can be overcome and damage to the relationship can be repaired, reassures him or her that love will prevail over hate and that loving relationships can be maintained (Klein 1932, 1975a, 1975b; Segal 1946).

Two Views of the Major Developmental Challenge of Childhood: Anna Freud Versus Melanie Klein

If we pause for a moment to compare the views of Melanie Klein with those of Anna Freud, we see that for Klein, the major developmental challenge facing children is the integration of contradictory feelings about the object, whereas for Freud, the major developmental challenge facing children is the achievement of relative independence from the object with the internalization of regulation in the form of a strong ego. These two theorists had other disagreements as well. Indeed, the struggle between Anna Freud and Melanie Klein and their followers for dominance and influence in psychoanalysis in the aftermath of Sigmund Freud's death is legendary in the history of psychoanalysis in Great Britain, where they both lived and worked (King and Steiner 1991). Nowadays, however, we do not have to be caught up in their conflict but can draw upon the best from both these theories in our view of the mind.

Wilfred Bion and D. W. Winnicott: The Container/Contained, the Good-Enough Mother, and the Holding Environment

Among the students of Melanie Klein were two other British psychoanalysts, Wilfred Bion (1897–1979) and D.W. Winnicott (1896–1971). Bion is known for his concept of the container and the contained. In this view, the mother must help the child manage intolerable and painful experience. Through the mother's caretaking acts, which include soothing and verbalizing (or what Bion called *reverie*), the infant's chaotic, unbearable experience is transformed into something more tolerable, so that the child can successfully move from the paranoid to the depressive position. In Bion's terms, the mother acts as a *container* for the infant's chaotic experience, which must be *contained.* Bion's theory has obvious implications for the theory of therapeutic action (Bion 1962,

1963, 1967, 1970), which we will touch on later in this chapter (see section "Object Relations Theory and Psychodynamic Treatment"). In Chapter 12 ("Self Psychology"), we will revisit Bion's theories about the role of the containing mother in helping the child to develop affect tolerance and other key capacities.

Winnicott proposed a theory of object relations that also describes the infant's capacity to relate to others, which develops in interaction with the mother. Winnicott is famous for his concepts of the *good-enough mother* (who provides the infant with the optimal amount of comfort and frustration) and the *holding environment* (created by a caregiver who is "good enough"). This holding environment is necessary for development of the child's capacity to experience *concern for the object* instead of merely using the object as a repository for the projection of bad experience (Winnicott 1954/1958, 1958, 1965, 1971). Like Klein, Winnicott saw successful development as representing the ability to integrate feelings of love and hate toward the object. Unlike Klein, Winnicott placed emphasis (as did Bion) on the role of the mother in providing the environment where this can happen.

Later in this chapter we will examine the contribution of the concept of the holding environment to the theory of therapeutic action in psychodynamic psychotherapy (see section "Object Relations Theory and Psychodynamic Treatment"). We will also discuss Winnicott's ideas in greater detail in Chapter 12 ("Self Psychology"), when we look at his theories about how the interactions between infant and mother are important for the development of an authentic sense of self in the child, as well as for the development of the child's capacity for play, fantasy, and a rich inner life.[2]

Margaret Mahler: Separation-Individuation

Meanwhile, in America, a psychoanalyst named Margaret Mahler (1897–1985) was doing important work based on her observations of young children and their mothers. Although Mahler saw herself as writing within the tradition of Ego Psychology and the Structural Model, her ideas drew from those of both Anna Freud and Melanie Klein and have contributed a great deal to our understanding of the

---

[2]Winnicott was heavily influenced by his studies with Klein. Working in the United Kingdom at the time of the Freud–Klein controversies, Winnicott helped to found the British Middle School, later known as the Independent Group (King and Steiner 1991).

child's interaction with caregivers. Mahler is best known for her most important idea, the process of *separation-individuation.*

In Mahler's theory, *separation* is a psychological process by which the child forms a representation of the self that is distinct or separate from the representation of the object. *Individuation* is a psychological process by which the child develops specific characteristics, so that the self becomes not only distinct from the object but also unique and autonomous (Mahler et al. 1975). In Mahler's view, the process of separation-individuation occurs between the ages of 9 months and 4 years. Mahler delineated four subphases of the separation-individuation process: *differentiation, practicing, rapprochement,* and *on the way to object constancy.* She proposed two other, earlier phases: the autistic phase (birth to 2 months), in which the infant is unresponsive to external stimuli, and the symbiotic phase (2–9 months), in which the infant is attached to the mother but imagines him- or herself to be merged with the mother. The autistic phase and the symbiotic phase have been largely discredited by studies indicating that even the youngest infants have highly developed capacities that allow for both contact with the outside world and differentiation between self and object (Stern 1985).[3] However, Mahler's views about separation-individuation have stood the test of time.

According to Mahler, the separation-individuation process begins with the *differentiation* subphase (6–9 months). In this subphase, the infant begins to take more interest in his or her surroundings and starts to

---

[3]Mahler's autistic and symbiotic stages of development, now no longer in use, represent a common and serious problem in some psychodynamic theory making in which adult psychopathology is seen as reflecting difficulty at an early stage of development. In this case, Mahler posited that "autistic schizophrenia" was the result of difficulties in the autistic stage of development and that "symbiotic schizophrenia" was the result of difficulties in the symbiotic stage of development. Mahler's work in this area is related to some of the most damaging errors in psychodynamic theory making, in which the difficulties of psychotic patients were blamed on problematic or "schizophrenogenic" mothering (Fromm-Reichmann 1950). Nowadays, schizophrenia is no longer conceptualized as reflecting difficulties in mother–infant interactions (Willick 2001). (In addition, as we have seen, infants are no longer thought to be either "autistic" or "symbiotic" in the first months of life.) Reexamination of these and other errors highlights the need for theory makers to avoid the "genetic fallacy" in which present-day functioning is conceptualized as reflecting difficulties in development, often in parent–child interactions (Willick 1983) (see also Chapter 7 ["The Oedipus Complex"] for a discussion of errors made in thinking about female development and about homosexuality).

interact more and more with the environment. The relationship to the mother is firmly established, as indicated by the frequent use of the social smile and the appearance of stranger anxiety (Mahler 1972; Mahler et al. 1975).

In the *practicing* subphase (10–15 months), the child experiments with distance by moving away from the mother, enjoying his or her newly developed capacities for crawling and walking. In this subphase, the child explores his or her expanding world at increasingly greater distances but still requires the mother to be available for *emotional refueling,* especially when the child is tired or upset. The practicing subphase is characterized by feelings of omnipotence and elation, because the child seems to be in a "love affair with the world" (Mahler 1972; Mahler et al. 1975).

The practicing subphase is followed by the *rapprochement* subphase (15–24 months). During rapprochement, the child experiences conflicting feelings brought on by a new awareness of him- or herself as a separate individual. In this subphase, the child begins to feel increasingly vulnerable, often showing intense separation anxiety. In the face of feeling more vulnerable and anxious, the child returns to the mother, often in a demanding and controlling way. At the same time, the child's clingy behavior arouses the fear that his or her newfound separateness and independence will be lost. The conflict between the wish to depend on the mother and the wish for autonomy from her creates a *rapprochement crisis.* This crisis is accompanied by feelings of anger and hostility; it is also accompanied by wide fluctuations in mood, as feelings of omnipotence alternate with feelings of vulnerability (Mahler 1972; Mahler et al. 1975). Indeed, anyone who has spent time with a young child in the rapprochement stage of development knows why this stage has been called "the terrible twos."

The Importance of Object Constancy

Mahler called the final subphase of separation-individuation by the term *on the way to object constancy. Object constancy* is one the most important concepts in the psychoanalytic model of the mind. It is defined as the ability to maintain a positively tinged feeling toward the mother (or anyone else) in the face of feelings of frustration, anger, and/or disappointment. A related concept is *self constancy,* defined as the ability to maintain a positive self representation in the face of failure or threats to self-esteem. Object constancy depends on the achievement of *object permanence* (usually by 6 months), defined as the ability to maintain a representation of an object (animate or inanimate) even when it is not within perceptual awareness (Piaget 1954/1990; Schacter et al. 2011,

p. 477). Object constancy, an emotional capacity, is often confused with object permanence, a purely cognitive capacity. Mahler borrowed the term *object constancy* from fellow ego psychologists Anna Freud and Heinz Hartmann, the latter of whom coined the term to describe object representations that remain stable and permanent "independent of the state of needs" (Hartmann 1953, p. 180). In other words, as we have seen, prior to the achievement of object constancy, the object is experienced as *need-satisfying,* or as existing only to meet the infant's needs (Hartmann 1952, 1953). In Klein's terms, the need-satisfying object is a *part object,* meaning that only one aspect of the relationship is experienced (and represented) by the child, as opposed to a *whole object,* which is experienced as complete, or integrated with respect to all its qualities, both good and bad. Mahler, like Klein, believed that the capacity for object constancy is achieved when the child is able to integrate bad representations of the mother with good representations of the mother, so that the object can retain its identity as a "good person" even when the mother does something that the child finds frustrating. In other words, Mahler's final stage of separation-individuation is roughly equivalent to the depressive position as described by Klein.

While Mahler argued that object constancy is fairly firmly established in the normal 3-year-old child, she called this final stage in the separation-individuation process *on the way to object constancy,* reflecting her feeling that the attainment of object constancy is a lifelong process. Klein also understood that the attainment of object constancy waxes and wanes throughout life. Although in her view, maturity is reflected in the movement from the paranoid to the depressive position, the two positions fluctuate in everyone. Indeed, in Klein's view, retreat to the paranoid position is often a defense against unbearable depressive anxiety, or the fear that one's own aggression will destroy the object.

Indeed, throughout the life cycle we face continual threats to object constancy posed by any event that causes separation from loved ones or feelings of vulnerability and anger. Actually, object constancy can be threatened by just about any strong feeling. Obvious examples of such threats include adolescence (often called "the second separation-individuation"), when we face the challenges of leaving home and finding new people with whom to identify (Blos 1967); parenthood, when we face the many feelings that come with having a baby (Anthony and Benedek 1970); the *midlife crisis,* when we face the fact that life does not go on forever (Jacques 1965); and many others (Akhtar 1994). When we discuss the contributions of the Object Relations model to psychoanalytic theories of psychopathology and therapeutic action (see sections "Object Relations Theory and Adult Psychopathology" and "Object Relations

Theory and Psychodynamic Treatment" later in this chapter), we will see that the concept of object constancy—including failures of object constancy (and of self constancy)—is at the root of all kinds of severe personality disorders.

John Bowlby: Attachment Theory

While Anna Freud and Melanie Klein were locked in struggles over Sigmund Freud's legacy and Margaret Mahler was studying babies and their mothers in New York City, the British psychoanalyst John Bowlby (1907–1990) was developing a different kind of object relations–based theory called *attachment theory* (Bowlby 1969/1982, 1973, 1980). Attachment theory is another theory of early development based on the study of interactions between infant and caregiver. Bowlby defined *attachment* as "lasting psychological connectedness between human beings" (Bowlby 1969/1982, p. 194). The central premise of attachment theory is that the infant's motivation to develop an attachment with the caregiver is an innate feature of the human mind dictated by evolutionary pressure, or by the survival needs of the species. The quest for attachment precedes—and is not reducible to—the quest for libidinal gratification (Auchincloss and Samberg 2012, pp. 20–22).

Bowlby argued that the motivation for attachment is realized through an inborn *attachment behavioral system* operating between infant and mother. He identified five components of the attachment behavioral system that regulate distance between infant and mother: sucking, smiling, clinging, crying, and following. When the infant becomes distressed (either by an internal stimulus, such as feeling hungry, or by an external stimulus, such as distraction in the mother), the attachment system is activated and the infant seeks physical contact with the mother. In return, the mother responds to the infant's signals with behaviors that increase closeness and nurturing. By contrast, when the infant feels secure, the attachment system is deactivated; attachment behaviors in both infant and mother cease.

For Bowlby, the nature of the child's earliest tie to the mother establishes the child's basic attitude toward others and the child's basic sense of self. The bond with the mother is represented in what Bowlby called *internal working models of attachment*, which are established by 1 year of age. Internal working models of attachment are analogous to the object relations that we have seen in the theories of Klein and Mahler in that they include a self representation, an object representation, and a representation of the interaction between the two. As with object relations, these internal models serve as a template for all future interactions with others. Internal working models of attachment also play a role in the development of cognitive capacities, affect regulation, impulse control, and other ego functions that we explored in the Structural Model. However, internal working models of attachment differ from object relations in that theories about their development place less emphasis on the emotional state of the child and more emphasis on the interactions between child and caregiver. As we have seen, Klein and Mahler both emphasized the influence of the young child's inner experiences of love and hate in the development of his or her object relations. In contrast, Bowlby placed greater emphasis on the nature of the interaction with the actual mother (Fonagy 2001; Johnson et al. 2007).

In the development of his theories, Bowlby was heavily influenced by work from a variety of neighboring disciplines, including biology, evolution, and ethology. He was influenced by Darwin's theory of evolution, understanding that the attachment behavior that links the dependent infant to the caretaking mother improves survival. Bowlby was also inspired by Konrad Lorenz's (1903–1989) research on *imprinting* in geese (Lorenz 1949/1979) and by Harlow's research on maternal deprivation in primates (Harlow and Zimmermann 1958), as both of these investigators explored aspects of inborn needs for a relationship. Indeed, because Bowlby's theory emphasized the importance of inborn behavioral patterns and of real relationships, he was often at odds with other psychoanalysts of the time, who tended to emphasize the internal workings of the mind rather than external behaviors (Coates 2004).

Mary Ainsworth and Mary Main: The Strange Situation and the Adult Attachment Interview

In any case, attachment theory did not enter the psychoanalytic mainstream until the 1970s and 1980s, with the important research of Mary Ainsworth (1913–1999) and Mary Main (1943–) (Fonagy 2001). Ainsworth developed a research procedure called the Strange Situation, which she used to assess individual differences in attachment organization. In the Strange Situation, the child is observed playing while caregivers and strangers enter and leave the room. An independent observer rates the child's behavior on several factors, including the following: the amount of exploration engaged in by the child, the child's reaction to the departure of the caregiver, the amount of stranger anxiety shown by the child when alone with the stranger, and the child's reunion behavior with the caregiver. Ainsworth described distinct patterns of attachment that she called *secure attachment, anxious-avoidant attachment,* and *anxious-resistant attachment* (Ainsworth et al. 1978). A fourth pattern, *disorga-*

nized/disoriented attachment, was added by Mary Main (Main and Solomon 1986). Main developed what she called the Adult Attachment Interview, used to investigate patterns in adult recollections of early childhood experience related to attachment. She described similar patterns, including the following: secure-autonomous, dismissing, preoccupied, and unresolved/disorganized (Main et al. 1985). The Adult Attachment Interview has been used by dozens of investigators to study the many complex effects of patterns of attachment.

Object Relations Theory and Adult Psychopathology

All psychodynamic clinicians agree that the quality of object relations, including a secure internal working model of attachment, is an important parameter along which to evaluate mental health. In general, object relations are assessed as mature when an individual is able to sustain loving attachments. This ability requires recognition that the object is distinct from the self and that one's own needs may sometimes conflict with those of the object. It also requires the capacity to accept some degree of dependence on the object, as well as some separation from the object. Mature object relations additionally require the acknowledgement, acceptance, and tolerance of *ambivalence* toward the object. Finally, mature object relations are marked by self and object constancy, allowing for the feeling that the self and the object are "good enough."

Using empirical research techniques, investigators have shown that disruptions in infant–caregiver relationships correlate with psychopathology both in early life and later on (Beebe and Lachmann 2003; Beebe and Stern 1977; Beebe et al. 1992, 2008; Bowlby 1944; Cassidy 2008; Deklyen and Greenberg 2008; Lyons-Ruth and Jacobvitz 2008; Spitz 1945; Spitz and Wolf 1946; Tronick 1989). In addition, investigators have explored the complex correlates in many mind/brain systems of these disruptions. For example, Allan Schore (1994) has summarized work investigating the development of affect regulation in the context of infant–caregiver relationships, integrating this work with findings from neurobiology (Eisenberg 1995; Hofer 1984, 1995). Schore (1994) posited that the function of emotion regulation, which develops in interaction with the parents, is eventually taken over by mental representations—internalized aspects of the caretaking environment that enable the child to independently regulate affect states. Drew Westen and others have attempted to integrate Object Relations Theory with aspects of attachment theory, social psychology, and cognitive neuroscience (Bandura 1986; Blatt and Lerner 1983; Calabrese et al. 2005; Smith et al. 2013; Wegner and Vallacher 1977; Westen 1990, 1991). More recently, in studies that promise to revolutionize our understanding of mental health, Avshalom Caspi and colleagues have reported that the experience of early deprivation and loss may interact with genetic vulnerability to produce psychopathology in later life (Uher et al. 2011; Zimmerman et al. 2011). Finally, Barbara Milrod and colleagues have suggested that "separation anxiety and its treatment could provide an important window to neural circuits and other biological processes associated with internalization of social supports" (Milrod et al. 2014, p. 40). Object Relations Theory interfaces with the National Institute of Mental Health Research Domain Criteria domain "Social Processes" and with the construct "Affiliation and Attachment" (Cuthbert and Insel 2013).[4] (Readers interested in a recent summary of correlations between neurobiology and Object Relations Theory are referred to Kernberg 2014.)

In the clinical situation we see disturbances in object relations in many kinds of adult psychopathology (Nigg et al. 1992). In healthier patients, establishment of mature object relations during the preoedipal period of development is a necessary forerunner to successful navigation of the oedipal stage (Klein 1945). For example, the young woman who was "afraid to be left on the shelf," whom we discussed in Chapters 6 ("The World of Dreams") and 7 ("The Oedipus Complex"), suffered terrible loss at the time of her mother's death, leaving her even more afraid than usual that strong feelings of competition aroused in the oedipal stage would lead to abandonment. As we have seen, this young woman treated most romantic opportunities with a feeling of being "above it all." The young doctor who was obsequious in the presence of authority, whom we discussed in Chapter 10 ("Conflict and Compromise"), was also raised in difficult circumstances by parents whose own struggles with illness led them to demand that their son be a "good boy" who showed little aggression. As a result, he came into the oedipal stage already afraid of confrontation and competition.

In more seriously ill patients, failure to successfully differentiate self from object is reflected in psychotic experiences of all kinds, including those resulting from severe mental illness (e.g., schizophrenia, affective disorder) or from organic conditions, toxic states, or trauma. Although it is possible to describe psychotic experience in terms of ego weakness

---

[4]See nimh.nih.gov/research-priorities/rdoc/index.shtml (accessed January 12, 2014).

(such as disturbances in reality testing and/or the use of denial), many aspects of psychosis are best described in terms of self and object representations. For example, in the case of hallucinations or delusions, the patient may be unable to tell whether thoughts or voices originate in his or her own mind or the minds of other people.

Inability to tolerate ambivalence, or to maintain object constancy, is reflected in severe personality disorders, including borderline, paranoid, and some narcissistic conditions. Again, although it is possible to describe serious personality disorders in terms of ego weakness (such as impulse dyscontrol and affect intolerance), a better way of understanding these disorders may be to conceptualize them as reflecting an inability to maintain loving relationships in the face of frustration. Many patients with severe personality pathology do not form attachments at all because they are afraid of the intense feelings that will be stirred up by an intimate attachment; others are unable to tolerate separation and loss. Many suffer from problems with both attachment and separation.

Otto Kernberg: Integration of Object Relations Theory With the Structural Model

The American psychoanalyst Otto Kernberg has done important work integrating many of the best aspects of Object Relations Theory with the best aspects of the Structural Model. For example, although Kernberg adheres to a concept of *drive*, which he uses to describe the peremptory, superordinate search for pleasure (or impulse for aggression) guiding all behavior, he conceptualizes drive somewhat differently than do many who adhere more fully to the Structural Model. In Kernberg's view, the experience of drive results not from the body's innate demand for pleasure but rather from an innate disposition to experience pleasure in the context of relationships, which leads people to seek similar pleasurable relationships in an ongoing way. In other words, pleasurable (or good) experiences in the context of relationships become organized as drives.

Kernberg developed an important system for classifying personality organization (Kernberg 1970) and a theory for understanding borderline personality disorder (Kernberg 1975). These theories reflect his efforts to integrate Ego Psychology with Object Relations Theory (Kernberg 1976) and have been highly influential in the field of mental health.

Kernberg's Classification of Personality Disorders

According to Kernberg, in the development of healthy object relations, every individual must succeed at two basic tasks. The first task is the ability to differentiate self from object, or to construct self and object representations with clear boundaries. The second task is the ability to integrate self and object representations with respect to their good (pleasurable) and bad (frustrating) aspects. Kernberg saw the successful development of object relations as the attainment of object constancy, or the ability to maintain a positive attachment to an object even in the face of frustration or anger. Included in Kernberg's concept of *object constancy* is the concept of *self constancy*.

The twin tasks of separating self from object and of integrating good and bad aspects of self and object are closely related. This relationship is seen in many instances of psychological stress. For example, in the common experiences that involve separation from loved ones, we all face difficulty managing feelings, which often include frustration and anger. We must be able to withstand these feelings without losing either the capacity for self and object differentiation (task 1) or the capacity for object constancy (task 2). According to Kernberg's classification of personality disorders, patients who frequently fail at the task of differentiating self from object (task 1) are prone to psychotic pathology; patients who frequently fail at the task of integrating good and bad experience (task 2) but who mainly succeed at the task of differentiating self from object (task 1) are prone to borderline psychopathology; and patients who usually succeed at tasks 1 and 2 are prone to neurotic psychopathology (Kernberg 1970). Kernberg is most famous for his descriptions of the second group, or those with borderline personality organization (Kernberg 1975).

Kernberg's Conceptualization of Borderline Personality Organization

Kernberg's borderline personality organization (BPO) is a psychoanalytic diagnosis marked by nonspecific ego weaknesses (such as poor impulse control and affect intolerance) and by disturbances in object relations. In Kernberg's view, BPO is characterized by object relations in which there are poorly integrated good and bad self and object representations. BPO is also characterized by the use of defense mechanisms based on *splitting*, such as *projective identification* and *omnipotent control*. These defenses are based on a need to separate positive from negative experience, get rid of negative experience through projection onto the object, and control the object, who is now experienced as bad and potentially dangerous. In other words, the defenses characteristic of BPO reflect the underlying disturbances in object relations. As described by Kernberg, BPO corresponds to Klein's concept of the paranoid position, which (as we recall) is characterized by the splitting off and projection of all-bad experiences onto the object, in contrast to Klein's depressive position, where love and hate are integrated.

In BPO, a failure to integrate good and bad aspects of experience underlies the inability to experience a coherent picture of oneself and/or of others. Patients with BPO often manifest wide fluctuations in mood, which represent the activation of self and object representations that are split apart or experienced as all-good or all-bad. The patient's mood fluctuates according to which part of this poorly integrated representation is activated. An incoherent picture of the self, which Kernberg (borrowing from Erikson 1956) called *identity diffusion,* leaves patients with BPO at risk for extreme swings in self-experience and self-esteem. An incoherent picture of others leaves patients with BPO at risk for misinterpretation of the actions of others and interpersonal chaos. BPO is found in borderline personality disorder as defined by DSM-5 (American Psychiatry Association 2013), as well as in other severe personality disorders, such as paranoid personality disorder, schizoid personality disorder, and some types of narcissistic personality disorder.

Other Perspectives on the Etiology of Borderline Psychopathology

As we saw in Chapter 10 when we discussed differing ways of understanding ego weakness (see section "Theories of Ego Weakness: Defense Versus Deficit"), a key debate among psychoanalytic theorists focuses on whether psychopathology is best explained as resulting from defenses against intrapsychic conflicts (i.e., the defense/conflict model) or as resulting from deficits due to failure of the early environment to provide the necessary ingredients for optimal psychological development (i.e., the deficit/developmental failure model). Kernberg's view of BPO emphasizes the role of aggression in distorting internalized object relations, as "all good" and "all bad" self and object representations are actively kept apart by defenses based on splitting. In other words, Kernberg's theory of BPO is a *defense/conflict model.* In contrast to Kernberg's emphasis on defense as the cause of BPO, other theorists argue that failures in infant–caregiver interactions during childhood are the major cause of deficits in the psychic structure of patients with borderline personality disorder. In other words, these theorists hold to a *deficit/develop-*

mental failure model of psychopathology. For example, some have argued that experiences of abandonment by parents lead to the borderline individual's inability to tolerate aloneness (Adler and Buie 1979; Masterson 1981) or failure to achieve object constancy (Akhtar 1992, 1994). More recently, Peter Fonagy and Mary Target (1996) have proposed that borderline psychopathology results from deficits in the capacity for self-reflection and/or *mentalization,* which in turn result from impaired infant–caregiver interactions (Auchincloss and Samberg 2012, p. 28; Fonagy and Target 1996; Fonagy et al. 1993b, 2002). We will see another example of the defense/conflict versus the deficit/developmental failure debate in Chapter 12 when we explore differences in how Kernberg and Kohut conceptualized narcissistic problems.

Contemporary understanding of borderline psychopathology is informed by research from many fields, including social cognitive psychology and cognitive neuroscience (Depue and Lenzenweger 2001/ 2005; Donegan et al. 2003; Fertuck et al. 2006; Graham and Clark 2006; Lenzenweger et al. 2004; Minzenberg et al. 2006; Posner et al. 2002). This research supports a view of borderline psychopathology as resulting from the interaction of temperament and environmental risk factors, including abuse or neglect, which leads to an incoherent sense of self and other, insecure working models of attachment, deficits in mentalization, and poor systems of self-control.

Object Relations Theory and Psychodynamic Treatment

Object Relations Theory has made major contributions to our understanding of how psychodynamic psychotherapy works. We see these contributions most obviously in the specific psychodynamic psychotherapies developed for the treatment of borderline personality disorder. For example, Kernberg's own treatment for borderline personality disorder, called Transference-Focused Psychotherapy (TFP) (Clarkin et al. 2006), is based on his Object Relations Theory of borderline personality disorder. TFP is based on the premise that underlying object relations are activated in patient–therapist interactions. Therefore, it emphasizes work in the transference as offering the most effective means of addressing these underlying object relations. A primary task of the TFP therapist is to observe and interpret pathological object relations as they are activated in the patient–therapist relationship (Clarkin et al. 2006). In contrast to Kernberg's TFP, Anthony Bateman and Peter Fonagy have developed Mentalization-Based Treatment (MBT) for psychotherapy with patients with borderline personality disorders, which focuses on developing mentalizing capacity in these patients (Bateman and Fonagy 2004, 2006).

However, we see the influence of Object Relations Theory in all psychodynamic psychotherapies, not just those designed for severe personality disorders (Caligor et al. 2007). The most obvious influence is a change in the goals of therapy to include not just the aim of understanding wishes, prohibitions, and ideals and the habitual modes of managing conflict (Structural Model) but also the aim of building strong relationships with other people. Therapists using Object Relations Theory are very interested in how each patient finds attachments and intimate connections that are sustaining and how each patient maintains a sense of separateness. They are also interested in how each patient does (or does not) have internal structures marked by self and object constancy, which support a sense of being "good enough."

In addition, we see the influence of Object Relations Theory on how psychotherapy is conducted. For example, we see this influence in the strong emphasis on use of *countertransference* (defined as the therapist's feelings about the patient) as a primary source of information about the patient's inner life (Heimann 1950, 1956). We also see the influence of Object Relations Theory on theories of therapeutic action (Blatt et al. 1994; Fonagy et al. 1993a; Mayes and Spence 1994). For example, over time, theories have begun to emphasize the importance of the patient–therapist relationship not just as a source of information but also as a force for change. In general, over the years, we have seen a shift from early theories of therapeutic action emphasizing change resulting from *insight* derived from *interpretation* to more recent theories emphasizing change resulting from the relationship with the therapist. Various theorists have emphasized different aspects of the therapeutic relationship using different terminology, including the following: *corrective emotional experience* (Alexander and French 1946), *new object* (Loewald 1960); *real relationship* (Greenson and Wexler 1969), *therapeutic alliance* (Zetzel 1956), *holding environment* (Modell 1976), and *container/contained* (Bion 1963, 1970). Indeed, in our Preface and Introduction to this book, we mentioned the importance of the *therapeutic alliance* in all psychoanalytic treatments, a concept that has been increasingly well understood as a result of Object Relations Theory (Krupnick et al. 1996; Zetzel 1956).

A relatively recent school of psychoanalysis called Relational Psychoanalysis emphasizes that the meaning of the patient–therapist interaction is "co-created" and urges exploration of this co-creation process as a major emphasis of the work (Greenberg and Mitchell 1985). We will not discuss Relational Psychoanalysis in this book, as it consists mainly of theories about the clinical situation and how best to understand what goes on between patient and therapist. Many relational theorists have so stressed the phenomenon of co-created meaning that the concept of a model of the mind unique to the patient rather than co-created in the clinical situation is difficult to grasp.

The debate continues over which aspect of psychotherapy—the therapist's interpretations or the relationship between patient and therapist—is more important to therapeutic change. However, according to Glen Gabbard and Drew Westen (2003), this debate is of less relevance today than it was in the past. Nowadays, we must integrate many theories of therapeutic action, including the role of interpretation and the role of the relationship, which work together. Nevertheless, readers should keep this debate in mind as we move on to Chapter 12 ("Self Psychology"), where we will explore yet another model of the mind with a somewhat different view on how the therapeutic relationship helps the patient.

Chapter Summary and Chart of Core Dimensions

Table 11–1 introduces our Object Relations Theory chart of core dimensions, in which we have placed the following key concepts:

- **Topographic point of view:** Object relations are largely unconscious.
- **Motivational point of view:** People are object seeking from birth; object seeking is not secondary to other motivations. Wishes for *separation* from the object and for autonomy (*individuation*) are also inborn. There is inevitable conflict between wishes for affiliation and wishes for separation, accompanied by ambivalent feelings of love and hate for the object. If successful compromises are forged between these wishes and feelings, the individual acquires the ability to experience gratitude toward the object, along with growing confidence that envy can be overcome and damage to the relationship can be repaired.
- **Structural point of view:** The basic unit of experience is the *object relation*—an intrapsychic structure consisting of a self representation, an object representation, and the representation of an affectively charged interaction between self and object. Object relations can be either fleeting or enduring. Enduring object relations serve as templates for all psychic structures (such as ego, id, and superego) and for all future relationships. Related concepts include need-satisfying object, object constancy, self constancy, attachment behavioral system, internal working models of attachment, and mentalization.

- **Developmental point of view:** Object relations are largely formed in interaction with caregivers during childhood. Anna Freud, Klein, Bion, Winnicott, Bowlby, Mahler, Fonagy, and Kernberg have offered overlapping developmental models for object relations. Each of these developmental models ends in attainment of the capacity for *object constancy*, or the ability to maintain strong, positive ties to an object even in the face of separation, frustration, or anger.
- **Theory of psychopathology:** The quality of object relations serves as an index of mental health/illness. Strong, realistic object relations marked by object constancy are the hallmark of mental health. In contrast, disturbed object relations manifested by an inability to maintain object constancy are seen in many kinds of adult psychopathology, including severe personality disorders such as borderline, paranoid, and some narcissistic conditions, or any disorder characterized by borderline personality organization.
- **Theory of therapeutic action:** In psychodynamic psychotherapy, object relations are activated in the therapist–patient relationship, which is then used to understand them. As a result, Object Relations Theory leads to therapies that emphasize the transference, and especially the *countertransference*. It also leads to theories of therapeutic action that emphasize the role of *the therapist as a new object* (as opposed to theories that emphasize insight). Two well-known psychodynamic psychotherapies developed specifically for the treatment of borderline personality disorder are Kernberg's Transference-Focused Psychotherapy and Bateman and Fonagy's Mentalization-Based Treatment.

TABLE 11–1.   Object Relations Theory

Topography	Motivation	Structure/Process	Development	Psychopathology	Treatment
Object relations are largely unconscious	Conflicting wishes for affiliation and for separation-individuation	Object relation Self representation Object representation Representation of interaction between the two	Attachment Separation of self from other	The quality of object relations serves as an index of mental health/illness	Activation of object relations in the therapist–patient relationship
	Love/hate/ambivalence Envy/gratitude/repair	Need-satisfying object	Paranoid position and depressive position	Borderline personality organization (BPO)	Countertransference The therapist as a new object
		Object constancy Self constancy	Container/contained Good-enough mother Holding environment		Transference-Focused Psychotherapy
		Attachment behavioral system	Separation-individuation Differentiation Practicing		Mentalization-Based Treatment
		Internal working models of attachment	Rapprochement On the way to object constancy		
		Mentalization	Parenthood Midlife crisis		
			Development of mentalization		

References

Adler G, Buie DH: Aloneness and borderline psychopathology: the possible relevance of Child Dev issues. Int J Psychoanal 60:83–96, 1979

Ainsworth MDS, Blehar MC, Waters E, et al: Patterns of Attachment: A Psychological Study of the Strange Situation. Hillsdale, NJ, Lawrence Erlbaum, 1978

Akhtar S: Broken Structures: Severe Personality Disorders and Their Treatment. Northvale, NJ, Jason Aronson, 1992

Akhtar S: Object constancy and adult psychopathology. Int J Psychoanal 75:441–455, 1994

Alexander F, French T: Psychoanalytic Therapy: Principles and Application. New York, Ronald Press, 1946

American Psychiatric Association: Diagnostic and Statistical Manual of Mental Disorders, 5th Edition. Arlington, VA, American Psychiatric Publishing, 2013

Anthony EJ, Benedek T (eds): Parenthood: Its Psychology and Psychopathology. Boston, MA, Little, Brown, 1970

Auchincloss EL, Samberg E: Psychoanalytic Terms and Concepts. New Haven, CT, Yale University Press, 2012

Bandura A: Social Foundations of Thought and Action: A Social Cognitive Theory. Englewood Cliffs, NJ, Prentice-Hall, 1986

Bateman A, Fonagy P: Psychotherapy for Borderline Personality Disorder: Mentalization-Based Treatment. Oxford, UK, Oxford University Press, 2004

Bateman A, Fonagy P: Mentalization-Based Treatment for Borderline Personality Disorder: A Practical Guide. Oxford, UK, Oxford University Press, 2006

Beebe B, Lachmann F: The relational turn in psychoanalysis: a dyadic systems view from infant research. Contemporary Psychoanalysis 39:379–409, 2003

Beebe B, Stern DN: Engagement-disengagement and early object experience, in Communicative Structure and Psychic Structures. Edited by Freedman M, Grenel S. New York, Plenum, 1977, pp 33–55

Beebe B, Jaffe J, Lachmann F: A dyadic systems view of communication, in Relational Perspectives in Psychoanalysis. Edited by Skolnick N, Warshaw S. Hillsdale, NJ, Analytic Press, 1992, pp 61–81

Beebe B, Jaffe J, Buck K, et al: Six-week postpartum depressive symptoms and 4-month mother-infant self- and interactive contingency. Infant Mental Health Journal 29:442–471, 2008

Bion W: Learning from Experience. London, Heinemann, 1962

Bion W: Elements of Psycho-Analysis. London, Heinemann, 1963

Bion W: Second Thoughts: Selected Papers on Psycho-analysis. London, Heinemann, 1967

Bion W: Attention and Interpretation: A Scientific Approach to Insight in Psycho-analysis and Groups. London, Tavistock, 1970

Blatt S, Lerner H: Investigations in the psychoanalytic theory of object relations and object representations, in Empirical Studies of Psychoanalytic Theories. Edited by Masling F. Hillsdale, NJ, Lawrence Erlbaum, 1983, pp 189–249

Blatt S, Ford R, Berman W, et al: Therapeutic Change: An Object Relations Perspective. New York, Plenum, 1994

Blos P: The second individuation process of adolescence. Psychoanal Study Child 22:162–186, 1967

Bowlby J: Forty-four juvenile thieves: their characters and home life. Int J Psychoanal 25:107–128, 1944

Bowlby J: Attachment and Loss, Vol 1: Attachment (1969). New York, Basic Books, 1982

Bowlby J: Attachment and Loss, Vol 2: Separation: Anxiety and Anger. New York, Basic Books, 1973

Bowlby J: Attachment and Loss, Vol 3: Loss: Sadness and Depression. New York, Basic Books, 1980

Calabrese M, Farber B, Westen D: The relationship of adult attachment constructs to object relational patterns of representing self and others. J Am Psychoanal Assoc 33:513–530, 2005

Caligor E, Kernberg OF, Clarkin JF: Handbook for Dynamic Psychotherapy for Higher-Level Personality Pathology. Washington, DC, American Psychiatric Publishing, 2007

Cassidy J: The nature of the child's ties, in The Handbook of Attachment Theory and Research, 2nd Edition. Edited by Cassidy J, Shaver P. New York, Guilford, 2008, pp 3–22

Clarkin JF, Yeomans FE, Kernberg OF: Psychotherapy for Borderline Personality: Focusing on Object Relations. Arlington, VA, American Psychiatric Publishing, 2006

Coates SW: John Bowlby and Margaret S. Mahler. J Am Psychoanal Assoc 52:571–601, 2004

Cuthbert BN, Insel TR: Toward precision medicine in psychiatry: the NIMH research domain criteria project, in The Neurobiology of Mental Illness, 4th Edition. Edited by Charney DS, Sklar P, Buxbaum JD, et al. New York, Oxford University Press, 2013, pp 1076–1088

Deklyen M, Greenberg M: Attachment and psychopathology in childhood, in Handbook of Attachment Theory, Research and Clinical Applications, 2nd Edition. Edited by Cassidy J, Shaver P. New York, Guilford, 2008, pp 637–665

Depue R, Lenzenweger M: A neurobehavioral dimensional model of personality disturbance (2001), in Handbook of Personality Disorders. Edited by Livesley W. New York, Guilford, 2005, pp 136–176

Donegan N, Sanislow C, Blumberg H, et al: Amygdala hyperreactivity in borderline personality disorder: implications for emotional dysregulation. Biol Psychiatry 54:1284–93, 2003

Eisenberg L: The social construction of the human brain. Am J Psychiatry 152:1563–1575, 1995

Erikson E: The problem of ego identity. J Am Psychoanal Assoc 4:56–121, 1956

Fairbairn W: An Object-Relations Theory of the Personality. New York, Basic Books, 1954

Fertuck E, Lenzenweger M, Clarkin J, et al: Executive neurocognition, memory systems, and borderline personality disorder. Clinical Psychology Review 26:346–375, 2006

Fonagy P: Attachment Theory and Psychoanalysis. New York, Other Press, 2001

Fonagy P, Target M: Playing with reality, I: theory of mind and the normal development of psychic reality. Int J Psychoanal 77:217–233, 1996

Fonagy P, Moran G, Edgcumbe R, et al: The roles of mental representations and mental processes in therapeutic action. Psychoanal Study Child 48:9–48, 1993a

Fonagy P, Steele M, Moran G, et al: Measuring the ghost in the nursery: an empirical study of the relation between parents' mental representations of childhood experiences and their infants' security of attachment. J Am Psychoanal Assoc 41:929–989, 1993b

Fonagy P, Gergely G, Jurist E, et al: Affect Regulation, Mentalization, and the Development of the Self. New York, Other Press, 2002

Freud A: The concept of developmental lines. Psychoanal Study Child 18:245–265, 1963

Fromm-Reichmann F: Principles of Intensive Psychotherapy. Chicago, IL, University of Chicago Press, 1950

Gabbard G, Westen D: Rethinking therapeutic action. Int J Psychoanal 84:823–841, 2003

Graham S, Clark M: Self-esteem and organization of valenced information about others: The "Jekyll and Hyde"-ing of relationship partners. J Pers Soc Psychol 90:652–665, 2006

Greenberg J, Mitchell S: Object Relations in Psychoanalytic Theory. Boston, MA, Harvard University Press, 1983

Greenson R, Wexler M: The nontransference relationship in the psychoanalytic situation. Int J Psychoanal 50:27–39, 1969

Harlow HF, Zimmermann RR: The development of affective responsiveness in infant monkeys. Proc Am Philos Soc 102:501–509, 1958

Hartmann H: The mutual influences in the development of ego and id. Psychoanal Study Child 7:9–30, 1952

Hartmann H: Contribution to the metapsychology of schizophrenia. Psychoanal Study Child 8:177–198, 1953

Heimann P: On counter-transference. Int J Psychoanal 31:81–84, 1950

Heimann P: Dynamics of transference interpretations. Int J Psychoanal 37:303–310, 1956

Hofer MS: Relationships as regulators: a psychobiologic perspective on bereavement. Psychosom Med 46:183–197, 1984

Hofer M: Hidden regulators: implications for a new understanding of attachment, separation and loss, in Attachment Theory: Social, Developmental, and Clinical Perspectives. Edited by Goldberg S, Muir R, Kerr J. Hillsdale, NJ, Analytic Press, 1995, pp 203–230

Jacques E: Death and the mid-life crises. Int J Psychoanal 46:502–514, 1965

Johnson SC, Dweck CS, Chen FS: Evidence for infants' internal working models of attachment. Psychol Sci 18:501–502, 2007

Kernberg O: A psychoanalytic classification of character pathology. J Am Psychoanal Assoc 18:800–822, 1970

Kernberg O: Borderline Conditions and Pathological Narcissism. New York, Jason Aronson, 1975

Kernberg O: Object Relations Theory and Clinical Psychoanalysis. New York, Jason Aronson, 1976

Kernberg O: Neurobiological correlates of object relations theory: the relationship between neurobiological and psychodynamic development. International Forum of Psychoanalysis 2014. Available at: http://www.tandfonline.com/doi/abs/10.1080/0803706X.2014.912352#.VJsSAv8OS80. Accessed December 24, 2014.

King P, Steiner R (eds): The Freud–Klein Controversies 1941–45. London, Tavistock/Routledge, 1991

Klein M: The Psycho-Analysis of Children. London, Hogarth Press, 1932

Klein M: The Oedipus complex in the light of early anxieties. Int J Psychoanal 26:11–33, 1945

Klein M: Love, Guilt and Reparation, and Other Works, 1921–1945. London, Hogarth Press, 1975a

Klein M: Envy and Gratitude, and Other Works, 1946–1963. London, Hogarth Press, 1975b

Krupnick JL, Sotsky SM, Elkin I, et al: Therapeutic alliance in psychotherapy and pharmacotherapy outcome: findings in the National Institute of Mental Health treatment of depression collaborative research program. J Consult Clin Psychol 64:532–539, 1996

Lenzenweger M, Clarkin J, Fertuck E, et al: Executive neurocognitive functioning and neurobehavioral systems indicators in borderline personality disorder: a preliminary study. J Pers Disord 18:421–438, 2004

Loewald H: On the therapeutic action of psychoanalysis. Int J Psychoanal 41:16–33, 1960

Lorenz K: King Solomon's Ring (1949). New York, Harper-Collins, 1979

Lyons-Ruth K, Jacobvitz D: Attachment disorganization: genetic factors, parenting contexts, and developmental transformation from infancy to adulthood, in The Handbook of Attachment Theory and Research, 2nd Edition. Edited by Cassidy J, Shaver P. New York, Guilford, 2008, pp 666–697

Mahler M, Pine F, Bergman A: The Psychological Birth of the Human Infant. New York, Basic Books, 1975

Main M, Solomon J: Discovery of an insecure disorganized/disoriented attachment pattern: procedures, findings and implications for the classification of behavior, in Affective Development in Infancy. Edited by Brazelton TB, Yogman MW. Norwood, NJ, Ablex, 1986, pp 95–124

Main M, Kaplan N, Cassidy J: Security in infancy, childhood and adulthood: a move to the level of representation, in Growing Points of Attachment Theory and Research. Edited by Bretherton I, Waters E. Monographs of the Society for Research in Child Development 50(1–2):66–104, 1985

Masterson J: The Narcissistic and Borderline Disorders. New York, Brunner/Mazel, 1981

Mayes LC, Spence DP: Understanding therapeutic action in the analytic situation: a second look at the developmental metaphor. J Am Psychoanal Assoc 42:789–816, 1994

Milrod B, Markowitz JC, Gerber AJ, et al: Childhood separation anxiety and the pathogenesis and treatment of adult anxiety. Am J Psychiatry 171:34–43, 2014

Minzenberg M, Poole J, Vinogradov S: Adult social attachment disturbance is related to childhood maltreatment and current symptoms in borderline personality disorder. J Nerv Ment Dis 194:341–348, 2006

Modell AH: "The holding environment" and the therapeutic action of psychoanalysis. J Am Psychoanal Assoc 24:285–307, 1976

Nigg J, Lohr N, Westen D, et al: Malevolent object representation in borderline personality disorder and major depression. J Abnorm Psychol 101:61–67, 1992

Piaget J: Construction of Reality in the Child (1954). London, Psychology Press, 1990

Posner M, Rothbart M, Vizueta N, et al: Attentional mechanisms of borderline personality disorder. Proc Natl Acad Sci U S A 99:16366–16370, 2002

Schacter DL, Gilbert DT, Wegner DM (eds): Psychology, 2nd Edition. New York, Worth, 2011

Schore A: Affect Regulation and the Origin of the Self: The Neurobiology of Emotional Development. Hillsdale, NJ, Lawrence Erlbaum, 1994

Segal H: An Introduction to the Work of Melanie Klein. London, Karnac, 1946

Smith AS, Kelly L, Wang Z: The neurobiology of social attachment, in The Neurobiology of Mental Illness, 4th Edition. Edited by Charney DS, Sklar P, Buxbaum JD, et al. New York, Oxford University Press, 2013, pp 1112–1126

Spitz R: Hospitalism—an inquiry into the genesis of psychiatric conditions in early childhood. Psychoanal Study Child 1:53–74, 1945

Spitz R, Wolf K: Anaclitic depression—an inquiry into the genesis of psychiatric conditions in early childhood. Psychoanal Study Child 2:313–342, 1946

Stern DN: The Interpersonal World of the Infant: A View from Psychoanalysis and Developmental Psychology. New York, Basic Books, 1985

Tronick E: Emotions and emotional communication in infants. Am Psychol 44:112–119, 1989

Uher R, Caspi A, Houts R, et al: Serotonin transporter gene moderates childhood maltreatment's effect on persistent but not single-episode depression: replications and implications for resolving inconsistent results. J Affect Disord 135:56–65, 2011

Wegner DM, Vallacher RR: Implicit Psychology: An Introduction to Social Cognition. New York, Oxford University Press, 1977

Weinberger J, Weiss J: Psychoanalytic and cognitive conceptions of the unconscious, in Cognitive Science and the Unconscious. Edited by Stein DJ. Washington, DC, American Psychiatry Publishing, 1997, pp 23–54

Westen D: Towards a revised theory of borderline object relations: contributions of empirical research. Int J Psychoanal 71:661–693, 1990

Westen D: Social cognition and object relations. Psychol Bull 109:429–455, 1991

Willick M: On the concept of primitive defenses. J Am Psychoanal Assoc 31 (suppl):175–200, 1983

Willick M: Psychoanalysis and schizophrenia: a cautionary tale. J Am Psychoanal Assoc 49:27–56, 2001

Winnicott DW: The depressive position in normal emotional development (1954), in Through Paediatrics to Psycho-Analysis: Collected Papers. New York, Basic Books, 1958, pp 262–277

Winnicott DW: The Maturational Processes and the Facilitating Environment. New York, International Universities Press, 1965

Winnicott DW: Playing and Reality. New York, Basic Books, 1971

Winnicott DW: Through Paediatrics to Psycho-Analysis: Collected Papers. New York, Basic Books, 1958

Zetzel E: Current concepts of transference. Int J Psychoanal 37:69–375, 1956

Zimmermann P, Brückl T, Nocon A, et al: Interaction of FKBP5 gene variants and adverse life events in predicting depression onset: results from a ten-year prospective community study. Am J Psychiatry 168:1107–1116, 2011

CHAPTER 12

Self Psychology

This chapter introduces Self Psychology. It explains how this model of the mind works and what it contributes to our understanding of psychopathology and treatment. Vocabulary introduced in this chapter includes the following: *affect mirroring, alien self, core sense of self, disorder of the self, emergent sense of self, empathy, false self, grandiose self, idealized parental imago, idealized selfobject, idealizing transference, identity diffusion, mirror transference, mirroring selfobject, narcissism, narcissistic rage, narrative sense of self, pathological grandiose self, pathological narcissism, self, selfobject, selfobject transference, self–selfobject matrix, subjective sense of self, transitional object, transitional phenomena, true self, twinship transference,* and *verbal or categorical sense of self.*

As with the Topographic Model and the early Structural Model, Self Psychology was largely the work of one man—Heinz Kohut (1913–1981) developed this model in the 1960s, 1970s, and 1980s. In common with Melanie Klein and others who developed Object Relations Theory, Kohut was initially schooled in the Structural Model (or Ego Psychology) but came to feel that that model was insufficient to describe or treat the patients and problems that he saw. However, Kohut did not work with object relations theorists but instead proposed his own model of the mind.

The Self and Its Development

Self Psychology is a theory of the mind based on a structure at the core of the personality—the *self*. In this theory, the *self* is a mostly unconscious structure that is defined as the center of initiative and a source of the coherent experience of sameness. The self is made up of an individual's ambitions, ideals, and talents. The self is healthy if it is characterized by feelings of cohesion and continuity; feelings of energy and initiative; mature self-assertion, self-esteem, and pride; and investment in a stable set of ideals and goals. The self is also considered healthy if it is characterized by the ability to regulate affects and to make use of interactions with selfobjects. When an individual has psychopathology, or a *disorder of the self*, the self feels weak, incoherent, ineffective, and bad, or it cannot find meaning in goals or ideals (Auchincloss and Samberg 2012, pp. 234–238).

Developmental theory describes the growth of the self in detail and is very important in Self Psychology. Self Psychology asserts that the individual is born with an innate set of *narcissistic strivings* that serve as the major force for motivation in the personality. *Narcissism* is defined as an investment in the self. These innate narcissistic strivings include needs for aliveness, authenticity, coherence, mastery, safety, autonomy, uniqueness, creativity, a sense of agency and purpose, and self-esteem. The self develops from an admixture of innate factors and interactions with caregivers. Among the inborn needs of the infant is a need for recognition from caregivers, who must respond with *empathy* to infant's growing self. *Empathy* is defined as the capacity to feel or to understand the subjective experience of another person. Empathic responsiveness in caregivers, usually the mother and the father, is vital to the development of the self. These empathic caregivers are the child's first *selfobjects*. A *selfobject* is defined as another person who is experienced as part of the self and who fulfills the needs of the self. Indeed, in Self Psychology, the self cannot be conceptualized outside of the *self-selfobject matrix*.

According to Self Psychology, there are two major narcissistic lines of development, or components of the self that develop in the child in interaction with caregivers. One component is the *grandiose self*, which expresses innate strivings for power and recognition. The grandiose self develops in interaction with a *mirroring selfobject* who validates and takes pleasure in the child's exhibitionism and accomplishments. The other component of the self is the *idealized parental imago*, which results from the child's attributions of omnipotence and perfection to caregivers. The idealized parental imago develops in interaction with an *ideal-*

ized selfobject who provides the strength and calm needed for the child to feel safe and to develop affect regulation.

In the course of development, both of these components of the self grow stronger through gradual internalization of empathic selfobject experiences. In other words, internalization occurs in the context of the caregiver's empathic responsiveness to the child's selfobject strivings. Over time, the grandiose self matures into stable self-esteem, assertion, and realistic ambition. The idealized parental imago matures into enduring ideals. The mature and healthy self then is able to pursue ideals with assertion and energy.

In Self Psychology, dreams often reflect the state of the self, in what Kohut and his followers have called *self-state dreams* (Kohut 1971, 1977, 1984) (see Chapter 6, "The World of Dreams"). We can also see here that Kohut has elaborated on Freud's concept of the *ego ideal* (see Chapter 9, "The Id and the Superego") in his theory of the development of the self and its ideals or goals.

Kohut's Theory of Adult Psychopathology: Disorders of the Self

According to Kohut's theory, disorders of the self result when a caregiver does not mirror the child's grandiosity—or reflect back to the child the needed recognition, validation, and joyful acceptance of this grandiosity. Disorders of the self also result when a caregiver does not help the child to modulate his or her grandiosity. In both of these cases, the *grandiose self* is repressed or disavowed, or is poorly integrated within the adult personality. It retains its childish quality and fails to mature into healthy self-esteem and self-assertion. In serious cases or under severe stress, individuals with disorders of the self may have trouble managing aspects of reality, as in borderline conditions or addictions. Disorders of the self also result when a caregiver does not allow the child to develop and/or modulate the *idealized parental imago.* Failures such as this occur when the caregiver either seriously disappoints the child or fails consistently to meet the child's expectations. In such cases, wishes for an idealized parent may persist in their childish form, or the child may give up on such wishes. In either case, the child is not able to develop lasting ideals and goals.

In other words, in disorders of the self, clinicians may see a weakening of either the grandiose self or the idealized parental imago. The clinician may also see compensatory structures developed to make up for a weak self, such as aloofness, addiction, or perversion, to mention a few. Disorders of the self include what is called narcissistic personality disorder in DSM-5 (American Psychiatric Association 2013). Disorders of the self may also be accompanied by *narcissistic rage* (Kohut 1972/1978). Narcissistic rage is understood as a consequence of a perceived threat to the self and is triggered and accompanied by experiences of shame, humiliation, and/or disappointment. Narcissistic rage can range from trivial irritation to fanatical fury and is characterized by the need for revenge and justice. Easy susceptibility to narcissistic rage makes for relationships with others that are volatile and unstable (Kohut and Wolf 1978).

Kohut's Theory of Therapeutic Action: Mobilization of Selfobject Transferences

In Self Psychology, treatment consists of guiding patients with disorders of the self as they experience a reactivation of the original needs of the self in the form of a variety of selfobject transferences. In fact, Kohut first began to sketch out his model of Self Psychology because he felt that the Structural Model of the mind did not help him to understand the transferences of his patients, which he called *narcissistic transferences*. With mobilization of a *mirror transference*, the patient's archaic grandiose self is revived. In these transferences, the patient wants the therapist to behave in ways that validate or recognize the self. With mobilization of an *idealizing transference,* the patient's idealized parental imago is revived. In these transferences, the patient wants the therapist to behave in ways that are experienced as perfect. The patient may also develop a *twinship transference,* in which he or she assumes or demands that the patient and the therapist are exactly the same. This transference serves to make a weak self stronger.

Mobilization of these selfobject transferences serves as an opportunity for renewed development of the self. Indeed, in Self Psychology, psychodynamic therapy is approached from a developmental point of view. The therapist focuses on the selfobject function of the transference, linking the transference to selfobject functions that the patient experiences as having been missing during his or her childhood. In this way, the transference is seen as expressing a longing for these selfobject functions to be taken over by the therapist, so that a weakened self can be repaired. In other words, the therapist emphasizes the patient's felt need rather than the patient's feelings of having unacceptable wishes.

In Self Psychology, examination of moments of disruption between patient and therapist is central for therapeutic action. These moments, in which the therapist fails to understand the patient's need, are inevitable. They provide an opportunity for patient and therapist to better understand what is felt to be missing in the present and in the past and to better understand what is felt to be required for repair.

Although Kohut argued that the therapist's empathy is not in itself part of the therapeutic action, he considered empathic communication and interpretation to be a requisite ingredient for psychological change (Kohut 1984). Furthermore, the therapist's ongoing effort to be empathic plays an important role in treatment by diminishing the patient's need for defenses and expanding the patient's capacity for introspection, promoting the emergence of warded-off feelings and memories, which can then be explored.

Comparison of Self Psychology With the Structural Model and Object Relations Theory

A brief comparison of several of the basic tenets of Self Psychology with those of the Structural Model and Object Relations Theory may be useful in clarifying how Self Psychology differs from those earlier models:

- **Topographic point of view**—Self Psychology does not differ significantly from the Structural Model or from Object Relations Theory in that the self has both conscious and unconscious aspects.
- **Motivational point of view**—In Self Psychology, the strivings of the self, or *narcissistic needs*, are the driving force in the personality, in contrast to unacceptable wishes for bodily pleasure (Structural Model) (Ornstein 1993) or needs for attachment/separation (Object Relations Theory). Indeed, if other wishes are too evident, in Self Psychology they are conceptualized as the result of threats to the self. Narcissistic strivings have their own line of development and cannot be reduced to other needs (Structural Model); in Self Psychology, aggression, or *narcissistic rage*, is a consequence of a perceived threat to the self rather than an inborn striving (Structural Model and some kinds of Object Relations Theory).
- **Structural point of view**—In Self Psychology, the self is the superordinate of structure in the mind, as opposed to ego, id, and superego (Structural Model) or object relations (Object Relations Theory). When evident, other structures (such as the id or superego) are conceptualized as the result of threats to the self.
- **Developmental point of view**—Whereas all models affirm that empathic responses from caregivers serve an important selfobject func-

tion that is crucial to development, in Self Psychology it is the actual behavior of the caregiver, especially *empathic behavior,* that is spotlighted as the major contributor to the child's experience of self, as opposed to the thoughts, feelings, and fantasies within the child's own mind (Structural Model and Object Relations Theory). Selfobject needs persists throughout the life cycle; narcissistic strivings are never outgrown but instead develop into mature forms, such as creativity, humor, and wisdom.

- **Theory of psychopathology and theory of therapeutic action**—In Self Psychology, psychopathology is the result of arrested development, or selfobject failures on the part of caregivers, rather than the result of conflict (Structural Model and most kinds of Object Relations Theory). In Self Psychology, the oedipus complex is not the predominant conflict in psychopathology (Structural Model) (Terman 1984/1985); instead, *disorder of the self* is the most important diagnostic concept in psychopathology, replacing *neurosis* (Structural Model) and/or *borderline personality organization* (Object Relations Theory). In Self Psychology, the reactivation of selfobject needs in the transference is conceptualized as the expression of frustrated needs from childhood, as opposed to being conceptualized as representing conflict, defense, and compromise (Structural Model and most kinds of Object Relations Theory). Finally, the empathic understanding offered by the therapist is crucial to therapeutic action, as opposed to insight gained through interpretation (Structural Model and some kinds of Object Relations Theory).

Narcissistic Personality Disorder: Kohut Versus Kernberg

A good way to deepen one's understanding of Self Psychology is to consider the controversy between Heinz Kohut and Otto Kernberg about how best to conceptualize narcissistic personality disorder. These thinkers agree on the description of a certain kind of individual who is preoccupied with fantasies of success and power, who expects to be seen as special or superior, who is demanding of constant attention, who is envious of others who have more than he or she does, who is intent on being seen as powerful and perfect, who is arrogant and prone to rage and depression, and who is lacking in empathy for others. Such people are described as having narcissistic personality disorder (NPD) (American Psychiatric Association 2013).

Kohut's View

In Kohut's view, patients with NPD show the persistence of a grandiose self left over from childhood in situations in which caregivers failed to meet selfobject needs during the childhood. In cases such as these, the child's grandiose self has failed to mature and still seeks selfobject recognition from others in an intense form. When selfobject recognition cannot be found, narcissistic rage ensues because the self feels threatened.

According to Kohut's treatment model, the therapist must allow the patient's thwarted selfobject needs to emerge in the transference. The therapist must then handle this selfobject transference with empathic understanding. Finally, inevitable empathic failures in the treatment must be explored so as to promote growth. Ultimately, the remobilized grandiose self can resume maturation and be integrated into the patient's personality.

Kernberg's View

In Kernberg's view (see Chapter 11, "Object Relations Theory"), the patient with NPD does not show the persistence of a normal grandiose self left over from childhood; instead, this individual shows a new pathological structure that Kernberg calls the *pathological grandiose self,* which forms the center of what Kernberg terms *pathological narcissism.* This pathological grandiose self serves to ward off dependency on another person, who is experienced as important only when giving praise. Rather than having any other needs, the individual with NPD prefers to see him- or herself as self-sufficient. In other words, for Kernberg, the pathological grandiose self is a defense against dependency. If an individual with NPD were to experience true dependency, that individual would immediately experience him- or herself to be in the *paranoid position* (see Chapter 11) and would feel *persecutory anxiety* (see Chapter 11). This is because underneath, the individual with NPD is unable to integrate bad and good experiences of the object (see Chapter 11), because his or her angry feelings at this object feel too strong.

According to Kernberg's treatment model, the therapist must allow the patient's pathological grandiose self to emerge in the transference. The therapist must then interpret the patient's defenses against dependency (and the paranoid position). Finally, the therapist must help the patient to understand that his or her paranoid fears are a reflection of the patient's own aggression toward the object (and the therapist). When this aggression becomes more manageable, the patient will develop the ability to integrate good and bad experiences toward the therapist, thereby overcoming the paranoid position (Kernberg 1975, 1976).

Discussion

Although this comparison is highly oversimplified, it does serve to highlight some of the differences between Self Psychology (Kohut) and the Structural Model/Object Relations Theory (Kernberg) toward NPD. The differences lie in 1) the extent to which the grandiose self is seen as either a normal vestige of childhood (Kohut) or a pathological structure (Kernberg); 2) the extent to which the grandiose self is conceptualized as either a *deficit* due to empathic failures in caregivers during childhood (Kohut) or a *defense* against dependency (Kernberg); and 3) the extent to which aggression is seen as either the result of threats to the self (Kohut) or the underlying cause of the whole problem, making integration of experience impossible (Kernberg). Many clinicians use both models (see Chapter 13, "Toward an Integrated Psychoanalytic Model of the Mind"), emphasizing Self Psychology with some kinds of patients and Kernberg's model with other kinds of patients. Many also use both models with the same patient at different times, employing a more empathic stance at some times and a stance that includes confrontation of the patient's aggressive feelings at other times. Many use a more empathic stance early in the treatment, when the patient feels more vulnerable to criticism and less trusting of the therapist.

Influence of Self Psychology on Psychodynamic Psychotherapy

Self Psychology has influenced psychodynamic treatment in several important ways, even if the clinician does not adhere to the whole of Self Psychology in every situation. First of all, Self Psychology emphasizes the empathic immersion of the therapist in the patient's experience as being important for all psychodynamic treatment. In addition, Self Psychology provides a developmental rationale for why empathic immersion is crucial to the patient, and Self Psychology alerts the therapist to watch for the consequences of empathic failure. Self Psychology also alerts the therapist to watch for specific selfobject transferences in all patients and to manage these transferences properly. In addition, Self Psychology alerts the therapist to look for a history of empathic failures on the part of caregivers and other significant objects and to look for ways in which patients manage ongoing selfobject needs. Finally, Self

Psychology reminds the therapist that narcissistic strivings are inborn and natural and pursue their own line of development and that patients may be highly self-critical and/or ashamed of these strivings. We see the influence of Self Psychology when the clinician works with the patient to help the patient become the center of his or her own life story, lived with meaning, and to develop goals that are invested with interest and pursued with energy and creativity.

Other Conceptions of the Self: Contributions From Ego Psychology and Object Relations Theorists

We have seen that although both the Structural Model and Object Relations Theory include a concept of self, the conception of self in these models is very different from the conception of self in Self Psychology. For example, in Chapter 8 ("A New Configuration and a New Concept: The Ego") we explored Erikson's theories on *ego identity* (Erikson 1950, 1956), and in Chapter 11 ("Object Relations Theory") we examined Mahler's theories on *individuation* and her concept of *practicing* (Mahler et al. 1975). Certainly both of these theorists were aware of the need for individuals to develop a coherent and strong self, defined in various ways. Also in Chapter 11, we saw that Kernberg's theory includes the concept of *identity diffusion* (borrowed from Erikson), an incoherent experience of the self evinced in patients with borderline personality organization (but not in those with NPD; Kernberg argues that patients with NPD are protected against identity diffusion by the organization provided by the pathological grandiose self). However, Kernberg contends that identity diffusion is caused by the individual's failure to integrate good and bad experiences of the self (i.e., *self inconstancy*) rather than by empathic failures of the original selfobjects. Nevertheless, Self Psychology and other models of the mind, especially Object Relations Theory, overlap in that most models are interested in how interactions with caregivers promote the growth or dysfunction of the self. Let us look some more at several important theorists from other models to see better what we mean.

Winnicott, whose ideas were explored a bit in Chapter 11, was also very interested in the role of the mother in promoting aspects of the infant's self. For example, he wrote extensively about the good-enough mother, the holding environment, and the mirroring function of the mother's face. He also wrote about the *transitional object,* defined as a teddy bear, blanket, or some other important object that the child experiences as both "me" and "not me" simultaneously, and about *transitional phenomena* in general as being important in the development of the child's capacity for play, fantasy, and a complex inner life. Finally, Winnicott wrote about how children who were deprived of a facilitating maternal environment develop a *false self* that is displayed in response to the caregiver's expectations and demands while the *true self* lies buried deep within (Winnicott 1953, 1965, 1971).

Winnicott's ideas were very influential on the development of Self Psychology and also on the work of two other psychoanalytic "baby watchers": Daniel Stern and Peter Fonagy. Stern wrote about development of the self in interaction in the first relationship with the mother, describing the stages of self development as *emergent sense of self* (birth to 2 months), *core sense of self* (2–6 months), *subjective sense of self* (beginning around 9 months), *verbal or categorical sense of self* (beginning around 18 months), and *narrative sense of self* (beginning in the third or fourth year) (Stern 1985, 1989). By placing the narrative sense of self as the final stage of development, Stern is putting the capacity to tell a story about the self at the center of his concept of full development. Here Stern is in agreement with cognitive psychologists, who increasingly use what they call *scripts* as probes for investigation (Tomkins 1986). He is also in agreement with Damasio (see Chapter 1, "Overview: Modeling the Life of the Mind") and others from the field of neuroscience, who stress the importance of narrative, arguing that the self is a story that the mind tells itself in a high level of self-monitoring (Damasio 1984, 1999). Finally, Stern is in agreement with clinicians who emphasize the self as being at the center of storytelling in the treatment situation.

Fonagy likewise has written extensively about the development of the self in terms of the capacity for *mentalization* (see Chapter 1 and Appendix C, "Glossary"), which always develops in interaction with the mother (see Chapter 11). Fonagy describes in detail how the mother's *affect mirroring* of the child lays the groundwork for the child's development of mentalization, as she helps the child become confident that he or she can manage intense feeling states and can tell the difference between self and other, and between reality and fantasy. If the mother's affect mirroring is mistuned, insensitive, or otherwise defective, the child may go on to develop an *alien self*, which is similar to Winnicott's *false self* (Fonagy et al. 2002). We have already seen in Chapter 11 how these children may also go on to develop borderline personality disorder.

In Fonagy's work, we find that the development of affect tolerance, mentalization, and the self are closely related. We also hear echoes of Bion (see Chapter 11), who stressed the mother's important role in helping the child to develop affect tolerance (Bion 1962, 1963, 1967, 1970). Indeed, many self psychologists have argued for a reworking of the view of therapeutic action posited by Self Psychology to include not only the therapist's empathic mirroring of the patient (per Kohut's views) but also the therapist's additional function of taking on the role of the containing mother (per Bion's views) in helping the patient to manage intense feelings that may otherwise be difficult for the patient to handle and may lead to continued psychopathology (Newman 2007; Socarides and Stolorow 1984). We can see here that clinicians in the office often draw from several models of the mind in their work with patients. As we move on to Chapter 13 ("Toward an Integrated Psychoanalytic Model of the Mind"), where we consider how to develop a psychoanalytic model that incorporates the best features of all models, readers should keep in mind the idea that in this case, clinicians are melding the views of Kohut and Bion.

The Study of the Self: Contributions From General Psychology and Neuroscience

Meanwhile, as psychodynamic psychotherapists are working out how to use Self Psychology in their work with patients, investigators from many branches of general psychology, including personality theory, developmental psychology, and social psychology, are studying concepts of the self, using methodologies appropriate to these fields. Areas of study include the following: self-concept (an individual's explicit knowledge of his or her own behaviors, traits, or characteristics) (Baumeister 1998); self-narrative (the stories that individuals tell about themselves) (McAdams 1993; McLean 2008); self-schema (traits used by individuals to define themselves) (Markus 1977); self-relevance (an individual's enhanced awareness of phenomena relating to him- or herself) (Rogers et al. 1977); self-concept and memory (Kihlstrom et al. 2002); self-verification (an individual's tendency to seek evidence to confirm his or her self-concept) (Swann et al. 2003); the feeling of agency (an individual's sense of initiative) (Haggard and Tsakiris 2009); locus of control (an individual's habitual tendency to locate the cause of events either within or outside of him- or herself) (Rotter 1966); self-consistency (the need for and extent of feelings of coherence) (Lecky 1945); self-esteem (the extent to which an individual likes, values, or accepts him- or herself) (Baumeister et al. 2003; Brown 1993); self-discrepancy (the extent to which an individual's self-schema matches his or her preferred self-schema) (Higgins 1987); the relationship between self-esteem and status (Barkow 1980); the relationship between self-esteem and a sense of belonging (Leary and Baumeister 2000); self-efficacy (the extent to which an individual feels effective) (Bandura 1977); and self-serving bias (the tendency for individuals to take credit for their successes but to downplay responsibility for their failures) (Miller and Ross 1975; Shepperd et al. 2008). Efforts are also being made to integrate findings from general psychology with psychoanalysis (Andersen et al. 2005; Westen 1992). Neuroscientists, too, are investigating the neural structures that underlie the self (Damasio 1984, 1999; Feinberg 2001; LeDoux 2002; Macrae et al. 2004; Mitchell et al. 2002; Morin 2002). Empathy is receiving a great deal of attention from both psychologists and neuroscientists (Carr et al. 2003; Decety and Ickes 2009). In addition, the concept of *self* interfaces with the National Institute of Mental Health Research Domain Criteria, domain "Social Processes"; construct "Perception and Understanding of Self"; and subconstructs "agency" and "self-knowledge" (Cuthbert and Insel 2013).[1]

The Self
in the Psychoanalytic Model of the Mind

The self is so important in the study of psychology that it may seem odd that Self Psychology, the last of the psychoanalytic models of the mind to be presented here, was not fully developed until late in the twentieth century. In fact, some theorists, like Kohut himself, have argued that Freud ignored the self, or perhaps took the self for granted, in the development of his models. In any case, we need not take a position on this debate, because we have the advantage of psychoanalytic models of the mind that include both those developed by Freud and those that came after. If we can integrate these models into a single model of the mind, we need not decide which we prefer. The challenge of Chapter 13 will be to propose an approach to using all of the models of the mind together as an integrated whole.

---

[1]See nimh.nih.gov/research-priorities/rod/index.shtml (accessed January 12, 2014).

Chapter Summary and Chart of Core Dimensions

Table 12–1 introduces our Self Psychology chart of core dimensions, in which we have placed the following key concepts:

- **Topographic point of view:** The self and the selfobject are largely unconscious.
- **Motivational point of view:** The individual is born with an innate set of *narcissistic strivings* that serve as the major force for motivation in the personality. These strivings include needs for aliveness, authenticity, coherence, mastery, safety, autonomy, uniqueness, creativity, a sense of agency, and self-esteem. Narcissistic strivings develop in interaction with selfobjects, and so are often called *selfobject strivings*. These strivings are never outgrown; instead, they develop into mature forms.
- **Structural point of view:** The *self* is the superordinate structure in the mind at the core of the personality. It is the center of initiative and the source of the coherent experience of sameness. A *selfobject* is the internal experience of another person who is part of the self and who serves the needs of the self. *Dreams* may reflect the *self-state* of the dreamer.
- **Developmental point of view:** The self develops from an admixture of innate factors and interactions with caregivers, who must respond with *empathy* to the infant's growing self. These empathic caregivers are the child's first selfobjects, and development occurs in the context of this *self-selfobject matrix*. There are two major components of the developing self: 1) the *grandiose self*, which forms in interaction with the *mirroring selfobject*, and 2) the *idealized parental imago*, which forms in interaction with the *idealized selfobject*. Over time, the grandiose self matures into stable self-esteem, and the idealized parental imago matures into enduring ideals.

    Stern wrote about development of the self in interaction in the first relationship with the mother, describing five stages of self development: *emergent sense of self* (birth to 2 months), *core sense of self* (2–6 months), *subjective sense of self* (beginning around 9 months), *verbal or categorical sense of self* (beginning around 18 months), and *narrative sense of self* (beginning in the third or fourth year).

- **Theory of psychopathology:** The health of the self—in terms of cohesion and continuity, feelings of energy and initiative, mature self-assertion, self-esteem, and investment in a stable set of ideals—serves as an index of mental health. Psychopathology is conceptualized as a *disorder of the self*—as reflected by an experienced lack of strength, cohesion, effectiveness, or goodness and/or an inability to find meaning in goals and ideals. Disorders of the self result from selfobject failures on the part of caregivers, such as when a caregiver does not mirror the child's grandiosity or does not let the child develop an idealized parental imago. Compensatory structures develop to make up for a weak self.

  Narcissistic personality disorder, as defined by DSM-5, has been conceptualized by Kohut as reflecting the *persistence of infantile narcissism* in cases where there has been a failure of empathy in caregivers, and by Kernberg as expressing a *pathological grandiose self* (in the form of *pathological narcissism*) that serves as a *defense against dependency.*

  Winnicott wrote about how children who were deprived of a facilitating maternal environment develop a *false self* that is displayed in response to the caregiver's expectations and demands while the *true self* lies buried deep within. Fonagy wrote about how the mother's affect mirroring of the child lays the groundwork for the child's development of mentalization. If the mother's affect mirroring is mistuned, insensitive, or otherwise defective, the child may go on to develop an *alien self,* which is similar to Winnicott's *false self.*

- **Theory of therapeutic action:** In psychodynamic psychotherapy, disorders of the self are treated through *mobilization of narcissistic transferences,* creating an opportunity for renewed development of the self. *Exploration of inevitable empathic failures*—moments of disruption between patient and therapist—is also central to the therapeutic action.

TABLE 12–1.	Self Psychology				
Topography	Motivation	Structure/Process	Development	Psychopathology	Treatment
Self and selfobject are largely unconscious	Narcissistic or selfobject strivings	Self Selfobject Self-state dreams	Development of the self Self-selfobject matrix Empathic caregivers Grandiose self forms in interaction with mirroring selfobject Idealized parental imago forms in interaction with idealized selfobject Emergent sense of self Core sense of self Subjective sense of self Verbal/categorical sense of self Narrative sense of self	The health/maturity of the self serves as an index of mental health Psychopathology is conceptualized as a disorder of the self Narcissistic personality disorder (NPD) Persistence of infantile narcissism (Kohut) Defense against dependency (Kernberg) Pathological grandiose self Pathological narcissism False self (vs. true self) Alien self	Mobilization of narcissistic transferences Exploration of inevitable empathic failures

References

American Psychiatric Association: Diagnostic and Statistical Manual of Mental Disorders, 5th Edition. Arlington, VA, American Psychiatric Publishing, 2013

Andersen SM, Reznik I, Glassman NS: The unconscious relational self, in The New Unconscious. Edited by Hassin RR, Uleman JS, Bargh JA. New York, Oxford University Press, 2005, pp 421–481

Auchincloss EL, Samberg E: Psychoanalytic Terms and Concepts. New Haven, CT, Yale University Press, 2012

Bandura A: Self-efficacy mechanisms in human agency. Am Psychol 37:122–147, 1977

Barkow K: Prestige and self-esteem: a biosocial interpretation, in Dominance Relations. Edited by Omark DR, Stayer FF, Freedman DG. New York, Garland, 1980, pp 319–322

Baumeister RF: The self, in The Handbook of Social Psychology, Vol 2. Edited by Gilbert DT, Fiske ST. New York, McGraw-Hill, 1998, pp 680–740

Baumeister RF, Campbell JD, Krueger JI, et al: Does high self-esteem cause better performance, interpersonal success, happiness, or healthier lifestyles? Psychological Science in the Public Interest 4:1–44, 2003

Bion W: Learning From Experience. London, Heinemann, 1962

Bion W: Elements of Psycho-analysis. London, Heinemann, 1963

Bion W: Second Thoughts: Selected Papers on Psycho-Analysis. London, Heinemann, 1967

Bion W: Attention and Interpretation: A Scientific Approach to Insight in Psycho-Analysis and Groups. London, Tavistock, 1970

Brown JD: Self-esteem and self-evaluation: feeling is believing, in The Self in Social Perspective: Psychological Perspectives on the Self, Vol 4. Hillsdale, NJ, Lawrence Erlbaum, 1993, pp 27–58

Carr L, Iacoboni M, Dubeau M, et al: Neural mechanisms of empathy in humans: a relay from neural systems for imitation to limbic areas. Proc Natl Acad Sci U S A 100:5497–5502, 2003

Cuthbert BN, Insel TR: Toward precision medicine in psychiatry: the NIMH research domain criteria project, in The Neurobiology of Mental Illness, 4th Edition. Edited by Charney DS, Sklar P, Buxbaum JD, et al. New York, Oxford University Press, 2013, pp 1076–1088

Damasio A: Descartes' Error: Emotion, Reason, and the Human Brain. New York, Putnam, 1984

Damasio A: The Feeling of What Happens: Body and Emotion in the Making of Consciousness. New York, Harcourt, Brace, 1999

Decety J, Ickes W (eds): The Social Neuroscience of Empathy. Cambridge, MA, MIT Press, 2009

Erikson E: Childhood and Society. New York, WW Norton, 1950

Erikson E: The problem of ego identity. J Am Psychoanal Assoc 4:56–121, 1956

Feinberg TE: Altered Egos: How the Brain Creates the Self. New York, Oxford University Press, 2001

Fonagy P, Gergely G, Jurist E, et al: Affect Regulation, Mentalization, and the Development of the Self. New York, Other Press, 2002

Haggard P, Tsakiris M: The experience of agency: feelings, judgments, and responsibility. Curr Dir Psychol Sci 18:242–246, 2009

Higgins ET: Self-discrepancy theory: a theory relating self and affect. Psychol Rev 94:319–340, 1987

Kernberg O: Borderline Conditions and Pathological Narcissism. New York, Jason Aronson, 1975

Kernberg O: Normal and pathological development, in Object Relations Theory and Clinical Psychoanalysis. New York, Jason Aronson, 1976, pp 55–83

Kihlstrom JF, Beer JS, Klein SB: Self and identity as memory, in Handbook of Self and Identity. Edited by Leary MR, Tangney JP. New York, Guilford, 2002, pp 68–90

Kohut H: The Analysis of the Self. New York, International Universities Press, 1971

Kohut H: Thoughts on narcissism and narcissistic rage (1972), in The search for the self. Selected Writings of Heinz Kohut: 1950–1978, Vol 2. Edited by Ornstein PH. New York, International Universities Press, 1978, pp 615–658

Kohut H: The Restoration of the Self. New York, International Universities Press, 1977

Kohut H: How Does Analysis Cure? Chicago, IL, University of Chicago Press, 1984

Kohut H, Wolf ES: The disorders of the self and their treatment: an outline. Int J Psychoanal 59:413–426, 1978

Leary MR, Baumeister RF: The nature and function of self-esteem: sociometer theory, in Advances in Experimental Social Psychology, Vol 32. Edited by Zanna MP. San Diego, CA, Academic Press, 2000, pp 1–62

Lecky P: Self-Consistency: A Theory of Personality. New York, Island Press, 1945

LeDoux JE: The Synaptic Self: How Our Brains Become Who We Are. New York, Viking, 2002

Macrae CN, Moran JM, Heatherton TF, et al: Medial prefrontal activity predicts memory for self. Cereb Cortex 14:647–654, 2004

Mahler M, Pine F, Bergman A: The Psychological Birth of the Human Infant. New York, Basic Books, 1975

Markus H: Self-schemata and processing information about the self. J Pers Soc Psychol 35:63–78, 1977

McAdams D: The Stories We Live By: Personal Myths and the Making of the Self. New York, Morrow, 1993

McLean KC: The emergence of narrative identity. Social and Personality Psychology Compass 2:1685–1701, 2008

Miller DT, Ross M: Self-serving biases in the attribution of causality: fact or fiction? Psychol Bull 82:213–225, 1975

Mitchell JP, Heatherton TF, Macrae CN: Distinct neural systems subserve person and object knowledge. Proc Natl Acad Sci U S A 99:15238–15243, 2002

Morin A: Right hemisphere self-awareness; a critical assessment. Conscious Cogn 11:396–401, 2002

Newman K: Therapeutic action in self psychology. Psychoanal Q 76 (suppl): 1513–1546, 2007

Ornstein PH: Sexuality and aggression in pathology and in the clinical situation, in Progress in Self Psychology, Vol 9: The Widening Scope of Self Psychology. Edited by Goldberg A. London, Routledge, 1993, pp 109–125

Rogers TB, Kuiper NA, Kirker WS: Self-reference and the encoding of personal information. J Pers Soc Psychol 35:677–688, 1977

Rotter JB: Generalized expectancies for internal versus external locus of control of reinforcement. Psychological Monographs: General and Applied 80:1–28, 1966

Shepperd J, Malone W, Sweeny K: Exploring the causes of the self-serving bias. Social and Personality Psychological Compass 2:895–908, 2008

Socarides D, Stolorow R: Affects and selfobjects. Annual of Psychoanalysis 12:105–119, 1984

Stern DN: The Interpersonal World of the Infant: A View from Psychoanalysis and Developmental Psychology. New York, Basic Books, 1985

Stern DN: Developmental prerequisites for the self of a narrated self, in Psychoanalysis: Toward the Second Century. Edited by Cooper AM, Person E, Kernberg OF. New Haven, CT, Yale University Press, 1989, pp 168–178

Swann WB, Rentfrow PJ, Guinn JS, et al: Self-verification: the search for coherence, in Handbook of Self and Identity. New York, Guilford, 2003, pp 367–383

Terman D: The self and the Oedipus complex. Annual of Psychoanalysis 12/13:87–104, 1984/1985

Tomkins SS: Script theory, in The Emergence of Personality. Edited by Aranoff J, Rabin AI, Zucker RA. New York, Springer, 1986, pp 147–216

Westen D: The cognitive self and the psychoanalytic self: can we put our selves together? Psychol Inq 3:1–13, 1992

Winnicott DW: Transitional objects and transitional phenomena. Int J Psychoanal 34:89–97, 1953

Winnicott DW: The Maturational Processes and the Facilitating Environment. New York, International Universities Press, 1965

Winnicott DW: Playing and Reality. New York, Basic Books, 1971

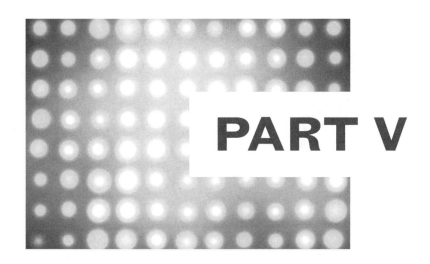

PART V

Integration
and Application

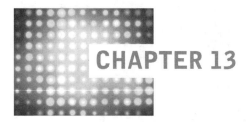

CHAPTER 13

Toward an Integrated Psychoanalytic Model of the Mind

This book has traced the evolution of efforts to conceptualize the nature of mental life, first in the work of Freud and then in the work of many other people. It has described four foundational psychanalytic models of the mind, looking at how each model thinks about the mind and about psychopathology and treatment. Our task for this final chapter is to discover how these four models of the mind can best be used to understand and help our patients.

To begin this task, let us refer to our composite chart (Table 13–1), which has grown throughout this book as each model has been introduced and its most important features discussed. We see that the chart is divided into six columns—labeled Topography, Motivation, Structure/Process, Development, Psychopathology, and Treatment—and has four rows, one for each model of the mind explored in this book. For each of these four models, many terms and concepts appear under the different column headings. There are lots of entries, and the sheer volume of these entries threatens to overwhelm us. How can we begin to make sense of so many separate terms and concepts, much less discover a way to use such a large number of ideas in an integrated way?

TABLE 13–1. Integrated Psychoanalytic Model of the Mind

Topography	Motivation	Structure/Process	Development	Psychopathology	Treatment
Topographic Model					
The mind is divided into three regions: Conscious Preconscious Unconscious	The unconscious mind consists of wishes always striving for expression	The unconscious operates according to primary process; the preconscious/conscious operates according to secondary process	Primary process is the earliest mode of mental functioning; secondary process develops later	Neurosis arises from conflict between the conscious/preconscious domains and the unconscious domain Return of the repressed Repetition compulsion	Free association ("fundamental rule")
	Unacceptable wishes are kept in check by forces of repression from the preconscious/conscious mind	A censor separates the unconscious and the conscious/preconscious mind	Wishes come from childhood and form the basis of infantile sexuality		Examination of transference and resistance
	Oedipal strivings Oedipal fears	Dreams	Oedipal strivings and fears persist into adolescence and adulthood		Therapeutic interpretation and reconstruction
		Complex Fantasy Narrative	Wishes become increasingly unacceptable		Insight ("Make the unconscious conscious")
		Conscience Identifications	Censoring capacity grows		Dream exploration

TABLE 13–1.   **Integrated Psychoanalytic Model of the Mind** *(continued)*

Topography	Motivation	Structure/Process	Development	Psychopathology	Treatment
Structural Model					
The ego and the superego have both conscious/preconscious and unconscious aspects	The ego, superego, and id each have separate aims: The ego—homeostasis and adaptation The superego—moral imperatives	The mind is divided into three structures: ego, superego, and id The ego Ego functions Defense Internalization Identification Signal affect Compromise formation Ego identity Character	Ego development Erikson's stages Superego development Development of the drives (id)	Ego strength/ego weakness serves as an index of mental health/illness Maladaptive compromise may lead to character disorders	Strengthening the ego Exploring conflict, defense, and compromise "Where id was, there ego shall be"
The id is entirely unconscious	The id—drives Libido Aggression Avoidance of danger situations Conflict is always present because of competing aims	The superego Ego ideal The id	Psychosexual phases (oral, anal, early genital [phallic], genital/oedipal, latency, adolescence) Fixation Regression	Defense versus deficit theories of psychopathology	

TABLE 13–1.   Integrated Psychoanalytic Model of the Mind *(continued)*

Topography	Motivation	Structure/Process	Development	Psychopathology	Treatment
Object Relations Theory					
Object relations are largely unconscious	Conflicting wishes for affiliation and for separation-individuation	Object relation Self representation Object representation Representation of interaction between the two	Attachment Separation of self from other	The quality of object relations serves as an index of mental health/illness	Activation of object relations in the therapist-patient relationship
	Love/hate/ambivalence Envy/gratitude/repair	Need-satisfying object	Paranoid position and depressive position	Borderline personality organization (BPO)	Countertransference The therapist as a new object
		Object constancy Self constancy	Container/contained Good-enough mother Holding environment		Transference-Focused Psychotherapy
		Attachment behavioral system	Separation-individuation Differentiation Practicing Rapprochement On the way to object constancy Parenthood Midlife crisis		Mentalization-Based Treatment
		Internal working models of attachment			
		Mentalization	Development of mentalization		

TABLE 13–1. Integrated Psychoanalytic Model of the Mind (*continued*)

Topography	Motivation	Structure/Process	Development	Psychopathology	Treatment
Self Psychology					
Self and selfobject are largely unconscious	Narcissistic or selfobject strivings	Self	Development of the self	The health/maturity of the self serves as an index of mental health	Mobilization of narcissistic transferences
		Selfobject	Self-selfobject matrix		
			Empathic caregivers		Exploration of inevitable empathic failures
		Self-state dreams			
			Grandiose self forms in interaction with mirroring selfobject	Psychopathology is conceptualized as a disorder of the self	
			Idealized parental imago forms in interaction with idealized selfobject	Narcissistic personality disorder (NPD)	
				Persistence of infantile narcissism (Kohut)	
			Emergent sense of self	Defense against dependency (Kernberg)	
			Core sense of self		
			Subjective sense of self		
			Verbal/categorical sense of self	Pathological grandiose self	
			Narrative sense of self	Pathological narcissism	
				False self	
				Alien self	

We believe that the best approach to using the different psychoanalytic models of the mind is two-pronged: 1) in some circumstances, treat all four models of the mind as a single model; and 2) when called for, use each model separately. How would this process work?

Let us reverse the axes of the chart, so that the rows become columns (Topographic Model, Structural Model, Object Relations Theory, and Self Psychology) and the columns become rows (Topography, Motivation, Structure/Process, Development, Psychopathology, and Treatment). With this new orientation of our chart (Table 13–2), we can begin to see how the four models might be used together, even while remaining distinct.

Can There Be a Unified Psychoanalytic Model of the Mind?

In Table 13–2, we can see at a glance what each model has to say about each of the core dimensions of mental functioning and mental illness/treatment. For example, if we look at the Motivation row, we see that the motivations emphasized in the Structural Model are those related to the body's quest for pleasure, whereas the motivations emphasized in Object Relations Theory are those related to needs for attachment and/or separation. These impelling forces for mental and/or physical activity are very different from each other, but they are not mutually exclusive. The same holds true for much of the content of the other core dimensions—Topography, Structure/Process, Development, Psychopathology, and Treatment—when compared across models. Writers who have attempted to delineate the common features of the various psychoanalytic views of the mind have used very similar dimensions (Cooper 1985a; Gedo and Goldberg 1973; Klein 1976; Michels 2005; Rothstein 1985; Wallerstein 2000). Let us take these dimensions one by one, in a search for common features among our four models.

Topography

When we look at the integrated psychoanalytic model of the mind along the dimension of Topography (see first row of Table 13–2), it is relatively simple to see a common theme: almost every component of the mind has a conscious and unconscious component, with a few exceptions (e.g., the concept of the id, which is rarely used in contemporary psychodynamic work). In other words, clinicians working from a unified psychoanalytic point of view must remember that there is always more to the story than what the patient is aware of and that patients do not *want* to know much of what is hidden. In fact, the most important feature of a unified psychoanalytic model of the mind is the concept of the dynamic unconscious.

Motivation

We have just been reminded that concerns about which contents of the mind should be allowed access to consciousness cannot be neatly separated from motivational concerns. Indeed, the dynamic unconscious is defined as the aspect of the mind that we avoid through the "motive of defense" (Breuer and Freud 1893/1895/1962, p. 285). Clinicians working with a unified model of the mind must remember that part of every patient wants to hide awareness of aspects of him- or herself, whatever else that patient may wish or fear. In fact, as they listen to a patient's story, clinicians will always ask what the patient does not want to know at any given moment. In addition, psychodynamic clinicians will work from a very strong motivational point of view with regard to many other phenomena, examining every behavior and experience with the aim of understanding what motivations this behavior/experience serves. In all models of the mind, when we talk about motivation, the pleasure principle and the reality principle are always in operation. In addition, a unified psychoanalytic model of the mind pays attention to many different motivations, including the search for bodily pleasure (libido), aggressive impulses, wishes for attachment to other people and for separation from them, and wishes for self-actualization (along with threats to all four), no matter what point of view predominates in either therapist or patient. We will explain more about how to think about differences in a moment.

Structure/Process

A unified psychoanalytic model has a structural view of the mind. In other words, psychodynamic clinicians always see the patient's mind as being organized in a stable way over time. The mind does not just consist of fleeting motivations, many of them outside of awareness, but also includes consistent configurations or patterns, along with the processes by which these configurations are modulated. In a unified psychoanalytic model of the mind, structures and processes are understood to be concerned with self-regulation (or homeostasis), adaptation, and defense. Psychodynamic clinicians also look at the importance of narrative structure, or of stories, in the organization of experience. Finally, psychodynamic clinicians always look at the structure of the whole person, or his or her *character*. Again, differences will be discussed below.

TABLE 13–2. Reverse Axis—Integrated Psychoanalytic Model of the Mind

	Topographic Model	Structural Model	Object Relations Theory	Self Psychology
Topography	The mind is divided into three regions: Conscious Preconscious Unconscious	The ego and the superego have both conscious/preconscious and unconscious aspects The id is entirely unconscious	Object relations are largely unconscious	Self and selfobject are largely unconscious

Motivation	The unconscious mind consists of wishes always striving for expression
	
	Unacceptable wishes are kept in check by forces of repression from the preconscious/conscious mind
	
	Oedipal strivings
	Oedipal fears
		The ego, superego, and id each have separate aims:
		The ego—homeostasis and adaptation
		The superego—moral imperatives
		The id—drives
		  Libido
		  Aggression
		
		Avoidance of danger situations
		
		Conflict is always present because of competing aims
			Conflicting wishes for affiliation and for separation-individuation
			
			Love/hate/ambivalence
			Envy/gratitude/repair
				Narcissistic or selfobject strivings

TABLE 13–2. Reverse Axis—Integrated Psychoanalytic Model of the Mind *(continued)*

	Topographic Model	Structural Model	Object Relations Theory	Self Psychology
Structure/Process	The unconscious operates according to primary process; the preconscious/conscious operates according to secondary process	The mind is divided into three structures: ego, superego, and id	Object relation Self representation Object representation Representation of interaction between the two	Self Selfobject Self-state dreams
	A censor separates the unconscious and the conscious/preconscious mind	The ego Ego functions Defense Internalization Identification Signal affect Compromise formation Ego identity Character	Need-satisfying object Object constancy Self constancy Attachment behavioral system Internal working models of attachment Mentalization	
	Dreams Complex Fantasy Narrative	The superego Ego ideal		
	Conscience Identifications	The id		

TABLE 13–2. Reverse Axis—Integrated Psychoanalytic Model of the Mind *(continued)*

	Topographic Model	Structural Model	Object Relations Theory	Self Psychology
Development	Primary process is the earliest mode of mental functioning; secondary process develops later	Ego development Erikson's stages	Attachment	Development of the self Self-selfobject matrix Empathic caregivers
		Superego development	Separation of self from other	
	Wishes come from childhood and form the basis of infantile sexuality	Development of the drives (id)	Paranoid position and depressive position	Grandiose self forms in interaction with mirroring selfobject
		Psychosexual phases (oral, anal, early genital [phallic], genital/oedipal, latency, adolescence)	Container/contained Good-enough mother Holding environment	Idealized parental imago forms in interaction with idealized selfobject
	Oedipal strivings and fears persist into adolescence and adulthood	Fixation Regression	Separation-individuation Differentiation Practicing Rapprochement On the way to object constancy Parenthood Midlife crisis	Emergent sense of self Core sense of self Subjective sense of self Verbal/categorical sense of self Narrative sense of self
	Wishes become increasingly unacceptable			
	Censoring capacity grows		Development of mentalization	

TABLE 13–2. Reverse Axis—Integrated Psychoanalytic Model of the Mind *(continued)*

	Topographic Model	Structural Model	Object Relations Theory	Self Psychology
Psychopathology	Neurosis arises from conflict between the conscious/preconscious domains and the unconscious domain	Ego strength/ego weakness serves as an index of mental health/illness	The quality of object relations serves as an index of mental health/illness	The health/maturity of the self serves as an index of mental health
	Return of the repressed	Maladaptive compromise may lead to character disorders	Borderline personality organization (BPO)	Psychopathology is conceptualized as a disorder of the self
	Repetition compulsion	Defense versus deficit theories of psychopathology		Narcissistic personality disorder (NPD)
				Persistence of infantile narcissism (Kohut)
				Defense against dependency (Kernberg)
				Pathological grandiose self
				Pathological narcissism
				False self
				Alien self

TABLE 13–2. Reverse Axis—Integrated Psychoanalytic Model of the Mind (*continued*)

	Topographic Model	Structural Model	Object Relations Theory	Self Psychology
Treatment	Free association ("fundamental rule")	Strengthening the ego	Activation of object relations in the therapist–patient relationship	Mobilization of narcissistic transferences
	Examination of transference and resistance	Exploring conflict, defense, and compromise	Countertransference	Exploration of inevitable empathic failures
	Therapeutic interpretation and reconstruction	"Where id was, there ego shall be"	The therapist as a new object	
	Insight ("Make the unconscious conscious")		Transference-Focused Psychotherapy	
	Dream exploration		Mentalization-Based Treatment	

Development

A unified psychoanalytic model of the mind has a developmental point of view, because no part of the mind can be understood apart from its history. This history will always include the story of childhood and will feature caretakers and family members, as well as sentinel events, both happy and sad. Clinicians working with a unified psychoanalytic model understand that the mind of the child lives on in the adult.

Theory of Psychopathology and Therapeutic Action (Treatment)

Clinicians working with a unified psychoanalytic model of the mind examine every patient from each of the above points of view, with an eye to understanding his or her psychopathology. Although this is not a book about psychopathology and/or psychodynamic treatment, psychodynamic clinicians working with different models of the mind have much in common. Psychodynamic treatment strategies may differ, but they share a commitment to understanding the patient's story, told to the therapist with as much candor as possible. Exploration of how the story is told will always be part of the therapeutic work, and exploration of the transference experience is always part of the process. Every treatment seeks to understand the patient's way of finding pleasure, managing aggression, negotiating attachments and separations, and expressing the self. Every treatment seeks to understand the feelings and fears associated with all of these aspects of the patient's mental life and the compromises forged among competing aims. This understanding will be shared with the patient so that he or she can find better ways to handle the challenges of being human.

Why Is Having Different Models Useful and Important?

Although models of the mind have much in common, they also have important differences. Indeed, a major aim of this book has been to make readers aware of the major differences among models. Which model is best? It is not clear. This is true partly because we lack methods good enough to answer the question empirically. It is also true because the mind is an immensely complex system, with many moving parts. Therefore, it should not be surprising that there are many ways to think about it and many ways to intervene. In other words, if we know that there is a dynamic interaction between many aspects of the mind, then we should expect the entire system to change in response to several different kinds of interventions.

For example, a stronger self might make a brash young man less annoying to others, who resent his constant demands for attention. At the same time, a stronger self might make this young man less likely to give in to his sadistic superego, which feels to him like a source of power. However, having a less sadistic superego might allow this man to display less passive aggression because of a reduced need to be defiantly rebellious against all authority. Less rebellion against authority might enable this same man to allow himself more kinds of pleasure, thereby becoming less resentful of those who are having fun, with less need to upstage them. Less rebellion might also make him more admiring of his father and therefore more comfortable with being idealistic himself. If this man is able to experience more feelings of real idealism instead of just cravings for attention, he might like himself better—and so on. Sometimes it will be best to conceptualize this young man as dealing with forbidden oedipal strivings by making himself into an "annoying boy"; at other times, it will be best to imagine him as needing to stay close to those he loves, even while struggling with aggression toward them; at still other times, it will be best to imagine him struggling with a self that feels weak and unrecognized, turning to aggression to help himself feel stronger. We can imagine many interventions at many points.

In a second example, let us return to the young woman with panic attacks, one of which was triggered by the suggestion that she visit a nail salon (see Chapters 5 and 6). Clearly this young woman becomes anxious whenever she is tempted to pursue embellishments to make herself more feminine or beautiful. Is she afraid of competitive oedipal wishes? Does she feel closer and more attached to her mother if she stays somewhat dowdy like her mother was? Maybe becoming more beautiful would represent a painful and terrifying separation from her mother. On the other hand, maybe this young woman cannot allow herself to express strivings to be noticed as beautiful because her mother, who was often depressed during the patient's childhood, failed to acknowledge and enjoy these strivings. Each of these ideas is true about the patient, and each represents a different model of the mind.

In this book we have seen how each model of the mind tries to correct shortcomings of previous models. However, each model also creates new problems and new blind spots. In fact, clinicians who use only one model of the mind to the exclusion of all others run the risk of ignoring important aspects of the patient's mind. For this reason, it is wise to use all four models, each of which emphasizes a different aspect of the mind and each of which has different strengths. Many theorists have written about how each model might be applied to different phenomena, different stages of life, and different kinds of patients (Gedo and Goldberg 1973; Pine 1988, 1989). We have also seen how models of the mind borrow from each other, as in the example of many so-called Self Psychology theorists who borrow the idea of the containing mother from Object Relations Theory (see Chapter 12).

Let us look at some more examples. In trying to help the young woman who dreamt about the doll on the shelf (see Chapters 6 and 7), would it be best to help her to talk about sexual and competitive wishes that have been driven underground because they are too frightening? Or would it be best to talk about her fear of loss, or her fear that her own angry feelings might have led to her mother's death? Maybe it is important to help this young woman deal with her feeling of superiority (feeling "above it all") as being a search for the praise she did not get as a child. Or are the patient's feelings of superiority a defense against feelings of vulnerability and dependency? Maybe it is best to help her deal with her envy of her sister so that she is less likely to punish herself for this envy and can allow herself to pursue her own deepest wishes. The best answer is that it is important to talk with the patient about all of these issues.

How can we best understand the timid young doctor who dropped his mobile phone in an obsequious rush to be helpful (see Chapter 10)? Should we help him to be more aware of his aggressive feelings toward his therapist? Or should we talk about his feeling that he needs to be compliant in order to be loved by others? His abject need for love only makes him hate himself more; perhaps we should talk about this feeling of self-hatred. Or perhaps we should talk about his related feeling of weakness and his warded-off wishes to be seen as smart and accomplished, which were never recognized by his busy, unhappy parents. Again, the best answer is that we should talk about all of these issues.

Choosing the most important issues to talk about at the right time requires experience. Patients differ on which model of the mind best suits the problem with which they are struggling. Patients also differ with respect to which model of the mind best describes their problems at any given moment. However, without our four models of the mind, we would not even be alert to the presence of many issues. Having all models in one's psychodynamic toolbox allows one to listen to each patient, making sense of his or her suffering and finding ways to help. In other words, the best way to help each patient is to borrow from all four models. Every patient needs to feel more comfortable with his or her bodily strivings, his or her wishes for affiliation and separation, and his or her wishes for self-expression and meaningfulness. Every patient needs to deal with fears associated with all of these. Finally, every patient must deal with the constraints of reality, which include conflict, limitation, and loss. Which of these issues predominates at any given time will vary. However, clinicians need all four models of the mind to listen for each of them.

Importance of the Biological Model of the Mind

A good clinician always uses many perspectives other than the psycho-dynamic perspective with each patient. Even the best psychodynamic clinician always uses a neurobiological understanding of mental illness, employing interventions that take this understanding into account. Indeed, the young woman with panic attacks may need biological treatment for her anxiety or a course of cognitive-behavioral treatment. Less anxiety will itself have a positive dynamic effect. For example, the patient may feel better about herself, have less need to cling to her mother, and be less afraid of autonomy.

As noted in the Preface/Introduction to this book, there need be no conflict between the psychoanalytic model of the mind and other important points of view, including neurobiological, cognitive, and cultural approaches to understanding mental illness. Clinical work should be informed by empirical study from all disciplines and be consistent with these disciplines. For example, we know from the work of developmental psychologists that the superego does not develop suddenly at the end of the oedipal period, as Freud taught, but instead develops slowly over time (Emde et al. 1988). This fact influences our listening in that it will help us to be alert to a patient's guilt and shame surrounding events that predate the oedipal period. We also know that rhesus monkeys raised by "supermoms" can have a normal outcome even when they carry a genetic liability for anxious or aggressive temperament (Suomi 2004a, 2004b). This fact likewise influences our work, making us think harder about the importance of the selfobject function in psycho-dynamic psychotherapy.

Throughout this book, we have tried to highlight areas of research linking the psychoanalytic model of the mind with both neuroscience and general psychology. We should all be partners in our quest to better understand patients. There have been many good efforts on all sides to build this partnership (Bucci 1997; Cooper 1985b; Gabbard 1992; Kandel

1998, 1999, 2005; Kihlstrom 1994; LeDoux 1999; Levin 1991; Mayes et al. 2007; Olds and Cooper 1997; Shapiro and Emde 1995; Solms and Turnbull 2002; Westen 1998).

Dangers of Integration: A Note for Psychoanalysts

Not everyone agrees that integration of the various psychoanalytic models of the mind is either possible or wise. Indeed, as we mentioned briefly in the Preface/Introduction to this book, the field of psychoanalysis has been beset by arguments over which model of the mind is the best or the most useful. A summary of these arguments would take us far afield. For now, it is enough to say that we live in an era of psychoanalytic pluralism and that efforts at integration can be seen as efforts to undo this pluralism with a proposed synthesis that is experienced as "too prescriptive."

Indeed, in the Introduction to our book *Psychoanalytic Terms and Concepts,* Eslee Samberg and I wrote about the problems and the dangers of writing a psychoanalytic dictionary in an era of pluralism and in a field marked by efforts to model what cannot be seen—the mind—and the unseen part of the unseen—the unconscious mind. In our Introduction, we tried to describe how we arrived at a way to handle these problems so that we could proceed with the work of editing a dictionary, which requires admitting that one has a point of view (Samberg and Auchincloss 2010). Arguably, the problem here is even more challenging, because the task of integrating the various psychoanalytic models of the mind requires even more condensation than does the writing of a dictionary; condensation, perforce, requires that complexity—and many points of view—be eliminated. In other words, many will be aware that important points of view have been given short shrift in this book's chapters.

Nevertheless, attempts at integration are important because every clinician needs to have a robust and workable psychoanalytic model of the mind, usable with every patient in every situation. Most students of mental health will not become psychoanalysts, daily immersed in the complexity of psychoanalytic theory, fascinated by the ways different theorists use different words, or intrigued by differences of opinion. For these reasons, integration is important, even at the risk of oversimplification. Future clinicians must be able to use our models of the mind to help patients. The aim of this book is to provide a starting point for those interested in understanding the complexity of theory either through further reading or through education. In a previous commentary, I argued that the clinical work of doing psychodynamic psychotherapy offers the best exposure to the psychoanalytic model of the mind (Auchincloss 2002). Here we are arguing that we need a psychoanalytic model of the mind to do good clinical work. Both of these statements are true.

Conclusion

Throughout this book we have tried to emphasize the fact that psychoanalytic model making should be an ongoing process. For example, readers must understand that the word *superego* is simply the name Freud gave to his observation that most people are strongly influenced by thoughts about right and wrong. Object relations gained traction when clinicians realized that it is difficult to talk about how some people function without thinking about how they organize their experience of self, other, and the interaction between the two. Self Psychology would not have survived if thinking in greater detail about the components of the self were not useful. Clinicians always face the same questions that challenged Freud and his followers: How can we understand patients, and how can we help them change? Our models of the mind are important and useful only to the extent that they help us to answer these questions.

Further Reading

Auchincloss EL, Samberg E: Psychoanalytic Terms and Concepts. New Haven, CT, Yale University Press, 2012

Gabbard GO, Litowitz BE, Williams P (eds): Textbook of Psychoanalysis, 2nd Edition. Washington, DC, American Psychiatric Publishing, 2012

Gilmore KJ, Meersand P: Normal Child and Adolescent Development: A Psychodynamic Primer. Arlington, VA, American Psychiatric Publishing, 2013

References

Auchincloss EL: Commentary on "The Place of Psychoanalytic Treatments Within Psychiatry," by Glen Gabbard, Peter Fonagy, and John Gunderson. Arch Gen Psychiatry 59:501–503, 2002

Breuer J, Freud S: Studies on hysteria (1893/1895), in The Standard Edition of the Complete Psychological Works of Sigmund Freud, Vol 2. Translated and edited by Strachey J. London, Hogarth Press, 1962, pp 1–335

Bucci W: Psychoanalysis and Cognitive Science: A Multiple Code Theory. New York, Guilford, 1997

Cooper AM: A historical review of psychoanalytic paradigms, in Models of the Mind: Their Relationship to Clinical Work. Edited by Rothstein A. Madison, CT, International Universities Press, 1985a, pp 5–20

Cooper A: Will neurobiology influence psychoanalysis? Am J Psychiatry 142:1395–1402, 1985b

Emde R, Johnson W, Easterbrooks M: The dos and don'ts of early moral development: psychoanalytic tradition and current research, in The Emergence of Morality. Edited by Kagan E, Lamb S. Chicago, IL, University of Chicago Press, 1988, pp 245–276

Gabbard GO: Psychodynamic psychiatry in the "decade of the brain." Am J Psychiatry 149:991–998, 1992

Gedo J, Goldberg A: Models of the Mind: A Psychoanalytic Theory. Chicago, IL, University of Chicago Press, 1973

Kandel E: A new intellectual framework for psychiatry. Am J Psychiatry 155:457–469, 1998

Kandel E: Biology and future of psychiatry: a new intellectual framework for psychiatry revisited. Am J Psychiatry 156:505–524, 1999

Kandel E: Psychiatry, Psychoanalysis and the New Biology of Mind. Washington, DC, American Psychiatric Publishing, 2005

Kihlstrom JF: Commentary: psychodynamic and social cognition—notes on the fusion of psychoanalysis and psychology. J Pers 62:681–696, 1994

Klein GS: Psychoanalytic Theory: An Exploration of Essentials. Madison, CT, International Universities Press, 1976

LeDoux J: Psychoanalytic theory: clues from the brain. Neuropsychoanalysis 1:44–49, 1999

Levin F: Mapping the Mind: The Intersection of Psychoanalysis and Neuroscience. Hillsdale, NJ, Analytic Press, 1991

Mayes L, Fonagy P, Target M (eds): Developmental Science and Psychoanalysis: Integration and Innovation. London, Karnac, 2007

Michels R: Basic principles of psychodynamic psychiatry, in Psychodynamic Concepts in General Psychiatry. Edited by Schwartz H, Bleiberg E, Weissman SH. Washington, DC, American Psychiatric Publishing, 2005, pp 3–12

Olds D, Cooper AM: Dialogue with other sciences: opportunities for mutual gain. Int J Psychoanal 78:219–225, 1997

Pine F: The four psychologies of psychoanalysis and their place in clinical work. J Am Psychoanal Assoc 36:571–596, 1988

Pine F: Motivation, personality organization, and the four psychologies of psychoanalysis. J Am Psychoanal Assoc 37:31–64, 1989

Rothstein A (ed): Models of the Mind: Their Relationship to Clinical Work. Madison, CT, International Universities Press, 1985

Samberg E, Auchincloss EL: Psychoanalytic lexicography: notes from two "harmless drudges." J Am Psychoanal Assoc 58:1059–1088, 2010 (published also as Introduction, in Psychoanalytic Terms and Concepts. New Haven, CT, American Psychoanalytic Association and Yale University Press, 2012)

Shapiro T, Emde R: Research in Psychoanalysis: Process, Development, Outcome. Madison, CT, International Universities Press, 1995

Solms M, Turnbull O: The Brain and the Inner World: An Introduction to the Neuroscience of Subjective Experience. New York, Other Press, 2002

Suomi SJ: How gene-environment interactions influence emotional development in rhesus monkeys, in Nature and Nurture: The Complex Interplay of Genetic and Environmental Influences on Human Behavior and Development. Edited by Coll CG, Bearer EL, Lerner RM. Mahway, NJ, Lawrence Erlbaum, 2004a, pp 35–51

Suomi SJ: How gene-environment interactions shape the development of impulsive aggression in rhesus monkeys, in Developmental Psychobiology of Aggression. Edited by Stoff DM, Susman EJ. New York, Cambridge University Press, 2004b, pp 252–268

Wallerstein R: Forty-Two Lives in Treatment: A Study of Psychoanalysis and Psychotherapy. The Report of the Psychotherapy Research Project of the Menninger Foundation, 1954–1982. New York, Other Press, 2000

Westen D: The scientific legacy of Sigmund Freud: toward a psychodynamically informed psychological science. Psychol Bull 124:333–371, 1998

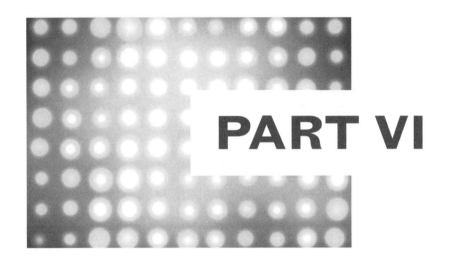

PART VI

Appendixes

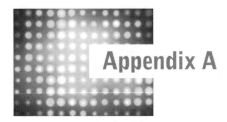

Libido Theory

Libido is the name that Freud gave to the drive for sexual pleasure. The word *libido* is derived from the Latin for "wish" or "desire." Ideas about the origins, transformations, and effects of libido have been collectively referred to as *libido theory*. For a full discussion of the illustration in this appendix, readers are referred to the section "Freud's Drive Theory" in Chapter 9 ("The Id and the Superego").

APPENDIX A.   Libido Theory

Libido	→	Transformation via defense	→	Outcome
	→	Repression of ideation but with excitement remaining	→	"Normal" sexuality and foreplay
	→	Repression of ideation and excitement	→	Sexual inhibition
	→	Direct expression of a component of libido	→	Atypical sexuality ("perversion")
	→	Repression with "the return of the repressed"	→	Neurosis
		Repression with partial "return"	→	Neurosis: anxiety disorder
		Conversion	→	Neurosis: conversion disorder
		Reaction formation	→	Neurosis: obsessive-compulsive disorder
		Projection	→	Neurosis: paranoid disorder
		Displacement	→	Neurosis: phobia
Infantile sexuality from the erotogenic zones Oral Anal Phallic Genital/oedipal	→	Repression, sublimation, and reaction formation	→	Character
		Fixation at the oral phase	→	Oral character
		Fixation at the anal phase	→	Anal character
		Fixation at the phallic phase	→	Phallic narcissistic character
	→	Repression and sublimation	→	Culture Art Science Religion Law

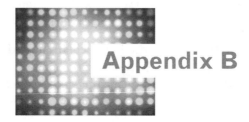

Appendix B

Defenses

Many theorists have made efforts to classify and organize the defenses. For example, Otto Kernberg (1970) has offered the most commonly used system for classifying psychopathology according to level of functioning, including psychotic, borderline, and neurotic levels. In addition, George Vaillant (1977, 1992; Vaillant et al. 1986) attempted to correlate defensive style with level of mental health, using data gathered from his longitudinal study of a large group of men. In this appendix, we will draw upon both of their systems. (See also Auchincloss and Samberg 2012; Dickerman and Auchincloss, in press; and Gabbard et al. 2012.)

Mature Defenses With Little Cost in Terms of Ego Functioning

Altruism: A defense in which an individual shows concern for the well-being of others in order to avoid painful feelings such as anxiety about his or her own well-being.

> *Example:* A wealthy woman satisfies her need to feel important and avoids unacceptable feelings of selfishness by donating large amounts of time and money to "worthy" causes.

Humor: A defense in which an individual treats a painful subject with a comic attitude, thereby diminishing the pain.

Example: A woman who is getting old and approaching her death puts everyone at ease by making humorous statements about her disabilities.

Reparation: A defense in which an individual attempts to relieve guilt or anxiety experienced for having had aggressive wishes toward a loved and needed object by making efforts to repair the imagined damage or harm done by those aggressive impulses.

Example: A young man shows his little brother how to play baseball, because he feels badly that he has often made fun of him.

Sublimation: A defense in which the individual deflects a wish from its original aim to one with a higher social value.

Example: A young man expresses his unacceptable aggressive impulses by engaging in competitive sports while expressing easy amiability in everyday life.

Suppression: A defense in which an individual consciously places unpleasant thoughts or feelings out of awareness.

Example: A middle-aged man in the cardiac intensive care unit maintains a positive attitude toward his prognosis and intentionally avoids thinking about his precarious condition.

Neurotic Defenses With Mild or Moderate Cost in Terms of Ego Functioning

Displacement: A defense in which an individual redirects interest or intensity attached to one idea toward another more acceptable idea.

Example: A young man who is angry at his boss for criticizing him becomes angry with his own son and shouts at the child with little provocation.

Idealization: A defense in which an individual sees another individual in an exaggeratedly positive light, so as to ward off disappointment or to enhance his or her own experience of self.

Example: A young man sees his father as good at everything, avoiding the painful awareness that his father let him down many times during his childhood.

Introjection: A defense in which an individual internalizes an aspect of the external world, usually an object, so as to avoid a painful feeling, such as loss or disappointment.

Example: A young woman whose mother has died develops an intense interest in cooking, in identification with an important aspect of her mother.

Isolation of affect: A defense in which an individual separates the affective meaning of an event or thought from his or her awareness of the event/thought in order to lessen the emotional impact. *Intellectualization* is a form of isolation of affect characterized by the use of excessive cognitive activity to control and ward off unacceptable feelings.

Example: A mother becomes an expert in the science behind her daughter's attention-deficit/hyperactivity disorder while being emotionally distant from her daughter and appearing to have no emotional response to her daughter's disability.

Projection: A defense in which an individual attributes an unacceptable or intolerable idea, impulse, or feeling to another individual.

Example: An aggressive, competitive young woman perceives others as "having it in for her."

Rationalization: A defense in which an individual resorts to seemingly reasonable explanations to account for feelings or actions, thereby avoiding recognition of more painful feelings and/or motivations.[1]

Example: A young man blames "time constraints at work" for often arriving late to sessions with his therapist, thereby avoiding feelings of anger toward his therapist.

Reaction formation: A defense in which an individual transforms a forbidden wish into its opposite.

Example: A young man expresses extreme homophobia in order to avoid awareness of his own homosexual interests.

---

[1]See also Tierney J: Go ahead, rationalize. Monkeys do it, too. *New York Times,* November 6, 2007.

Repression: A defense in which an individual excludes unacceptable thoughts and feelings from consciousness.

Example: A young woman is unaware that she feels sexually interested in her next-door neighbor but is anxious in his presence.

Undoing: A defense in which an individual negates unacceptable sexual, aggressive, or shameful feelings associated with a previous behavior by doing or saying the opposite.

Example: A young man who often makes hostile jokes about colleagues usually follows these interactions by saying, "I was just kidding!"

Primitive Defenses With Significant Cost in Terms of Ego Functioning

Denial/disavowal: A defense by which an individual repudiates aspects of external reality, thereby diminishing painful feelings.

Example: In the face of much evidence to the contrary, a middle-aged man in the cardiac intensive care unit asserts that his health is improving.

Dissociation: A disruption in the continuity of mental experience for the purpose of defense. *Splitting* is an example in which dissociation is applied to mutually contradictory conscious experiences.

Example: A young woman is outraged by the idea that she might be sexually interested in her best friend's husband, ignoring the fact of having flirted with him intensely the night before.

Primitive Idealization: A defense in which an individual splits apart exalted and devalued aspects of another individual, experiencing only the exalted aspect, so as to ward off feelings associated with the devalued aspect, or to enhance his or her own experience of self.

Example: Early in the treatment, a young woman who is afraid of her rage at those in authority sees her current therapist as "perfect," while recounting stories in which all the other therapists whom she knows or has seen are highly flawed.

Projective Identification: An interpersonal defense in which an individual transfers parts of the self onto an object in order to rid him- or herself of those parts and to control the object from inside. When using projective identification, the individual often behaves in a way that influences the other individual's behavior and experience to be consistent with the projection.

> *Example:* A young woman who vehemently denies that she is aggressive and intrusive resists her boyfriend's efforts to discuss emotionally troublesome issues, causing him to lose patience with her and make angry, intrusive efforts to engage her in a discussion of their interaction.

Somatization: A defense in which an individual expresses unacceptable feelings in the form of physical symptoms, so as to lessen their painful impact. *Conversion,* the symbolic transformation of unacceptable wishes into physical symptoms, represents the classic example of somatization.

> *Example:* A young man who does not "want to see" painful truths about his father's infidelity complains to his doctor about his own "intermittent blurred vision."

Splitting: A defense in which an individual separates contradictory, conflicting conscious experiences, thereby preventing their integration, so as to prevent the emotional impact of integration.

> *Example:* A young woman, who previously had nothing bad to say about her "perfect" therapist, states after a minor disappointment that her therapist is "a heartless person."

Other Defense Mechanisms

Altruistic surrender: A defense in which an individual can only achieve gratification of unacceptable wishes vicariously through extreme, selfless devotion to a proxy.

> *Example:* A teenage girl who finds her own interest in boys to be unacceptable works tirelessly to make her best friend more attractive.

Identification with the aggressor: A defense in which an individual takes on the characteristics or role of someone who had formerly tormented or abused him or her, so as to avoid painful feelings of passivity and shame.

> *Example:* A young gay man who has been teased by family members for being "too effeminate" treats himself with contempt.

Regression in the service of the ego: A form of regression that, although it may be originally instituted for defensive purposes, leads to a more innovative and adaptive mental function and organization (as in artistic creation).

Example: A successful female author is able to evoke the voice of a child in her writing.

Turning against the self: A defense in which an individual directs an unacceptable wish, usually aggressive, from another individual toward him- or herself.

Example: A man who finds his anger at his wife to be unacceptable often blames himself excessively for their altercations.

Turning passive into active: A defense in which an individual acts out an experience of having been a passive participant in an interaction by assuming the active role, thereby avoiding feelings and/or memories of being out of control or helpless.

Example: A middle-aged man who was physically abused by his own father during childhood enjoys a job in which he exercises control over others who work for him but avoids situations in which he feels powerless, as in seeking treatment for illness.

References

Auchincloss EL, Samberg E: Psychoanalytic Terms and Concepts. New Haven, CT, Yale University Press, 2012

Dickerman AL, Auchincloss EL: Psychodynamic psychotherapy, in Contemporary Theory and Practice of Counseling and Psychotherapy. Edited by Tinsley HEA, Lease SL, Wiersma NSG. Thousand Oaks, CA, Sage (in press)

Gabbard GO, Litowitz BE, Williams P (eds): Textbook of Psychoanalysis, 2nd Edition. Arlington, VA, American Psychiatric Publishing, 2012

Kernberg OF: A psychoanalytic classification of character pathology. J Am Psychoanal Assoc 18:800–822, 1970

Vaillant GE: Adaptation to Life. Boston, MA, Little, Brown, 1977

Vaillant GE (ed): Ego Mechanisms of Defense: A Guide for Clinicians and Researchers. Washington, DC, American Psychiatric Publishing, 1992

Vaillant GE, Bond M, Vaillant CO: An empirically validated hierarchy of defense mechanisms. Arch Gen Psychiatry 73:786–794, 1986

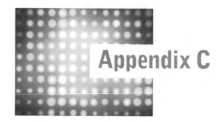

Glossary

Activation-synthesis hypothesis   A theory of DREAM formation introduced by Hobson and McCarley (see Chapter 6) in which the brain constructs a dream by synthesizing random sensorimotor information from the pons with information stored in memory.

Adaptation   The individual's ability to make changes and/or compromises so as to become better suited to his or her external environment.

Adaptational perspective   In the psychoanalytic model of the mind, the effort to understand aspects of behavior and mental life that serve the purpose of coping with the external world.

Adult Attachment Interview   An instrument developed by Main (see Chapter 11) to investigate patterns in adult recollections of early childhood experience related to attachment.

SMALL CAPS type indicates terms defined as main entries elsewhere in this glossary.

The reader is referred to Auchincloss and Samberg (2012) for more a more extensive exploration of terms and concepts.

Affect(s) The complex emotional/physical states—both pleasurable and painful—produced by and in the body as part of its system of evaluating the self in relationship to the environment for the purpose of survival. Commonly called *feelings.*

Affect mirroring The process by which the mother empathically reads and reflects back to the child his or her feeling states, thereby helping the child gain confidence in managing intense AFFECTS and learn to differentiate between self and other, and reality and FANTASY. The mother's affect mirroring of the child lays the groundwork for the child's development of MENTALIZATION.

Affect tolerance The ability to experience AFFECT states without having to ward them off through DEFENSE.

Aggression The WISH to subjugate, prevail over, harm, or destroy others, and the expression of such a WISH in thought, action, words, or FANTASY.

Aggressive drive In Freud's TOPOGRAPHIC MODEL, the source of PSYCHIC ENERGY deriving from the organism's aggressive WISHES.

Alien self In Fonagy's theory (see Chapter 12), an inauthentic sense of self that can develop when the mother's AFFECT MIRRORING is mistuned, insensitive, or otherwise defective. Similar to Winnicott's FALSE SELF.

Altruism A DEFENSE in which an individual shows concern for the well-being of others in order to avoid painful feelings such as ANXIETY about his or her own well-being.

Altruistic surrender A DEFENSE in which an individual can only achieve gratification of unacceptable WISHES vicariously through extreme, selfless devotion to a proxy.

Ambivalence The simultaneous existence of opposite feelings, attitudes, or tendencies toward another person, thing, or situation.

Anal character A personality style characterized by marked orderliness, stubbornness, and obstinacy, thought to be related to the predominant influence of LIBIDO arising from the anal EROTOGENIC ZONE.

Anal phase The second phase of psychosexual development (extending from 18 months to 3 years), during which LIBIDO deriving from the anal EROTOGENIC ZONE dominates the organization of psychic life.

Anxiety   An AFFECT characterized by a painful experience of apprehension and anticipation of danger.

Attachment   The biologically based bond between infant and caregiver.

Attachment behavioral system   A component of ATTACHMENT THEORY that includes inborn features of behavior in infant and caregivers that ensure the establishment of attachment.

Attachment theory   A view of ATTACHMENT proposed by Bowlby (see Chapter 11) that includes development, patterns in children and adults, and sequelae over the course of the life cycle.

Autoerotic   Libidinal aims directed toward the child's own body, as opposed to those directed toward another person.

Automatic thoughts   Unconscious mentation in COGNITIVE PSYCHOLOGY or in cognitive-behavioral therapy.

Autonomous ego functions   Inborn capacities of the MIND that develop independently (or autonomously) from CONFLICT and that include thought, memory, perception, cognition, and motility.

Average expectable environment   The caregiving situation within which an infant's capacities can develop in a predictable and progressive manner.

Behaviorism   A branch of PSYCHOLOGY that seeks to explain human (and animal) activity as a chain of stimulus-response connections, linked together by reinforcement.

Borderline personality organization   A psychoanalytic diagnosis introduced by Kernberg (see Chapter 11), marked by EGO WEAKNESSES and disturbances in OBJECT RELATIONS, including poorly integrated SELF and OBJECT REPRESENTATIONS.

Castration anxiety   The fear that unacceptable WISHES will lead to punishment in the form of loss of or injury to one's genitals or one's body.

Cathartic method   Breuer's technique (see Chapter 2) of treating patients with HYSTERIA, consisting of HYPNOSIS and the expression of AFFECTS associated with sequestered ideas.

Censor   In Freud's TOPOGRAPHIC MODEL, an agent of REPRESSION whose function is to keep from CONSCIOUSNESS mental content judged to be unacceptable.

Censorship   In Freud's TOPOGRAPHIC MODEL, the system by which WISHES are appraised as unacceptable to CONSCIOUSNESS and then repressed.

Character   An individual's stable and enduring traits, attitudes, cognitive styles, and moods.

Character disorder   A disturbance in the structure of an individual's personality in which there are rigidly held patterns of behavior that get the individual in trouble or lead to the defeat of his or her own aims but that cause him or her little subjective distress.

Co-created experience   A process that integrates the subjective experiences of two people in a relationship into a single experience.

Cognitive psychology   A branch of PSYCHOLOGY that focuses on the study of how people know things. Cognitive psychology posits the existence of stable, autonomous cognitive STRUCTURES, or REPRESENTATIONS, operating within an organism (and analogous to the software programs in a computer) that account for its behavior (or output).

Cognitive unconscious   Mentation that is not within awareness that mostly includes phenomena related to information processing.

Complex   A set of UNCONSCIOUS associated feelings and ideas that form a network or template in the MIND.

Compromise/compromise formation   A mental product that reflects the EGO's solution to a problem presented by the competing demands of ID, SUPEREGO, and external reality.

Computational model of the mind   The view that the human mind or the human brain (or both) is an information processing system (in the sense of a symbol manipulator that follows step-by-step functions to compute input and form output).

Condensation   A mental process by which a single idea is capable of representing many related ideas, linked by private associations.

Conflict   A struggle within the MIND between thoughts, feelings, or structures with opposing aims.

Conflict theory   A theory about how the EGO manages the competing aims of ID, SUPEREGO, and external reality by forging COMPROMISE.

Confrontation   A therapeutic intervention that directs attention to aspects of CONSCIOUS experience that are observable but that are avoided or disavowed.

Conscious   In Freud's TOPOGRAPHIC MODEL, that part of the MIND that is accessible to awareness.

Consciousness   A mental state characterized by awareness and self-awareness.

Container/contained   In Bion's theory (see Chapter 11), caretaking acts, including soothing and verbalizing, that serve to transform the infant's chaotic experience into something more tolerable.

Conversion   The symbolic transformation of unacceptable WISHES into physical symptoms.

Core sense of self   The second stage in the development of the SELF—from 2 to 6 months—in Stern's theory (see Chapter 12) about how the sense of self develops in interaction with the mother/caregiver.

Corrective emotional experience   In the theory of Alexander and French (see Chapter 11), therapeutic change that results from the therapist's specific efforts to be different from the patient's parents.

Countertransference   The therapist's responses to the patient, CONSCIOUS and UNCONSCIOUS, including responses that are mainly a reaction to the therapist's own inner life and those that are mainly a reaction to the patient.

Danger situations   Circumstances that trigger ANXIETY in all human beings, including loss of an important OBJECT, loss of an object's love, CASTRATION ANXIETY, and SUPEREGO disapproval (or GUILT).

Day residue   An event from the waking life in the day before the dream that appears in the DREAM as a symbol.

Defense   Any UNCONSCIOUS psychological maneuver used to avoid the experience of a painful state of mind.

Defense mechanism   A specific and well-delineated act of DEFENSE, such as REPRESSION, REACTION FORMATION, or SUBLIMATION.

Defensive style   An individual's characteristic mode of DEFENSE, a major constituent of CHARACTER.

Deficit   A weakness in psychic STRUCTURE caused by early deprivation.

Denial   A DEFENSE by which an individual repudiates aspects of external reality, thereby diminishing painful feelings. Also called *disavowal.*

Depressive anxiety   A fear that one's own angry feelings may threaten or harm a needed and loved OBJECT.

Depressive position   In Klein's theory (see Chapter 11), a stage of development marked by attainment of the ability to integrate good and bad aspects of the experience with an OBJECT.

Descriptive unconscious   Mentation that is not within awareness at any given moment but can easily be brought to awareness if attention is applied to it.

Developmental lines   Distinct developmental sequences of function and behavior, including WISHES, fears, self-regulation, morality, SELF and OBJECT REPRESENTATIONS, and narcissistic strivings.

Developmental point of view   An approach to understanding behavior and mental life as part of a meaningful progression from infancy to adulthood.

Differentiation   In Mahler's theory (see Chapter 11), a subphase of the SEPARATION-INDIVIDUATION process in which the infant begins to show interest in the external world.

Disavowal   See DENIAL.

Disorder of the self   In SELF PSYCHOLOGY, a type of psychopathology that is characterized by weakness in the self.

Displacement   A process whereby the interest or intensity attached to one idea is redirected onto another associated idea; often used as a DEFENSE.

Dissociation   A disruption in the continuity of mental experience for the purpose of DEFENSE.

Dream   A mental event occurring during sleep that consists of a collection of images, ideas, and emotions.

Dream work   The process of transforming the LATENT DREAM THOUGHTS into the MANIFEST DREAM.

Drive   A psychological REPRESENTATION of a motivational force that emerges from the body as a result of an individual's biological needs.

Drive theory   A theory about the role of DRIVE in development, normal functioning, and psychopathology.

Dynamic   A state of continuous interplay of multiple psychological forces or motivations.

Dynamic unconscious   Mentation that is actively denied access to CONSCIOUSNESS by the force of REPRESSION.

Ego   In Freud's STRUCTURAL MODEL, the executive agency of the MIND, responsible for mediating among the demands of the DRIVES (the ID), the external world, and the SUPEREGO.

Ego dystonic   Behaviors that are experienced by the individual as incompatible with the dominant view of the self.

Ego function(s)   Specific capacities of the EGO employed in the service of self-regulation and/or ADAPTATION, such as cognition, perception, memory, motility, AFFECT, thinking, language, SYMBOLIZATION, REALITY TESTING, evaluation, judgment, CENSORSHIP, impulse control, AFFECT TOLERANCE, DEFENSE, and CONFLICT mediation.

Ego ideal   A repository of standards, values, and images of perfection by which an individual measures him- or herself.

Ego identity   In Erikson's theory (see Chapter 8), the consolidation of a stable sense of oneself as a unique individual in society.

Ego psychology   The branch of PSYCHOANALYSIS, roughly equivalent to the STRUCTURAL MODEL, that emphasizes the concept of the EGO and its role in the psychological functioning.

Ego strength   In the STRUCTURAL MODEL, a state of psychological health characterized by the ability to efficiently fulfill EGO FUNCTIONS required for self-regulation and/or ADAPTATION, including REALITY TESTING and social judgment, abstract thinking, AFFECT TOLERANCE, impulse control, and the flexible utilization of appropriate DEFENSE MECHANISMS.

Ego syntonic   Behaviors that are experienced by the individual as compatible with his or her dominant view of the self.

Ego weakness   In the STRUCTURAL MODEL, a state of psychopathology characterized by the inability to fulfill EGO FUNCTIONS required for self-regulation and/or ADAPTATION.

Embodiment   The idea that the MIND is intrinsically shaped by its connection to the body.

Emergent property   A property of any system that is dependent on another system (as MIND is to brain) but that cannot be described in terms appropriate to that system, so that the new (or emergent) property must be described in new terms.

Emergent sense of self   The first stage in the development of the self—from birth to 2 months—in Stern's theory (see Chapter 12) about how the sense of self develops in interaction with the mother/caregiver.

Empathy   The capacity to feel, imagine, or sense the experience of another person.

Empiricism   The belief that the only source of true knowledge about the universe comes from the evidence of the senses.

Envy   A feeling of wishing to have something that another person has, often accompanied by destructive feelings toward that person.

Epigenesis   The view that development proceeds in a series of successive transactions between the individual and the environment, with the outcome of each phase dependent upon the outcomes of all previous phases.

Erotogenic zone   A body part that serves a source of libidinous excitement or gratification. Sigmund Freud postulated a developmental series of erotogenic zones: oral, anal, phallic, and genital.

False self   In Winnicott's theory (see Chapter 12), the self experience that emerges in response to another person's needs, expectations, and demands (as opposed to the TRUE SELF that emerges in response to one's own needs, expectations, and demands).

Fantasy   An imagined scenario in narrative form in which the imagining person is featured in a major role and often in an emotionally charged situation.

Fixation   The persistent and overwhelming influence of a particular stage of development on adult functioning.

Free association   A technique of PSYCHODYNAMIC PSYCHOTHERAPY in which a patient suspends CONSCIOUS control over his or her thought processes, thereby revealing UNCONSCIOUS influences on the patient's subjective experience.

Functionalism   A branch of PSYCHOLOGY that explores the function, or purpose, of mental life.

Fundamental rule   A request made by therapist to patient to report whatever comes to mind, speaking with as little CENSORSHIP as possible.

Genetic perspective   In the psychoanalytic model of the mind, the effort to understand the adult patient's report of his or her development as an important determinant of experience.

Genital phase   The fourth phase of psychosexual development, following the oral, anal, and phallic phases. The genital phase is sometimes combined with the OEDIPAL STAGE and called the *genital/oedipal phase.*

Good-enough mother   In Winnicott's theory (see Chapter 11), a mother who provides nurturing, optimal responsiveness, and safety so that the infant can thrive.

Grandiose self   In SELF PSYCHOLOGY, a component of the self that represents the earliest expression of inborn narcissistic strivings to be omnipotent and special.

Guilt   A feeling of badness and ANXIETY linked to thoughts of moral transgression.

Hedonic principle   A principle from general psychology that asserts that behavior and mental activity seek always to maximize feelings of pleasure and minimize feelings of pain.

Holding environment   In Winnicott's theory (see Chapter 11), a situation created by a GOOD-ENOUGH MOTHER (or caregiver).

Homeostasis   A state of stable intrapsychic equilibrium or self-regulation.

Humor   A DEFENSE in which an individual treats a painful subject with a comic attitude, thereby diminishing the pain.

Hypnosis A state of altered CONSCIOUSNESS (accompanied by changes in brain waves) induced by special techniques and often used for the purpose of treatment.

Hysteria A type of psychopathology characterized by somatic symptoms that are unrelated to demonstrable anatomical or physiological pathology.

Id In Sigmund Freud's STRUCTURAL MODEL, the seat of the DRIVES, including sexual and aggressive urges. The content of the id is always UNCONSCIOUS.

Idealization The attribution of exalted qualities to someone or something. A DEFENSE in which one individual sees another individual in an exaggeratedly positive light, so as to ward off disappointment or to enhance his or her own experience of self.

Idealized parental imago In SELF PSYCHOLOGY, a component of the self that represents the inborn need for perfection in the primary caregivers.

Idealized selfobject In SELF PSYCHOLOGY, a caregiver who can be experienced as perfect, thus allowing for healthy development of the IDEALIZED PARENTAL IMAGO.

Idealizing transference In SELF PSYCHOLOGY, a patient's exalted view of the therapist, which represents a revival of the IDEALIZED PARENTAL IMAGO in the person of the therapist.

Identification A process in which the individual's SELF REPRESENTATION is modified to resemble an OBJECT REPRESENTATION.

Identification with the aggressor A DEFENSE in which an individual takes on the characteristics or role of someone who had formerly tormented or abused him or her so as to avoid painful feelings of passivity and SHAME.

Identity The stable sense of oneself as a unique individual in society.

Identity diffusion Lack of coherence in SELF REPRESENTATION, resulting from failure to integrate all aspects of the SELF.

Imprinting According to Lorenz's theory (see Chapter 11), the act by which a newborn animal recognizes another animal as a parent.

Individuation In Mahler's theory of SEPARATION-INDIVIDUATION (see Chapter 11), the process by which children develop the feeling of autonomy and uniqueness.

Infantile sexuality Sexual and/or romantic feelings in children, especially as expressed in the psychosexual phases.

Insight Knowledge about the UNCONSCIOUS, often gained through INTERPRETATION.

Instinct In general biology, a species-specific, inherited pattern of behavior that does not have to be learned.

Intellectualization A defensive process in which an individual uses excessive cognitive activity to control and ward off unacceptable feelings.

Internalization A group of processes whereby an individual takes aspects of the external world into the psyche.

Internalized homophobia A process whereby a homosexual individual responds to homophobia in the surrounding culture by treating him- or herself in a homophobic way or by identifying with the aggressor.

Internal working models of attachment In Bowlby's theory (see Chapter 11) theory, psychological REPRESENTATIONS that include a REPRESENTATION of SELF, OBJECT, and the interaction between them, pertaining to ATTACHMENT.

Interpersonal Between two or more individuals in the external world.

Interpretation An explicit inference made by the therapist to the patient about the workings or the contents of the UNCONSCIOUS MIND.

Intersystemic conflict Struggle in the mind between opposing WISHES, thoughts, or feelings in different regions of the MIND, as between ID and SUPEREGO.

Intrasystemic conflict Struggle in the mind between opposing WISHES, thoughts, or feelings in the same system, as within the ID.

Introjection A DEFENSE in which an individual internalizes an aspect of the external world, usually an OBJECT, so as to avoid a painful feeling, such as loss or disappointment.

Introspection   The process of examining one's inner psychological experience.

Introspectionism   A branch of PSYCHOLOGY associated with Wundt (see Chapter 3) and characterized by the close examination of subjective experience in order to understand its most fundamental elements.

Isolation   A DEFENSE in which an individual separates events, thoughts, or parts of mental experience from one another in order to lessen their emotional impact.

Isolation of affect   The most commonly used form of ISOLATION, in which an individual separates an idea, experience, or memory from the feelings connected with it in order to lessen its emotional impact.

Latency   A developmental phase of childhood (roughly between 5 and 12 years of age), originally identified by Sigmund Freud as the period between the OEDIPAL STAGE and puberty, that is characterized by a lull in active libidinal and aggressive DRIVES and an apparent relative reduction in sexual interest.

Latent dream thoughts   The underlying content of the DREAM, made up of unacceptable thoughts and feelings.

Libido   The source of PSYCHIC ENERGY deriving from the organism's sexual WISHES, drawn from all levels of psychosexual development.

Libido theory   Sigmund Freud's theory about the origins, transformations, and effects of LIBIDO in the psychology of the individual and of culture (see Chapter 9 and Appendix A).

Manifest dream   The DREAM as recalled and narrated by the dreamer upon awakening.

Materialism   The belief that everything in the universe can be understood in terms of the properties of matter and energy, and reduced to descriptions expressed in measurements.

Mentalization   The ability to understand the behavior of others in terms of mental states such as beliefs, desires, feelings, and memories; the ability to reflect upon one's own mental states; and, the ability to understand that one's own states of mind may influence the behavior of others. Also called *reflective function*.

Mentalization-Based Treatment A therapy developed by Bateman and Fonagy (see Chapter 11) that aims to treat severe personality disorders through efforts to increase MENTALIZATION.

Mesmerism A theory and practice developed by Franz Anton Mesmer (see Chapter 2) based on his belief that disease was caused by disturbances in the free flow of hypothesized invisible fluids in the body and that the blocked flow could be corrected through magnetic force ("animal magnetism"). Mesmer's theory of cure proposed that the therapist, or "magnetizer," induce in the patient a trance-like state and then transmit his own stronger and better fluid to the patient through the channel of the rapport.

Metacognition The process of thinking about one's own thinking.

Midlife crisis A turning point in an individual's life, occurring in middle age, accompanied by emotional turmoil.

Mind An individual's experience, CONSCIOUS or UNCONSCIOUS, of perceiving, feeling, thinking, willing, and reasoning.

Mind–body dualism The view that the MIND and the body are two entirely and essentially different things.

Mirroring selfobject In SELF PSYCHOLOGY, a caregiver who offers recognition, validation, and enjoyment of the child's GRANDIOSE SELF, so that it can develop and mature properly.

Mirror neurons Neurons that fire when an individual performs an action and when he or she sees someone else perform the same action.

Mirror transference In SELF PSYCHOLOGY, a situation in PSYCHOTHERAPY in which the GRANDIOSE SELF is revived, so that the patient needs the therapist to respond to him or her with recognition and validation.

Model An imaginary construction that represents a complex system that cannot be observed directly in its entirety.

Motivational point of view In the psychoanalytic model of the mind, the effort to understand the interplay of psychological forces, or aims and strivings.

Narcissism An individual's investment in him- or herself or an aspect of the self.

Narcissistic rage   In Kohut's theory regarding DISORDERS OF THE SELF (see Chapter 12), an extreme affective state—ranging from irritability to fury and accompanied by feelings of SHAME, humiliation, and/or disappointment—triggered by a perceived threat to the self.

Narrative sense of self   The fifth stage in the development of the self—beginning in the third or fourth year—in Stern's theory (see Chapter 12) about how the sense of self develops in interaction with the mother/caregiver.

Narrative structure of the mind   In the psychoanalytic model of the mind, the understanding that mental life is shaped by stories.

Nature versus nurture   The ongoing controversy about whether a given phenomenon results from qualities that are intrinsic to the individual (nature) or from the effects of the external caregiving environment (nurture).

Need-satisfying object   The infant's initial experience of the maternal OBJECT, in which the OBJECT is experienced as existing only to meet the infant's needs.

Negative oedipus complex   An oedipal interaction between child and parents in which the child takes the same-sex parent as the love object and the opposite-sex parent as the rival.

Neurosis   A type of psychopathology characterized by inflexible, maladaptive behavior that represents a solution to UNCONSCIOUS CONFLICT.

Object   A person who is the focus of one's WISHES and needs.

Object constancy   The ability to maintain a positively tinged feeling toward the mother (or anyone else) in the face of feelings of frustration, anger, and/or disappointment.

Object permanence   The cognitive ability to know that an OBJECT (animate or inanimate) exists even when it cannot be perceived.

Object relations   A psychological configuration consisting of three parts: a SELF REPRESENTATION, an OBJECT REPRESENTATION, and a REPRESENTATION of an affectively charged interaction between the two.

Object Relations Theory   A model of the mind characterized by efforts to understand how OBJECT RELATIONS develop in childhood, how they are maintained throughout life, how they interact with other

STRUCTURES and motivations, and how they influence psychic functioning and behavior.

Object representation The individual's mental image of an OBJECT in his or her life. The REPRESENTATION contains aspects of the actual external OBJECT but is also colored by the individual's FANTASIES about the OBJECT.

Object seeking Libidinal aims that are directed toward another person, as opposed to those directed toward the child's own body (AUTOEROTIC).

Observing ego The part of the CONSCIOUS MIND that is capable of self-reflection and is activated in treatment.

Oedipal period/stage The period (between the ages of 3 and 6 years) during which the OEDIPUS COMPLEX emerges.

Oedipal victor A boy's experience of having triumphed over his father in obtaining his mother's special affection, or a girl's experience of having triumphed over her mother in obtaining her father's special affection.

Oedipus complex A set of feelings and thoughts about the role of the individual as a child in relation to his or her two parents, which includes the WISH for romantic union with one parent, along with a WISH to be rid of the other, competing parent.

On the way to object constancy In Mahler's theory (see Chapter 11), the final stage of SEPARATION-INDIVIDUATION in which the child learns to integrate positive and negative feelings/thoughts about the mother.

Oral character A personality style characterized by greed, dependency, demandingness, and impatience, thought to be related to the predominant influence of LIBIDO arising from the oral EROTOGENIC ZONE.

Oral phase The first phase of psychosexual development (consisting of approximately the first 18 months of life), during which LIBIDO deriving from the oral EROTOGENIC ZONE dominates the organization of psychic life.

Overdetermination The observations that any given manifestation of mental life can be given multiple psychological explanations.

Paranoid position   In Klein's theory (see Chapter 11), the earliest organization of the psyche, characterized by active SPLITTING of good and bad aspects of experience, accompanied by PROJECTION (later, PROJECTIVE IDENTIFICATION) of the bad aspects of experience onto the OBJECT.

Parapraxis   A symptomatic act, is one of a number of cognitive or functional errors such as slips of the tongue, forgetting of names or words, slips of the pen, or bungled actions.

Part object   In Klein's theory (see Chapter 11), the experience of only one aspect or attribute of an OBJECT, such as an all-good object or an all-bad object.

Pathological grandiose self   In Kernberg's theory of narcissistic personality disorder (see Chapter 12), an organization of the SELF that serves the defensive need to avoid dependency.

Pathological narcissism   In Kernberg's conceptualization (see Chapter 12), the name given to narcissistic psychopathology, the core feature of which is a structure called the PATHOLOGICAL GRANDIOSE SELF.

Penis envy   According to Sigmund Freud, a girl's or woman's feeling of discontent with her genitals, accompanied by a longing to have the genitals of a male.

Persecutory anxiety   In Klein's theory (see Chapter 11), an individual's fear that he or she is in danger of being destroyed by the bad OBJECT, who has become the repository for all of his or her own projected AGGRESSION.

Phallic narcissistic character   A personality style characterized by exhibitionism and extreme gender role behavior, thought to be related to the predominant influence of LIBIDO arising from the phallic EROTOGENIC ZONE.

Phallic phase   The third phase of psychosexual development (beginning at about 2 years of age and culminating in the OEDIPAL STAGE), during which LIBIDO deriving from the phallus (penis or clitoris) dominates the organization of psychic life. The phallic phase is often called the *early genital phase.*

Physical determinism   The belief that events in the material world are caused by other events in the material world.

Pleasure/unpleasure principle   A principle that asserts that behavior and mental activity seek always to maximize feelings of pleasure and minimize feelings of unpleasure or pain.

Position   In Klein's theory (see Chapter 11), a stable configuration of SELF and OBJECT REPRESENTATIONS resulting from the combined influence of WISHES, thoughts, and feelings as well as interactions with caregivers.

Positive oedipus complex   An oedipal interaction between child and parents in which the child takes the opposite-sex parent as the love object and the same-sex parent as the rival.

Positivism   A program for systematizing all knowledge of the world based on undeniable truths and often empirical methods as well.

Practicing   In Mahler's theory (see Chapter 11), a subphase of the SEPARATION-INDIVIDUATION process in which the child experiments with distance by moving away from the mother, enjoying his or her newly developed capacities for crawling and walking.

Preconscious   In Freud's TOPOGRAPHIC MODEL, one of the three components (with CONSCIOUS and UNCONSCIOUS) of the mental apparatus. Elements of the preconscious are not conscious but are easily brought into conscious awareness through focusing attention on them.

Preoedipal period/stage   The period of development from birth to the onset of the OEDIPAL PERIOD (between the ages of 3 and 6 years).

Primal scene   The childhood perception of parental sexual intercourse, whether actually observed, actually overheard, or only imagined, and the meaning the child attaches to it.

Primary femininity   A view of female development that asserts that the earliest sense of being female is not based on CONFLICT or is not a response to feeling inferior.

Primary process   A primitive form of thinking linked with the PLEASURE PRINCIPLE and characterized by reliance on SYMBOLIZATION, DISPLACEMENT, and CONDENSATION, as well as by a disregard for logical connections, for contradictions, and for the realities of time. The content of primary process is dominated by WISHES, AFFECTS, CONFLICT, and/or UNCONSCIOUS FANTASY. In Freud's TOPOGRAPHIC MODEL, primary process is associated with the UNCONSCIOUS domain of the MIND.

Primitive idealization   A DEFENSE in which an individual splits apart exalted and devalued aspects of another individual, experiencing only the exalted aspect, so as to ward off feelings associated with the devalued aspect, or to enhance his or her own experience of self.

Projection A DEFENSE in which an individual attributes an unacceptable or intolerable idea, impulse, or feeling to another individual.

Projective identification An INTERPERSONAL DEFENSE in which an individual transfers parts of the SELF onto the OBJECT in order to rid him- or herself of those parts and to control the OBJECT from inside.

Psychic determinism The belief that psychological events are caused by other psychological events, transformed according to natural laws, or that psychological life is lawfully determined.

Psychic energy In Sigmund Freud's theory, the force behind all mental activity.

Psychic reality Subjective psychological experience, understood as the result of the continuous interaction between inner WISHES and fears and the external world.

Psychoanalysis A branch of PSYCHOLOGY, introduced by Sigmund Freud, which includes a MODEL of the MIND, a treatment, and a method for exploring inner life. The psychoanalytic model of the mind explores mental life along topographic, motivational, structural, and developmental parameters, and examines the contributions of this model to the understanding of psychopathology and treatment.

Psychodynamic Pertaining to mental forces or motivations.

Psychology The study of MIND and behavior.

Psychosexual phases The phases of development introduced as part of LIBIDO THEORY, which posits a series of sequential, overlapping phases in the developing infant and child—oral, anal, phallic, and genital—each representing predominant sensual investment in a different EROTOGENIC ZONE.

Psychotherapy The treatment of mental disorder by psychological rather than medical means.

Rapprochement In Mahler's theory of SEPARATION-INDIVIDUATION (see Chapter 11), a subphase marked by conflicting feelings of dependence and outrage, brought on by new awareness of SEPARATION from the mother.

Rapprochement crisis In Mahler's theory of SEPARATION-INDIVIDUATION (see Chapter 11), the CONFLICT felt by the child during the subphase of RAPPROCHEMENT between WISHES to depend upon the mother and WISHES for autonomy, often accompanied by feelings of anger and wide fluctuations in mood.

Rationalization   A DEFENSE in which an individual resorts to seemingly reasonable explanations to account for feelings or actions, thereby avoiding recognition of more painful feelings and/or motivations.

Reaction formation   A DEFENSE in which an individual transforms a forbidden WISH into its opposite.

Reality principle   A principle that asserts that behavior and mental activity will take the constraints of the external world into account, even when seeking pleasure.

Reality testing   The capacity to understand aspects of external reality, beginning with the capacity to differentiate between reality and FANTASY.

Reconstruction   In INTERPRETATION made by the therapist that makes an inference about a forgotten or repressed aspect of the past.

Reflective function   See MENTALIZATION.

Regression   A change in psychological phenomena in a direction that is the reverse of its usual, progressive direction. For example, an individual may substitute a pleasure from an earlier stage of development for one from a later stage, as a DEFENSE against the danger felt to be part of the later stage.

Regression in the service of the ego   A form of REGRESSION that, although it may be originally instituted for defensive purposes, leads to a more innovative and adaptive mental function and organization (as in artistic creation).

Reparation   In Klein's theory (see Chapter 11), an individual's attempts to relieve GUILT or ANXIETY experienced for having had aggressive WISHES toward a loved and needed OBJECT by making efforts to repair the imagined damage or harm done by those aggressive impulses.

Repetition compulsion   A tendency to repeat patterns of behavior or to re-create situations that may be painful or self-destructive without recognizing the relationship of these behaviors/scenarios to early repressed WISHES or FANTASIES.

Representation   A stable psychological structure inside the mind that stands for something that is or was outside of the mind. In the psychoanalytic model of the mind, the term usually refers to internalized images of SELF, OBJECT, and interactions between self and object.

Repression   A DEFENSE in which an individual excludes unacceptable thoughts and feelings from CONSCIOUSNESS.

Resistance   A phenomenon in PSYCHODYNAMIC PSYCHOTHERAPY in which the patient evinces a noticeable discontinuity in the flow of association.

Return of the repressed   A phenomenon, thought to underlie NEUROSIS, in which unacceptable ideas that have been repressed reemerge in the form of symptoms.

Schema   In general PSYCHOLOGY, a word referring to a structure, or a relatively stable psychological configuration.

Schizophrenogenic mothering   In now-discredited theories, a quality of mothering thought to be the cause of schizophrenia.

Secondary process   A type of thinking linked with the REALITY PRINCIPLE and characterized by rationality, order, and logic. In Freud's TOPOGRAPHIC MODEL, secondary process is associated with the PRECONSCIOUS and CONSCIOUS domains of the MIND.

Seduction hypothesis   Sigmund Freud's early theory of HYSTERIA (see Chapter 7), which posited that symptoms are caused by sexual acts perpetrated on the child by caretakers.

Self   A psychic STRUCTURE, or REPRESENTATION, consisting of the individual's subjective sense of "I." In SELF PSYCHOLOGY, the superordinate STRUCTURE of the MIND.

Self constancy   The ability to maintain a positive SELF REPRESENTATION even in the face of failure or other threats to self-esteem.

Selfobject   In SELF PSYCHOLOGY, another person who serves the purpose of maintaining or supporting the SELF.

Selfobject transference   In SELF PSYCHOLOGY, any one of a number of TRANSFERENCES activated in PSYCHOTHERAPY in which SELFOBJECT needs are reactivated in relation to the therapist.

Self Psychology   A model of the mind based on the development and functioning of the self.

Self representation   The individual's mental image of himself or herself. This REPRESENTATION is made up of experiences of internal stimuli, FANTASIES about the SELF that are elaborated in relation to OBJECTS, and internalized perceptions of the way in which others experience the individual.

Self–selfobject matrix   In SELF PSYCHOLOGY, the combination of an individual and another person who serves the purpose of maintaining or supporting the SELF, originally the infant and the primary caregiver.

Self-state dreams   In SELF PSYCHOLOGY, DREAMS that represent the state of the self of the dreamer.

Separation   In Mahler's theory of SEPARATION-INDIVIDUATION (see Chapter 11), the process by which children form a mental REPRESENTATION of the SELF as distinct from the mental REPRESENTATION of the OBJECT.

Separation anxiety   A type of ANXIETY that appears in infants of about 6 months of age in response to being too far away from the mother or the primary caregiver.

Separation-individuation   A developmental process proposed by Mahler (see Chapter 11) in which the child must form a mental REPRESENTATION of the SELF as distinct from the mental REPRESENTATION of the OBJECT (SEPARATION) and must develop specific characteristics so that the SELF not only becomes distinct from the OBJECT but also becomes unique and autonomous (INDIVIDUATION).

Sexuality/psychosexuality   The search for sensual bodily pleasure in all its forms.

Shame   A feeling of badness or ANXIETY linked to an individual's awareness that others may see him or her to be bad or inferior.

Signal affect   An attenuated version of the experience of an AFFECT (either pleasure or pain) remembered from the past that is used by the EGO in appraisal of the current potential for danger. Also called *signal anxiety*.

Signal anxiety   See SIGNAL AFFECT.

Somatic marker hypothesis A hypothesis formulated by Damasio (see Chapter 10) that explains how emotional processes guide human behavior, choices, and decision making.

Somatization A DEFENSE in which an individual expresses unacceptable feelings in the form of physical symptoms, so as to lessen their painful impact.

Splitting A DEFENSE in which an individual separates contradictory, conflicting CONSCIOUS experiences, thereby preventing their integration, so as to prevent the emotional impact of integration.

Stranger anxiety A type of ANXIETY that appears in infants of about 6 months of age in response to the presence of persons who are not the mother or the primary caretaker.

Strange Situation An experimental situation designed by Ainsworth (see Chapter 11) in which the child is observed playing while caregivers and strangers who enter and leave the room, thus revealing his or her ATTACHMENT pattern.

Structuralism A branch on PSYCHOLOGY that attempts to delineate the structures of the CONSCIOUS MIND.

Structural Model Sigmund Freud's second psychoanalytic model of the mind (see Chapter 8), based on the division of the psyche into three parts: EGO, ID, and SUPEREGO.

Structural point of view In the psychoanalytic model of the mind, the effort to understand aspects of behavior and mental life by exploring the influence of three STRUCTURES: EGO, ID, and SUPEREGO.

Structure A relatively stable psychological configuration with a slow rate of change.

Subjective sense of self The third stage in the development of the self—beginning around 9 months—in Stern's theory (see Chapter 12) about how the sense of self develops in interaction with the mother/caregiver.

Sublimation A DEFENSE in which the individual deflects a WISH from its original aim to one with a higher social value.

Suggestion The phenomenon by which an idea proposed from outside the mind (or by one part of the mind) is taken up inside the mind (or by another part of the mind) and often then transformed into an action.

Superego   In Sigmund Freud's STRUCTURAL MODEL, one of three major agencies of the MIND and the seat of the individual's system of ideals and values, moral principles, and moral injunctions. Commonly called the *conscience.*

Suppression   A DEFENSE in which an individual consciously places unpleasant thoughts or feelings out of awareness.

Symbolization   A phenomenon in which an OBJECT or idea is represented by an image or something equally concrete.

Talking cure   A slang name for any type of therapeutic intervention, usually PSYCHOTHERAPY, that emphasizes shared narrative in an interaction.

Theory of mind   The capacity to understand that 1) others have beliefs, desires, and intentions, which constitute a "mind"; 2) this mind may be different from one's own; and 3) this mind causes others' actions.

Therapeutic alliance   The aspect of the relationship between patient and therapist that reflects the patient's capacity to sustain cooperative effort, independent of state of the TRANSFERENCE or RESISTANCE.

Topographic Model   Sigmund Freud's first psychoanalytic model of the mind (see Chapter 5), based on a division of the psyche into three parts: CONSCIOUS, PRECONSCIOUS, and UNCONSCIOUS.

Topographic point of view   In the psychoanalytic model of the mind, the effort to understand aspects of behavior and mental life by examining whether those aspects have access to CONSCIOUSNESS.

Transference   A phenomenon in which an UNCONSCIOUS WISH "transfers" some of its intensity to an unobjectionable PRECONSCIOUS thought so as to avoid CENSORSHIP. More commonly, the clinical phenomenon in which a patient transfers strong feelings from someone of emotional importance (often from childhood) to the therapist.

Transference-Focused Psychotherapy   A type of PSYCHOTHERAPY designed to treat BORDERLINE PERSONALITY ORGANIZATION, based on Kernberg's theory (see Chapter 11).

Transitional object   In Winnicott's theory (see Chapter 12), a treasured possession such as a teddy bear or a blanket that the child experiences as both "me" and "not me" simultaneously.

Tripartite Model Another name for Sigmund Freud's STRUCTURAL MODEL, emphasizing the fact that there are three structures: EGO, ID, and SUPEREGO.

True self In Winnicott's theory (see Chapter 12), the self experience—incorporating one's own needs, expectations, and demands—that emerges in the context of a facilitating maternal environment.

Turning against the self A DEFENSE in which an individual directs an unacceptable WISH, usually aggressive, from another individual toward him- or herself.

Turning passive into active A DEFENSE in which an individual acts out an experience of having been a passive participant in an interaction by assuming the active role, thereby avoiding feelings and/or memories of being out of control or helpless.

Twinship transference In SELF PSYCHOLOGY, a situation in PSYCHOTHERAPY in which the patient demands or expects that he or she and the therapist are exactly the same, thereby attempting to strengthen the self.

Unconscious That part of the MIND that is outside of awareness.

Undoing A DEFENSE in which an individual negates unacceptable sexual, aggressive, or shameful feelings associated with a previous behavior by doing or saying the opposite.

Verbal/categorical sense of self The fourth stage in the development of the self—beginning around 18 months—in Stern's theory (see Chapter 12) about how the sense of self develops in interaction with the mother/caregiver.

Whole object In Klein's theory (see Chapter 11), the experience of another person as complete and/or integrated, especially in terms of his or her good and bad aspects.

Wish An act of desire or a motivational aim.

Bibliography

Auchincloss EL, Samberg E: Psychoanalytic Terms and Concepts. New Haven, CT, Yale University Press, 2012

Gabbard GO, Litowitz BE, Williams P (eds): Textbook of Psychoanalysis, 2nd Edition. Washington, DC, American Psychiatric Publishing, 2012

Index

*Page numbers printed in **boldface** type refer to tables;
page numbers followed by "n" indicate note numbers.*